What works for children?

Effective services for children and families

DATE DUE			
15/7/14			
21/7/13			

What works for children?

Effective services for children and families

Edited by
DIANA McNEISH,
TONY NEWMAN and
HELEN ROBERTS

Open University Press

Open University Press
McGraw-Hill Education
McGraw-Hill House
Shoppenhangers Road
Maidenhead
Berkishire
SL6 2QL

email: enquiries@openup.co.uk
world wide web: www.openup.co.uk

and
Two Penn Plaza
New York, NY 10121-2289, USA

First Published 2002
Reprinted 2010

A catalogue record of this book is available from the British Library

ISBN-10   0 335 20938 6 (pb)   0 335 20939 4 (hb)
ISBN-13   978 0 335 20938 5 (pb)   978 0 335 20939 2 (hb)

Library of Congress Cataloging-in-Publication Data
What works for children? : effective services for children and families/edited by Diana
McNeish, Tony Newman, and Helen Roberts.
    p. cm.
  Includes bibliographical references and index.
  ISBN 0-335-20939-4 – ISBN 0-335-20938-6 (pbk.)
  1. Social work with children–Great Britain. 2. Family social work–Great Britain.
3. Child welfare–Great Britain. 4. Family services–Great Britain. I. McNeish,
Diana. II. Newman, Tony. III. Roberts, Helen.

HV751.A6 W45 2002
362.7'0941–dc21   2002022095

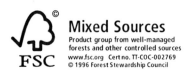

Mixed Sources
Product group from well-managed
forests and other controlled sources
www.fsc.org Cert no. TT-COC-002769
© 1996 Forest Stewardship Council

Typeset by Graphicraft Limited, Hong Kong
Printed in Great Britain by Bell & Bain Ltd., Glasgow

Contents

List of figures and tables   vii
Notes on contributors   viii
Preface   xiii

Introduction
Tony Newman, Helen Roberts and Diana McNeish   1

PART I   Services for adopted and looked after children   11

1   Family placement services   13
    Clive Sellick and June Thoburn

2   Promoting stability and continuity in care away from home   37
    Sonia Jackson

3   Leaving care   59
    Mike Stein

4   Residential care   83
    David Berridge

**PART 2   Preventing the social exclusion of children and
           young people**   105

5   Community development with children   107
    Gary Craig

6   Inclusive education   127
    Alan Dyson

7 Preventing the social exclusion of disabled children 147
Bryony Beresford

8 Young offenders in the community 165
David Utting, Julie Vennard and Sara Scott

9 Involving children and young people in decision making 186
Diana McNeish and Tony Newman

PART 3 Promoting and protecting children's health 205

10 Child protection 207
Geraldine Macdonald

11 Reducing inequalities in child health 232
Helen Roberts

12 Family support 252
Ann Buchanan

13 Last words: The views of young people 274
Diana McNeish and Tony Newman

Name index 288
Subject index 290

List of figures and tables

Figure 12.1   The 'spiral' effect   255
Figure 12.2   Children with significant emotional and behavioural
                problems some time in their childhood   256
Figure 12.3   The ecological framework   258
Figure 12.4   Percentages of boys and girls with maladjustment by
                family background   260

Table 4.1   Percentages of children and social workers attributing
                benefits to residential placements   92
Table 7.1   The Children Act 1989 and disabled children's rights
                to inclusion   159
Table 11.1   Interventions primarily aimed at children and
                adolescents   245
Table 12.1   Some possible consequences of emotional and
                behavioural problems   257
Table 12.2   Risk and protective factors   259
Table 12.3   Prevention projects   264
Table 12.4   Interventions for vulnerable children   266
Table 12.5   Effective individual interventions for children aged
                3–10 years   267
Table 12.6   Effective individual interventions for adolescents   269

Notes on contributors

Bryony Beresford has been doing research on issues related to disabled and chronically ill children and young people and their families for over ten years. Based at the Social Policy Research Unit at the University of York, her earlier work was concerned with looking at parents' needs and experiences. More recent projects have involved working directly with children and young people, looking at their housing needs, their information needs and their experiences of communicating with health professionals. Her current work is concerned with developing user-defined outcome measures of social care for disabled children and young people, for use by local authorities to evaluate the services they provide. Previous publications (some co-authored) include: *Personal Accounts: Involving Disabled Children in Research*; *Expert Opinions: A National Survey of Parents Caring for a Severely Disabled Child*; *On the Edge: Minority Ethnic Families Caring for a Severely Disabled Child*; *Unlocking Key Working: An Analysis and Evaluation of Key Worker Services for Families with Disabled Children*; and *Homes Unfit for Children: Housing, Disabled Children and their Families*.

David Berridge is Professor of Child and Family Welfare at the University of Luton and was previously Research Director at the National Children's Bureau and Research Fellow at the Dartington Social Research Unit. His career began as a residential social worker. He has been a child welfare researcher for 20 years with a particular focus on children living away from home. His most recent co-authored books are *Where to Turn? Family Support for South Asian Communities* (2000) and *Children's Homes Revisited* (1998).

Ann Buchanan is Reader in Social Work at the University of Oxford and a fellow of St Hilda's College. For more than 30 years her abiding interest has been working with, and researching into ways of helping troubled children and young people. She has published widely from books and research reports, to papers and articles.

Gary Craig worked for 20 years in the voluntary sector and in local government, mainly within large-scale community development projects. He returned to academic life in 1988 and, after periods at several universities, he is now Professor of Social Justice at the University of Hull. He was formerly editor of the *Community Development Journal* and secretary of the Social Policy Association and is now President of the International Association of Community Development. His research interests include community development and empowerment, local governance, poverty and inequality, and 'race' and ethnicity. He recently published *What Works in Community Development with Children?* and his next book is *Welfare Regimes in the Developed World* (edited with Pete Alcock). He has supported Fulham Football Club since he was 7.

Alan Dyson is Professor of Special Needs Education and co-Director of the Special Needs Research Centre in the Department of Education, University of Newcastle upon Tyne. His research interests are in special needs education and in the relationship between social and educational inclusion. This means that he has an interdisciplinary perspective (extending to broader social and economic policy) as well as a purely educational perspective. He has undertaken a great deal of funded research sponsored by ESRC, the Joseph Rowntree Foundation, DfEE, SOEID, DENI and LEAs, and other bodies. He was a member of the government's National Advisory Group on Special Educational Needs, is currently a member of the National Education Research Forum and has worked with TTA and Social Exclusion Unit task groups. He has an established international reputation, having worked in a consultative capacity with government departments and agencies in Chile, France, New Zealand, the Netherlands, Norway and South Africa. He is currently undertaking a writing project for UNESCO. He has published widely in both professional and research journals. Recent books (with colleagues) include *Schools and Special Needs* (2000), *Theorising Special Education* (1998), *New Directions in Special Needs* (1997) and *Towards Inclusive Schools?* (1995). His work on *The SENCO Guide* (1997) was distributed to all schools and he has recently produced (with colleagues) two reports for the Joseph Rowntree Foundation – *Housing and Schooling* and *School, Family and Community*. Alan Dyson has been at Newcastle University since 1988. Prior to that, he spent 13 years as a teacher, mainly as a Special Educational Needs Coordinator (SENCO) in urban comprehensive schools, though also with some special school experience.

Sonia Jackson was formerly Head and Professor of Applied Social Studies and Social Policy at the University of Wales Swansea. She trained as a clinical psychologist and has also worked as a teacher, educational adviser and local authority social worker. She now directs the By Degrees project at the Thomas Coram Research Unit, Institute of Education, University of London, providing support and tracking the progress of university students who have been in care. She has a longstanding interest in the education of children in care, first drawing attention to its neglect in 1983. She has published extensively on a broad range of child-related issues, including day care, child protection, social work education and child welfare outcomes. Her most recent publications are *Nobody Ever Told Us School Mattered*, *What Works in Creating Stability for Looked after Children* (with Nigel Thomas) and *Better Education, Better Futures* (with Darshan Sachdev).

Geraldine Macdonald is Professor of Social Work at the University of Bristol. She is also Visiting Professor at the Centre for Evidence-Based Social Services at the University of Exeter. She qualified as a social worker in 1979 and worked as a social worker and senior social worker for Oxfordshire Social Services, specializing in work with children and families. Her research interests include the evaluation of the effects of social interventions, particularly social work, decision making in child protection, and ethical issues in social work research and practice. She has recent publications in each of these areas.

She is actively involved in promoting the development, availability and use of systematic reviews of interventions relevant to health and social care. Between 1995 and 1999 she was Archie Cochrane Research Fellow at Green College, University of Oxford. Professor Macdonald is Coordinating Editor of the Cochrane *Developmental, Psychosocial and Learning Problems* review group. The Cochrane Collaboration seeks to prepare, maintain and make accessible systematic reviews of health care interventions. She is also convenor of the social welfare group within the Campbell Collaboration. The Campbell Collaboration is a sibling collaboration to Cochrane which aims to prepare, maintain and make accessible systematic reviews of interventions in education, social welfare and criminology.

Diana McNeish is currently Head of Research and Development with Barnardos. She spent ten years in local authority social work, team management and policy development before joining Barnardos research team in 1991. Her main research interests are children and young people's participation and the links between research, policy and practice.

Tony Newman spent ten years developing community based services for people with learning disabilities in South Wales before joining Barnardo's Research and Development Team in 1990. He has a particular interest in the promotion of childhood resilience, the impacts of parental disability on children and implementation strategies in evidence based practice. He holds honorary research fellowships at Oxford, Cardiff and Exeter Universities.

Helen Roberts is Professor of Child Health in the Institute of Health Sciences at City University, and before that, was Head of Research and Development at Barnardo's where she worked with colleagues to set up Barnardo's *What Works* series. She currently works on evidence-based health and social care for children, inequalities in child health and methods of consulting children effectively. Her methodological interests are in the synthesis of qualitative and quantitative research findings into systematic reviews which can be used by policy makers and practitioners.

Sara Scott is a principal research officer with Barnardo's. Her main research interests concern gender, violence and mental health. She was previously Director (1999–2001) of a Department of Health funded initiative developing training on gender issues for staff in the secure psychiatric sector. Her book *The Politics and Experience of Ritual Abuse: Beyond Disbelief* is published by Open University Press (2001). Her recent publications are concerned with contemporary discourse on child sexual abuse, developing a sociological understanding of dissociative identity and the need for gender sensitive mental health services.

Clive Sellick is a senior lecturer in social work at the University of East Anglia, Norwich and Director of the School's International Studies. He is a former social worker, manager of a fostering team, magistrate and guardian ad litem. He has written extensively about foster care including, with June Thoburn, *What Works in Family Placement?* in the Barnardo's 'What Works' series. His current research interest centres on the policy and practice of the much expanded independent fostering sector.

Mike Stein is Professor and Co-Director of the Social Work Research and Development Unit in the Department of Social Policy and Social Work at the University of York. For the last 20 years he has been researching the problems faced by young people leaving care and the way services respond to them. His research has also been concerned with the experiences of young people living on the streets and running away from home. He has been an adviser to local authorities, voluntary organizations and young people in care groups. He has been involved in the preparation of the guidance and training materials for the Children (Leaving Care) Act, 2000. He has published extensively in the area of leaving care and vulnerable young people.

June Thoburn is a professor of social work and Director of the Centre for Research on the Child and Family at the University of East Anglia. She is a qualified social worker and has taught and researched on child welfare issues since 1980. She has a particular interest in the interface between law and social work and is often called upon to be an expert witness in complex child care and adoption cases. She has published extensively in the area of child welfare. Of particular relevance to this book are *Permanent Family Placement for Children of Minority Ethnic Origin* (with L. Norford and S. Rashid) and *Child Welfare Outcome Research in the United States, the United Kingdom and Australia* (with A.N. Maluccio and F. Ainsworth).

David Utting is a writer on social policy and Head of Public Affairs at the Joseph Rowntree Foundation. He is author of the Foundation's report on

Family and Parenthood (1995) and co-author of *Crime and the Family* (1993) published by the Family Policy Studies Centre. His review of UK programmes relevant to *Reducing Criminality Among Young People* (1996) was published by the Home Office. In addition to *What Works With Young Offenders in the Community?* for Barnardo's (co-written with Julie Vennard) he is co-author of *Youth at Risk? A National Survey of Risk Factors, Protective Factors and Problem Behaviour Among Young People in England, Scotland and Wales*, published in 2002 by Communities that Care.

Julie Vennard is a research fellow in the Department of Law at the University of Bristol where she is currently co-directing a research project commissioned by the Home Office on the resettlement of short-term prisoners and collaborating in an evaluation of the new Victim Personal Statement scheme. Until February 1999 she was Head of the 'Dealing with Offenders Group' at the Home Office Research, Development and Statistics Directorate (RDSD), where she was responsible for planning and managing annual programmes of research on such topics as: effective interventions with offenders in custody and in the community; youth crime and the youth justice system; and risk/needs assessment. She has given many conference and seminar papers on the 'What Works' research and has published widely on many aspects of the criminal justice system. Recent publications include: *The Use of Cognitive-behavioural Approaches with Offenders: Messages from the Research* (1997); *Changing Offenders' Attitudes and Behaviour: What Works?* (1997); *Effective Interventions with Offenders* (1998); and *Learning Lessons from Serious Incidents* (with C. Hedderman, 1999).

Preface

Why 'what works?' When the editors of this volume, together with other colleagues, began an initiative in 1994 to promote evidence-based practice in social care with Barnardo's, the children's charity, the term seemed both fresh and challenging. It subsequently became the title of what was, and remains, a popular series of 'best evidence' reviews, the first of which was published in 1995 (Macdonald and Roberts 1995). This and many of the following publications in the series are cited by contributors to this volume. Our concern was, from the outset, value based as well as methodological. We posed the question:

> Experts have a duty not to intervene in people's lives on the basis of whim and intuition. But people at the receiving end of interventions are frequently vulnerable and powerless. How certain can they be that the services offered to them have been properly evaluated, that one service is better than another, or that any service is likely to be of greater benefit than no service at all?
>
> (Oakley and Roberts 1996: 1)

Although the phrase was undoubtedly used by others before us, and we make no claim for cause and effect, the term has entered public and professional discourse and is asked routinely by politicians when reviewing the possible range of welfare investment options. Although suffering from the inevitable effects of over-familiarity, asking 'what works?' has led to important ancillary questions being posed. What works for whom? Who decides what works? And, given the immense richness and complexity of human aspirations, how realistic is it to seek a body of knowledge that can assure us that what we are doing 'works' for most of the people most of the time? Let us reassure (or disappoint) the reader at the outset. What we hope to do in this book is to present a body of knowledge that represents, at this moment in time, reliable summaries – although not systematic reviews – of incomplete and often contradictory bodies of evidence that may guide social care practitioners towards strategies that are more likely to result in the kinds of outcomes that children and families want. A limited ambition, but one which we hope steers a middle path between prescriptive certainties and the 'do whatever works best for you' approach.

No intervention in health, education or social care works equally well for all people, in all communities, in all circumstances, all of the time. And even if it did, there is no guarantee that it would *remain* the most effective course of action, as techniques, policies, practice and, importantly, people's expectations change over time. In many cases, there is little variation in the effectiveness of different kinds of interventions, or the difference between intervening and doing nothing may be small. Clear evidence of the benefit of particular approaches may only emerge when data sets consisting of thousands or even millions of people are analysed. Small shifts at an individual level may, when aggregated, result in important overall benefits at a population level. However, the incentive to act on these data may be less compelling to a parent whose sole focus of concern is the 1.7 children in the average British family.

There is no single best way of helping a child learn to read, no single best treatment for depressive illnesses and no single best method of helping an anorexic child. The choice of approach will be guided by evidence, and an essential part of this evidence includes attention to the preferences of children and families, their environment, professional judgement, availability of skills, cost considerations and resource constraints. By a conscientious attention to the evidence base, we can increase the likelihood that the options we choose from are more rather than less effective, and ensure that the vulnerable people whom we serve are also able to make an informed choice. Increasing probabilities, not providing certainties, is the game we are in.

It will be evident to readers that, as the authors and editors of this book would be the first to acknowledge, the data presented as evidence are not all equally robust. Those of us in the evidence-based policy and practice community know that we have a long way to go, but there are many encouraging signs. These include the development of the Campbell Collaboration, an international organization that aims to prepare, maintain and disseminate high-quality, systematic reviews of studies of effectiveness in social and public policy (Petrosino *et al.* 2000; Campbell website at: http://campbell.gse.upenn.edu/). Funders are increasingly willing to consider proposals for systematic reviews, and policy makers are asking for them. The Economic and Social Research Council (ESRC) has established an evidence-based policy and practice network of which we are a part (www.evidencenetwork.org).

If we wait for the perfect reviews, if we believe that nothing can change until everything changes, we will have a long wait on our hands. This book, and the activities of a growing body of people in the evidence-based family, are making a start.

The editors would like to thank colleagues past and present for their assistance, advice and support.

REFERENCES

Macdonald, G. and Roberts, H. (1995) *What Works in the Early Years?* Ilford: Barnardo's.
Oakley, A. and Roberts, H. (eds) (1996) *Evaluating Social Interventions: A Report of Two Workshops Funded by the Economic and Social Research Council.* Ilford: Barnardo's.
Petrosino, A., Boruch, R.F., Rouding, C., McDonald, S. and Chalmers, I. (2000) The Campbell Collaboration Social, Psychological, Educational and Criminological Trials Register (C2-SPECTR) to facilitate the preparation and maintenance of systematic reviews of social and educational interventions, *Evaluation and Research in Education*, 14(3 & 4): 206–19.

TONY NEWMAN
HELEN ROBERTS
DIANA McNEISH

Introduction

I want a house with a pool
Shorter hours in school
And a room with my own private phone
I want to stay up all night
See the big city lights
No more trouble or words at home.
(Eddie Cochran, 1959, *Teenage Heaven*,
Jewel Music Publ. Co. Ltd)

Delivering effective social care services to children and families is an important and serious business. However, those of us who are preoccupied, professionally as well as personally, with the welfare of children need occasionally
to remind ourselves that *not* being at the centre of adults' attention is a major
part of growing up. Although we cannot claim to have our fingers firmly on
the pulse of contemporary music, we doubt that Eddie Cochran's vision of
teenage heaven is entirely obsolete. Much of what *matters* to children, rather
than what is effective, cannot be delivered by health and social care agencies,
however well-resourced they become. No professional has a magic wand that
can transform children's educational performance. We cannot mend their
parents' broken relationships, find them friends when they are lonely, make
them talented or endow them with riches. But we do know that some of the
things that practitioners and policy makers do *can* make a difference, even in
these tricky areas. Recognizing what we are unable to do (and the opportunity
costs involved in trying to do it) will leave us more time and resources to
devote to what we can do successfully.

   This book addresses many of the social care services delivered by statutory,
voluntary and, increasingly, private sector organizations to children in need.
Delivering effective services to the most vulnerable children is both a

professional and moral imperative, yet one curiously under-emphasized by both the UK and American social work associations (Myers and Thyer 1997). It is only recently that the *effectiveness* of social care services – that is, the extent to which interventions or strategies bring about the changes intended – has moved to the centre of the practitioner and policy arena. Research into social work practice has traditionally been preoccupied – if we judge this by the volume of publications – by descriptive studies and theoretical discussion. Publications that actually examine what social care workers do, and the effects their actions have on service users, account for, according to a recent review, only 14 per cent of articles in social work journals (Rosen *et al.* 1999). This is not, we would suggest, a satisfactory situation for a profession whose *raison d'être* is to provide a service.

The government has made it clear that social care services, in common with other professions, must base practice on 'the best evidence of what works' (Department of Health 1998a: 93). Major new investments in child care programmes have been accompanied by an increased emphasis on evidence-based practice, particularly interventions that have been validated by research methods featuring 'before' and 'after' measurements and comparison groups (for example, Sure Start 1999). Following the lead in health care, a growing range of consortia – for example, Research in Practice, Making Research Count and the Centre for Evidence Based Social Services – are making robust evidence available to an increasing number of social care workers. On the international front, the Campbell Collaboration, a sister organization to the Cochrane Collaboration in health care, has been established to review and disseminate evidence in the fields of educational, criminological and psychosocial interventions. In the UK, the Economic and Social Research Council has established an evidence-based policy and practice initiative in the social sciences. The establishment by the Department of Health of the Social Care Institute for Excellence is a clear recognition that the collection, appraisal, maintenance and dissemination of evidence now lies at the heart of a professional and accountable social care service.

Although some controversy surrounds the applicability of evidence-based practice to social care work, with some concerned that this will mean techno-cratic solutions to human problems, we believe that the empowering potential for end-point users, and for practitioners, in having access to interventions based on sound evidence is enormous. Whatever one's perspective, an under-standing of the issue has become of increasing relevance to all child welfare organizations and the practitioners they employ. What do we mean by evidence-based practice?

While accepting that no two situations – or children, or parents – are ident-ical, we suggest that social care workers should consider two basic proposi-tions. First, an approach should be chosen because a careful review of the evidence suggests that this course of action is more likely to result in the best outcome for the child than other approaches (and better than doing nothing at all). Second, we should attribute more confidence to some kinds of evidence than others. Drawing on several sources (e.g. Sackett *et al.* 1996; Sheldon and

Chilvers 2000), we offer a definition of evidence-based child care practice as *the process of systematically locating, critically reviewing and using research findings as the basis for decisions in child care practice.* The aim of this book is to provide, within most of the core areas of social care, a summary of what a wide range of research studies suggests are the most effective strategies and interventions for helping children and families.

Promoting evidence-based models of practice in social care organizations for children and families is not uncontroversial. Social care workers often feel uncomfortable with empirically based approaches and suspicious, often rightly so, of the 'research shows that . . .' argument. Practitioners may raise objections, including:

- Evidence-based practice is oppressive – why should one kind of knowledge be favoured over another?
- What about the experience and views of service users? Where do these fit in?
- Who decides what is 'best' evidence?
- Some things can't – and shouldn't – be measured. And not everything that counts can be counted.
- Social care is far too complicated to be researched and managed on this basis.
- Telling people what is 'best' practice interferes with professional autonomy.
- Evidence-based practice is an attempt to eliminate radical ideas by imposing conformity.
- There is so much information telling us what to do – and it often says completely different things. How do we know who to believe?

Although few would dissent from the proposition that the best possible evidence should guide child care practice, there is disagreement over what kinds of evidence are most relevant. Evidence-based practice in social care tends to be associated with empirical models of investigation and cognitive-behavioural methods of intervention. It has been argued that this kind of evidence is too narrow and other types of knowledge are correspondingly under-valued (Lewis 1998). The promotion of evidence-based practice has been associated with the elevation of managerialism over creativity (Trinder 1996; Webb 2001). Excessive emphasis on outcomes may diminish the importance of process (Sinclair 1998) and fail to influence practice if insufficiently grounded in the day-to-day experience of practitioners (Shaw and Shaw 1997). A more fundamental objection suggests that professional knowledge, far from being objective, constitutes a claim to power and that evidence-based practice, by failing to give equal status to the voices and views of users, is an essentially oppressive model (Everitt and Hardiker 1996; Witkin 1999).

These arguments share several common features. First, they all suggest that attempting to place the principles of the natural sciences in a more elevated position in social care is futile because, unlike health services, the messy texture of human relationships is more resistant to standardized interventions. We would argue, however, that this both exaggerates the extent to which anyone believes that 'evidence' *alone* can guide or legitimate a social care intervention and underestimates the 'messiness' of health service interventions. (If, for instance, your general practitioner prescribes the same analgesic in the same strength to all patients regardless of their age, preferences or medical history, then you would probably be looking for another doctor.) Second, there is a perception that evidence-based practice devalues the narratives of the powerless and privileges the good and the great. We do not hold this view. We would argue that those who believe that their chosen approach – whether based on 'knowledge', 'evidence', 'experience', 'intuition', 'practice wisdom' or simply an ideological conviction – is sufficient justification for their actions are adopting an authoritarian position (Chalmers 1983), one summed up more wittily than we could manage a century ago: 'First come I, my name is Jowett/ There is no knowledge but I know it/I am the Master of this college/What I don't know isn't knowledge'.

Although the collision between empiricism and intuition is not new (William Blake was on the case two centuries ago with his 'mind-forged manacles'), the dispute is more than a tedious argument between methodological anoraks. Important issues concerning the welfare of highly vulnerable people are at stake. Does the empirical investigation of social problems weaken our intuitive connection with those who are afflicted with poverty, impairment and disadvantage? To what extent can the human heart be moved by randomized controlled trials and systematic reviews? Are we artists or scientists? A glance through the 'books that have changed my life' feature in a leading journal for social care workers would seem to confirm the power of personal narrative as a vehicle for professional epiphanies. Volumes on spirituality, ethics and metaphysics loom large; no-one, to the best of our knowledge, has ever chosen the *Diagnostic and Statistical Manual of Mental Disorders* or the *Handbook of Empirical Social Work Practice*. The tension between promoting social change through appeals to both reason and emotion was well known to Thomas Barnardo. Although he based much of his early success on photographic images and detailed descriptions of children's misery, he also wished to establish a reputation as a serious social scientist. In an address to a social science convention in 1879, he provided an early example of a cost–benefit analysis. We could choose between expenditure, he suggested:

> in the shape of rates and taxes for the support of police, magistrates, justices, houses of detention, convict prisons . . . or in the form of donations to institutions like ours . . . every convict costs England upwards of £80 per head per annum. Every boy or girl taken from the streets costs but £16 per year.
>
> (*Night and Day*, September 1879; cited in Rose 1987: 85)

The notion that giving children the best possible start in life is sound economic sense was reiterated over a century later, in relation to the Perry Pre-School study: 'Over the lifetime of the participants, the pre-school program returns to the public an estimated $7.16 for every dollar spent' (Schweinhart *et al.* 1993:

to underestimate the contribution that can be made by temporary foster care placements. Stability in care is another Quality Protects objective, an issue explored in depth by Sonia Jackson, who notes that instability of residence may have serious effects on a child's health, educational performance and social relationships. Placement breakdown is not just distressing for the child and for all involved, it is also very expensive – investment in high-quality placement support is money well spent. Continuity of care, she suggests, should be the central aim of the whole care system. Mike Stein's review of leaving care research coincides with the implementation of the Children (Leaving Care) Act 2000, which introduces many of the duties to local authorities that campaigners in this area have argued for over many years. Although young people leaving care continue to face considerably more hardships and disadvantages than their peers, there is reason to believe that a period of decline in the attention given to this area has been reversed, and evidence continues to accumulate that well-resourced support programmes can make a real and tangible difference to the lives of these often very vulnerable young people. Concluding this section, David Berridge argues that effective residential care services are an essential placement option. Some children who, for a variety of reasons, do not want the more intimate experience of foster care, may be well-suited to a residential setting. In such settings, Berridge reminds us, the process of care and not just its outcomes are crucial. Children's views on good 'quality' care often focus on the personal attributes of the staff who care for them – reliability, a capacity and willingness to listen, respectful, informal but challenging. Recruiting and retaining staff with these qualities, he suggests, is as big a challenge as the more technocratic aspects of accumulating an evidence base.

Part 2, which looks at what works in relation to social exclusion, suggests that a prerequisite to social inclusion in a democratic society is social engagement. If young people are distanced from decision making – if, like the former prime minister Margaret Thatcher, they come to believe that there is no such thing as society – then inclusion will be an uphill struggle. McNeish and Newman's review of research and practice addressing 'what works' in involving children and young people points to several areas where work on engaging young people looks promising. Nevertheless, they also refer to issues often avoided by those looking at what works in social care – the potential to do harm through ill-conceived or poorly planned processes. They make no secret of the lack of systematic evaluation in this area. Although they raise potentially uncomfortable questions about the impact of participation on the *effectiveness* of services, they point out that participation is a basic human right. We do not need a systematic review of universal suffrage to know that it is a good idea. Utting, Vennard and Scott produce some of the stronger research evidence available to contributors to this book, but even so, they highlight considerable limitations of the evidence base, particularly in relation to work in Britain. Education, as a universal provision in the UK, clearly has enormous 'inclusion' potential, although in practice quite the reverse may happen, an issue that has taxed politicians and education policy makers. Dyson's review is appropriately cautious, while posing some of the prior questions that need to be answered to contextualize the effectiveness of inclusive education. The 'what works' question(s) cannot be answered by ignoring the issues of 'for whom' and 'in what circumstances'. It is an issue that also rests on matters of civil and human rights. As Beresford points out, in the context of disabled children's lives, exclusion from everyday mainstream activities has an impact on excluded children's ability to become included once the opportunity arises. Craig points out that it is not enough simply to assume that community development with children is a good thing. He suggests that, although there is evidence that direct engagement of children in a community development context brings benefits to them, there is not a strong evaluative base.

Part 3 reviews interventions and strategies that can reduce morbidity and mortality, focusing on three distinct but overlapping areas: the protection of children from abuse and neglect, the promotion of children's well-being through the reduction of health inequalities, and supporting families through addressing the single biggest challenge reported by parents and practitioners – how to help children with emotional and behavioural difficulties. The section begins with a review by Macdonald of effective interventions in child protection. While not devaluing the importance of social, political and economic strategies, Macdonald focuses on practitioner-led interventions, with an emphasis on what we can learn from randomized controlled trials and other robust studies. Adopting a structure of primary (population-based), secondary (children at risk) and tertiary (stopping more abuse) prevention, Macdonald argues that, in many areas, we already have compelling evidence that certain techniques and strategies, if used and authentically replicated, can reduce the exposure of children to many abusive experiences. Following the Acheson Report (Department of Health 1998b), which made the use of the term 'inequalities' politically respectable again, Roberts looks at links between poverty and ill health, arguing that the steep social class gradient for problems ranging from infant mortality to accidents can be reduced by a combination of good practice, political action and strategic decision making over resources. By treating parents and children as 'experts' in the art of keeping safe in their own environments, we can identify and rectify local dangers. Effective education, environmental change, technical solutions and effective and targeted social support all have a role to play. However, as Roberts points out, not all well-meaning health promotion activities work; in fact, some may do more harm than good. Sound evaluation is essential, especially where the intervention concerned is extensive and expensive. This section, and the book, concludes with Buchanan's discussion of how children with emotional and behavioural problems – which evidence suggests have become substantially more prevalent – may be helped. Family support services face difficulties in this area more than any other problem they encounter. However, there is a range of well-attested strategies that have proved to be effective in addressing many of these situations, and the evidence base is rather stronger in this field than in many other dimensions of child care practice. Buchanan reviews the range of childhood disorders, their genesis and maintenance, and explores how problems that cause so much distress to children and families may be reduced.

The final chapter highlights the views of young people themselves on the main themes in this book. The young people we spoke to were aged between 16 and 21 years and most had relied, to varying extents and in varying ways, on social care services for periods of their lives. Some of their observations make, albeit in different language, very similar points to those of our expert contributors; some are different, others express concerns not addressed in this volume at all. These commentaries are not meant to be a critique of the content. Rather, their inclusion is a recognition that the more remote the end-user becomes in any enterprise, the less likely it will be that their needs will remain paramount. Finding creative ways of introducing the voices of children and young people to otherwise adult debates is one way of keeping the end-users' welfare central to the task at hand.

In our collective experience and in our preparation for this volume, it has become clear that there is, in both the voluntary and statutory social care sectors, a hunger for robust, well-crafted, evidence-based research that has utility for day-to-day practice. We hope that this book goes a small way towards meeting this need.

REFERENCES

Chalmers, I. (1983) Scientific enquiry and authoritarianism in perinatal care and education, *Birth*, 10(3): 151–66.

Department of Health (1998a) *Modernising Social Services*, Cm. 4169. London: The Stationery Office.

Department of Health (1998b) *Independent Inquiry into Inequalities in Health* (Chair: Sir Donald Acheson). London: The Stationery Office.

Everitt, A. and Hardiker, P. (1996) *Evaluating for Good Practice*. Macmillan: Basingstoke.

Fagan, T.J. (1975) Nomogram for Bayes's theorem, *New England Journal of Medicine*, 293: 257.

Lewis, J. (1998) Building an evidence-based approach to social interventions, *Children and Society*, 12: 136–40.

Macdonald, G. and Roberts, H. (1995) *What Works in the Early Years?* Ilford: Barnardo's.

Myers, L.L. and Thyer, B.A. (1997) Should social work clients have the right to effective treatment?, *Social Work*, 42(3): 288–98.

Rose, J. (1987) *For the Sake of the Children*. London: Hodder & Stoughton.

Rosen, A., Proctor, E.K. and Staudt, M.M. (1999) Social work research and the quest for effective practice, *Social Work Research*, 23: 4–14.

Sackett, D.L., Rosenberg, W.M., Gray, J.H.M., Haynes, R.B. and Richardson, W.S. (1996) Evidence-based practice: what it is and what it isn't, *British Medical Journal*, 312: 71–2.

Schweinhart, L., Barnes, H. and Weikart, D. (1993) *Significant Benefits: The High/Scope Perry Pre-school Study through Age 27*. Ypsilanti, MI: High/Scope Press.

Sheldon, B. and Chilvers, R. (2000) *Evidence-Based Social Care: A Study of Prospects and Problems*. Lyme Regis: Russell House Publishing.

Shaw, I. and Shaw, A. (1997) Keeping social work honest: evaluating as profession and practice, *British Journal of Social Work*, 27: 847–69.

Sinclair, R. (1998) Developing evidenced based policy and practice in social interventions with children and families, *International Journal of Social Research Methodology*, 1(2): 169–86.

Sure Start (1999) *A Guide to Evidence Based Practice: 'Trailblazer' edition*, April. London: Sure Start Unit.

Trinder, L. (1996) Social work research: the state of the art (or science), *Child and Family Social Work*, 1: 233–42.

Webb, S. (2001) Some considerations on the validity of evidence-based practice in social work, *British Journal of Social Work*, 31: 57–79.

Witkin, S. (1999) Constructing our future (editorial), *Social Work*, 44(1): 5–8.

Zoritch, B. and Roberts, I. (1997) The health and welfare effects of day care for pre-school children: a systematic review of randomized controlled trials, *The Cochrane Library*, Issue 4. Oxford: Update Software.

PART I

Services for adopted and looked after children

In 2000, over 60,000 children in the UK were being looked after by local authorities at any one time, under the various provisions of the Children Act 1989 and its Scottish and Northern Ireland analogues. This represents about one-sixth of all children 'in need'. Although the number of children entering care has declined in recent years, the number of looked after children has increased by around 14 per cent over the past half-decade, largely because children who do enter care tend to stay longer. Although under 1 per cent of all children, this population includes some of our most troubled and, in some cases, most troublesome young people. Adoption has become a more widely used route to permanent care, with the number of children being placed for adoption increasing. Most looked after children are currently placed with foster carers, although residential placements still accommodate some children and many looked after children experience a period of residential care at some time in their lives.

The issues discussed in this section are various. The common theme that unites them is the way that state institutions and their representatives exercise parental responsibilities in many crucial areas of children's lives. Some of the material that follows is inevitably critical of the ways in which these duties are discharged. However, the enormity of the task that often confronts carers and social workers should not be underestimated. For most children, birth parents remain their most important emotional, maturational and financial resource, not just through childhood, but often into adulthood. Parents never forget their children's names; few social workers and carers can make this claim of all the children who pass through their hands. Providing intimate care in a professional context for children, especially for those who have suffered severe physical or emotional damage, is a uniquely challenging task. Where the contributors to this section highlight failures, fiscal, political and organizational factors play an important part. Where successes are noted, it is often due to the personal qualities of perseverance and dedication exhibited by professionals acting in parental roles and the resilience of the young people concerned. Most importantly, the voices and views of children themselves, as we are continually reminded, play an insufficiently elevated role in decision making about their own lives.

Looked after children face substantial obstacles. Although most children experience stability and continuity of care, environment, education and friendship, looked after children may find themselves on a roundabout of different carers, neighbourhoods and schools. When adulthood approaches, instead of a paced introduction to its stresses and responsibilities with a safety net of a stable family and community, looked after children may have to face the world with all its dangers and demands with little but their own natural assets. The chapters in this section describe some of the ways in which we can help make this journey more successful.

1

CLIVE SELLICK
JUNE THOBURN

Family placement services

KEY MESSAGES

- The maintenance of contact with birth families is increasingly recognized as a protective factor for children in alternative family placements.
- A well-resourced and well-supported range of temporary and longer-term foster placements is an essential dimension of an effective family placement service.
- Poor support and training will increase the likelihood of placement breakdown.
- Continuity of post-placement support from the worker or workers involved in the initial home assessment is preferred by foster carers.
- Local word-of-mouth recruitment continues to be the most fruitful source of foster carers, casting some doubt on the cost-effectiveness of large-scale advertising campaigns.
- Attracting and retaining foster carers is more successful when sound business principles are observed: targeted recruitment, preferably with the involvement of existing carers; sound assessment; effective and ongoing training.
- The importance of salaries is a growing issue, due to the increasing prominence of independent agencies, and this may be reflected in the rising number of male foster carers.
- There have been several important changes to the profile of foster care in recent decades, notably:

- an increased emphasis on placements with family and friends;
- the need to care for children with more difficult behaviours;
- more recruitment of carers from ethnic minorities;
- more recruitment of single carers;
- longer-term placements.

- Wanting to become a 'normal member of the family' is the clearest message from children. Where specialist therapeutic help is indicated, this should be negotiated with children and not undermine the child's relationship with the foster family.
- Although 'permanence' continues to be of paramount importance, contact with birth families and the need for a range of placement options are believed to be crucial mediating factors.

INTRODUCTION

The placement of a child with a supplementary or a substitute family is a highly complex intervention that brings with it particular problems when assessing effectiveness. In particular, time-scales are very important when trying to make sense of family placement research. At its simplest, the long-term outcomes of adoption of infants are measured 20 or more years after the child was placed, and the practice leading to these outcomes will have changed in the intervening period. Even for task-centred or respite care, many characteristics of the child, the two sets of parents and their parenting behaviours have to be taken into account as variables likely to have a stronger impact on outcome than the practice of individual social workers. Child placement practice comprises many elements. The decision to place and the choice of family will have the greatest influence on the long-term well-being of each child. Social work practice is complex, starting with recruitment and assessment and moving through intensive work at the time of placement to post-placement support and therapy with birth parents, the child, the new carers and the members of their families.

With such a complex research agenda, it is hardly surprising that there are many gaps in research-based knowledge on which to build child placement practice. Many of the 'certainties' that are often cited are actually value statements about what *should* be done rather than what has been shown by research to be effective. This chapter updates an earlier overview (Sellick and Thoburn 1996), separating out task-centred placements from those intended to provide permanent substitute families, although there are messages from research in each area that are relevant to the other.

TEMPORARY FOSTER CARE

Although we do refer to key research, the emphasis in this review is on recent studies that have not been considered together elsewhere. Over the past five years, government and non-government policy initiatives have had a significant influence on foster care practice. Some of the strongest messages to emerge from the Department of Health and the National Foster Care Association (NFCA) are related to the need to raise the standards of social work practice associated with foster care (Department of Health 1998; NFCA 1999a,b). The government's Quality Protects initiative laid down a series of priority areas and objectives. Introduced by the Department of Health in 1998, the Quality Protects programme enables local authorities to obtain funding for a wide range of practice developments, including those associated with supplementary foster care. Two areas in particular, placement choice and stability, are related to research messages about effectiveness. For example, increasing the choice of placements for looked after children is a major priority and is linked with objectives for recruiting a wider range and greater number of foster carers, areas where research studies have indicated a deficit (see, for example, Association of Directors of Social Services 1997; Warren 1997; Waterhouse 1997). Similarly, improving placement stability is linked to the objective of reducing the number of changes in main carers for children that are looked after, an issue that has also been researched extensively and which is discussed elsewhere in this section.

Until fairly recently, it was common to read about the paucity of foster care research (see, for example, Triseliotis *et al.* 1995; Berridge 1997), but this has now changed markedly. Several extensive studies have been undertaken across the UK over the past few years: Pithouse *et al.* (1994) and Pithouse and Parry (1997) reviewed fostering services and structures across the then eight Welsh county councils; Waterhouse (1997) examined fostering arrangements in 94 English local authorities; and a subsequent study of 32 Scottish local authorities by Triseliotis *et al.* (2000) completes a comprehensive account of family placement services in mainland Britain. The much enlarged independent fostering sector has been researched by Sellick (1999c), whose nationwide survey is in preparation. Other recent studies include those of Aldgate and Bradley (1999), who explored the use of short-term accommodation as a family support service to prevent long-term family breakdown, and of Sinclair *et al.* (2000), who examined over 500 foster placements in seven English local authorities. These and a number of smaller studies have much to say about supplementary and intermediate foster care practice in contemporary Britain. As we shall see, some of these recent research findings question established policy and practice, particularly regarding effective recruitment and retention methods.

In this part of the chapter on effectiveness in family placement, we describe foster care research in relation to the characteristics and circumstances of the children in placement, the contemporary profile and role of foster carers and the nature of the service itself. The following questions will be addressed:

- Are the children placed more challenging?
- Are their difficulties being addressed appropriately by the provision of social work and other services?
- Are the major players – the foster carers themselves – being recruited and retained to maximum effect?

THE CONTEMPORARY PROFILE OF SUPPLEMENTARY FOSTER CARE

KEY POINTS

- Foster care is the most common type of placement for looked after children.
- Lack of placement choice remains common.
- Independent fostering agencies are now used by most local authorities.
- Kinship care has grown in importance, notably in response to the need for culturally appropriate placements. More children are now in kinship care than in residential care; in some parts of the UK, numbers approach one-third of all placements.
- Up to half of children, depending on the area, are placed with single carers; a growing number are from ethnic minorities. Male carers are also growing in number and their value is increasingly stressed.
- Most placements are made in emergencies. In such cases, breakdown is common, especially in the first 12 months.
- Mean placement periods have become longer and the proportion of children presenting challenging behaviours has increased.

In our earlier review (Sellick and Thoburn 1996), we reported Stone's study of temporary foster placements in Newcastle, which provided a four-part framework of service provision (Stone 1995). Stone highlighted that the organization of fostering services, especially in terms of recruitment and training, should accurately reflect the nature and needs of the groups of children in placement, and that temporary fostering was as much about supporting families as about substitute parenting. The first point will always be relevant and stresses just how important research should be in the planning and provision of fostering services. It is clear from recent research studies that children are often presenting difficulties that challenge their foster carers and threaten their placements. Crucially, research has also clarified the importance of high-quality fostering and other services for children and the now widely acknowledged need for a range of support services for foster carers. Bringing all these together is at the heart of an effective family placement service. Recent studies also continue to shed light on the circumstances and needs of all the parties engaged in the fostering task. In doing so, they illustrate what endures (for example, the need for competent and responsive social workers) as well as what changes (for example, recognition of the need for specialist health and education services for looked after children).

Stone's second point, however, about the many children in very short-term care, needs to be revised in the light of subsequent studies and what these say about more children spending longer periods being looked after. This is an illustration of how research requires ongoing scrutiny and revision to assist in the maintenance or improvement of effective services. More recent research (e.g. Sellick 1999b) has shown the extent to which social work practice in foster care has been affected by policy changes. The following are the most important issues to have emerged:

1 Fostering is now the first (and often the only) choice of placement for many children, including teenagers. Recent annual reports from the Department of Health have consistently recorded as many as 65 per cent of looked after children being fostered.
2 Children and young people are offered little placement choice. Only 20 per cent of the English local authorities studied by Waterhouse (1997) reported that they could always offer a choice of placement for children under 10 years; this figure fell to only 3 per cent for children and young people over that age. In Scotland, a lack of placements meant that almost 30 per cent of children could not be placed and a further 14 per cent were not in a placement of first choice (Triseliotis *et al.* 2000).
3 Most English local authorities use agencies in the non-public sectors to provide foster placements. These grew from 11 in 1993 to 62 by the start of 1998 (Lord 1998). Current estimates put this number at 100. Although they developed from the teenage fostering schemes of the late 1970s, they now provide for a much more heterogeneous group of children. A former Chief Inspector of Social Services, commenting on the report of a government inspection of ten independent fostering agencies in 1994, stated that 'in some cases the inspectors thought that the children were amongst the most troubled children they had seen in foster care and in others they found it hard to believe that placements could not have been found nearer their homes' (Utting 1997: 41). Current research (Sellick and Connolly 2001) suggests that the balance has shifted towards meeting the needs of children who need a comprehensive range of educational and health services, in addition to a specialist fostering setting.
4 The use of kinship care has grown from 3 per cent more than a decade ago (Rowe *et al.* 1989) to 12 per cent in 1997 (Waterhouse 1997). In

some places, especially London, this figure is as high as 30 per cent. Some of these placements are made because of the shortage of stranger foster carers, but others are placements of choice because they meet the racial, cultural, language and religious needs of children from minority ethnic groups. The numbers of children accommodated in kinship foster placements are now higher than those in residential care (Department of Health 2000).

5 There are many more single foster carers than previously, the vast majority of whom are women. Fifty per cent of the carers in the study of Waterhouse and Brocklesby (1999) were single carers. Sinclair *et al.* (2000) reported single carers making up 24 per cent of carers across their sample from seven local authorities. Over one-third of boys were placed with single carers; half of these boys were aged over 10 years. Waterhouse and Brocklesby (1999) comment that, without substantial support networks for foster carers and appropriate services for children, this combination is very vulnerable to placement breakdown. Sinclair *et al.* (2000) highlighted another significant feature: 55 per cent of the single carers in their study were from ethnic minorities. Practice initiatives in the 1980s to recruit and approve black foster carers, many of whom were single women (described, for example, in Triseliotis *et al.* 1995), have clearly been effective. Methods for supporting them and retaining their services have, however, been less well scrutinized.

6 Considerable interest in the role and function of male foster carers is reflected in recently published accounts both in the UK (Gilligan 2000; Newstone 2000) and in the USA (Inch 1999). Male foster carers can provide positive and compensatory care to children whose experience of men has been distorted by harmful events as well as positive support to their (usually) female foster carer partners. Newstone argued that male carers can effectively contribute to better outcomes for foster children, especially in terms of the 'Looking after Children' dimensions of health, education and self-care (Department of Health 1995). In his evaluation of one independent fostering agency, Sellick (1999a) found that the fees paid to carers enabled men to be more evident, equal and effective foster care providers.

7 Most placements are unplanned or made in emergencies and often involve very young children. In the studies of Waterhouse and Brocklesby (1999) and Sinclair *et al.* (2000), 66 per cent of placements were in these categories; Waterhouse and Brocklesby noted that 75 per cent of these cases involved children under 5 years of age. In Scotland, over half the children studied by Triseliotis *et al.* (2000) were referred for placement in emergencies.

8 Many of these unplanned placements are made by a series of duty social workers and duty family placement workers, without first-hand knowledge of the child or the carer, and are provided by foster carers outside their approval range, a factor that Waterhouse and Brocklesby (1999) strongly associated with the risk of placement breakdown. Sinclair *et al.*

(2000) found that unplanned placements were as successful as planned ones once the child had been in placement for one year. Until then, however, they were likely to break down.

9 Children are remaining in care or accommodation for longer. Ten thousand or so children have been looked after in foster care for more than one year (Department of Health 2000). The studies of Rowe *et al.* (1989) and Stone (1995) painted a very different picture of placement length than the more recent study by Sinclair *et al.* (2000). A decade or so ago, somewhere between one-half and two-thirds of children, especially younger ones, were returning to live within their families of origin within weeks or at most months. In contrast, Sinclair *et al.* (2000) found that 30 per cent of foster carers who were approved as short term had children in placement for more than 12 months; a further 23 per cent of children in this study were in what their local authorities described as 'long-term' foster care.

10 One of the most striking and consistent findings from recent research is that, irrespective of their age, gender or ethnicity, children and young people in supplementary foster care are presenting behavioural difficulties that challenge and stretch their foster carers, often to their limits. In the study of Sinclair *et al.* (2000), over half of the children referred for placement were said to present behavioural or emotional problems; a further 10 per cent had a disability or health problem. The researchers described the range of children's behaviour as follows:

> They might steal, lie, break things, have tantrums, refuse to eat, smear walls, wet their beds, refuse to bath, continually defy their carers, set light to their bedding, take overdoses, make sexual advances to other children, expose themselves in public, make false allegations, attack others, truant, take drugs or get in trouble with the police.
>
> (Sinclair *et al.* 2000: 4)

School-excluded children, particularly boys, are especially difficult to manage without extensive support systems.

EFFECTIVE RECRUITMENT AND RETENTION

Research over the past five years has increased our knowledge base about successfully finding and keeping supplementary foster carers.

Recruitment

In a previous review (Sellick and Thoburn 1996), we highlighted three key recruitment messages from previous research studies.

> **KEY POINTS**
>
> - Success in recruiting an adequate number of high-quality foster carers is associated with targeted schemes.
> - Fostering agencies have to respond in an efficient and business-like way to sustain the interest of potential foster carers.
> - The retention of foster carers is associated with the initial recruitment process.

Recent research studies have continued to review effectiveness from the perspective of foster carers and have extended our knowledge base in this area.

Triseliotis and his colleagues (2000) found that the low profile of fostering within many Scottish local authorities had an adverse effect on policy development and resourcing. Twenty-five per cent of the agencies, including those serving the mostly highly populated areas, were experiencing serious carer shortages. Recruitment was largely one-off and unsystematic with no long-term direction or strategy. The most successful methods, however, were local. Fifty-three per cent of foster carers said they were attracted to fostering by word of mouth and another 22 per cent of existing carers were alerted to fostering by reading articles in the local press. This research finding does not sit well with the recent £2 million UK government funded foster care recruitment campaign. Results are being officially described as 'disappointing' (NFCA 2001). From a research perspective, this is unsurprising and fostering agency managers would do well to note that as many as 75 per cent of carers can be recruited cheaply and effectively through word of mouth and local press activities.

Sinclair *et al.* (2000) found that as many as 20 per cent of registered foster carers across seven local authorities were not currently fostering at the time of their study. Sellick and Connolly (2002) has found evidence of these dormant foster carers being recruited by independent agencies. Foster carers in the Scottish study felt that, if they played a central role in recruitment, they could address more effectively commonly held public fears and stereotypes of fostering and social work. This approach may make recruitment more successful, especially in urban areas, where the need is highest, yet where there is the lowest recruitment of foster carers.

Assessment

Assessing foster carer applicants has been influenced by different theoretical frameworks, ranging from the psycho-dynamic to the task-centred and to the competence-based approaches, with a mixed methodology usually incorporating individual, couple and group components. One approach relies on a systemic family therapy approach related to outcome research on what works and proposes a detailed six-session working model (McCracken and Reilly 1998). Earlier research (e.g. Triseliotis *et al*. 1995) described the interplay between the qualities and capacity of foster carers and the experiences and behaviour of children. The systemic approach has been adapted to take full account of family functioning, including the position of the applicants' children, and to supplement the traditional assessment features such as checks, references and medical examinations.

In research that explored the support provided to foster carers who had experienced an allegation of abuse against a member of their immediate family, Nixon (1997, 2000) recommended that, as early as the assessment stage, applicants should be made aware of the potential of such allegations. Although this may deter some applicants, others would see this as a good example of openness and honesty and as a first stage towards the later use of experienced foster carers in the training and support of carers.

Training

Based on data from their extensive sample, Triseliotis *et al*. (2000) concluded that foster carers who received a fee were more likely to support the idea of a salaried fostering service, attend training and support groups, and to recognize that there were benefits for children in seeing their parents. They were also more satisfied with the operation of the fostering service. Preparation and training were well received, but like carers in earlier studies, they wanted a more coherent and structured form of ongoing training. The issue of dealing with difficult behaviour emerged in the study of Sinclair *et al*. (2000), where foster carers commonly sought training on how to cope with anxious, depressed, aggressive or delinquent children and young people, or, as the researchers put it, 'training on issues which ordinary parents may not face' (Sinclair *et al*. 2000: 4). In a recent study (Minnis *et al*. 1999), a randomized control trial was conducted with the aim of assessing the impact of foster carer training on foster carer attitudes and children's behaviour. Although the authors' final conclusions have not yet been made available, an initial evaluation of the training programme of trained foster carers indicated success in terms of both the content of the programme in enabling them to understand and communicate more effectively with foster children and the process of joint training with social workers.

Foster carers in other studies have recommended that they become active participants in both preparation training, so as to expose unrealistic expectations (Butler and Charles 1999), and in ongoing training, so that they may share their practice knowledge with others.

Support

Recent research has provided new information, usually from the perspective of foster carers, about the importance of support. Although Sinclair *et al*.

(2000) were unable to show that support makes successful placements more likely, the combination of poor support, the complex needs of children and negative impacts upon foster carers does lead to a greater likelihood of placement breakdown, foster carer departure or both. It is clear from the wider literature that support is linked to foster carer retention. The role of the social worker – for the child, the family and the foster carers – remains pivotal. Good social workers 'talk and sort' (Sinclair *et al.* 2000: 4). Aldgate and Bradley (1999) defined this role in its relationship to carers and parents, where social workers 'engaged in the classic social work processes of assessment and intervention which are best described as social casework. This professional relationship was valued and used to good effect' (p. 207).

KEY POINTS

The literature identifies three main sources of satisfaction or dissatisfaction with social workers (Sellick 1999a; Fisher *et al.* 2000):

- their physical and emotional availability;
- teamwork and respect;
- help both of a practical nature and with the individual child.

Fisher *et al.* (2000) found that foster carers spoke positively of those social workers who exhibited the following qualities and skills:

- show an interest in how carers are managing;
- are easy to contact and responsive when contacted;
- do what they say they are going to do;
- are prepared to listen and offer encouragement;
- take account of the family's needs and circumstances;
- keep them informed and include them in planning;
- ensure that payments, complaints and so on are processed as soon as possible;
- attend to the child's interests and needs and involve foster carers where appropriate (Fisher *et al.* 2000: 231).

Where face-to-face support from social workers was not possible, Fisher *et al.* (2000) found that foster carers were satisfied with regular telephone contact with them.

In addition to the importance of good social worker support, the need for foster carer to foster carer support has been highlighted, to add a different dimension to the support needs of foster carers. Within the context of social work staff shortages and the prioritization of child protection and other crisis work, Pithouse and his colleagues (Pithouse *et al.* 1994; Pithouse and Parry 1997) have emphasized the importance of foster carer support and self-help groups. Similarly, Nixon (2000) highlighted the importance of carer to carer support when malpractice allegations are made, suggesting that this is particularly valued by foster carers under crisis-driven conditions.

Foster carer payment has been widely researched in the UK (e.g. Bebbington and Miles 1990; Sellick 1992). Pithouse et al. (1994) found that systems of remuneration were both 'confused and confusing' (p. 45) and were linked to the status of foster carers as employees, volunteers or professionals. One small-scale study of 20 female foster carers concluded that 'the place of payment within foster care is likely to remain complex and controversial' (Kirton 2001). Foster carers reported that payment did not motivate them to become foster carers, but that adequate and efficient payment systems kept them going when they felt dissatisfied by the children's behaviour or lack of progress.

Foster carers were found to perceive inadequate direct social work provision for children and foster carers as a key limitation of the overall social work service (Triseliotis et al. 2000). Sellick's (1999c) evaluation of one large independent fostering agency, which offered additional services for children, including therapy, special education and contact and leisure facilities, found that local authority social workers valued these highly and commented frequently how well these services compared in terms of quality and availability with those in their own authorities.

Another important type of support is that which foster carers receive from their partners and relatives. Sinclair et al. (2000) found that, without such support, foster carers were more likely to give up fostering. Some local authorities have applied this research message by approving a relative, often a female foster carer's mother or sister, to provide them with a respite service.

Although the turnover of carers reported by Sinclair et al. (2000) was low (about 10 per cent), the carers still experienced problems found in other research, including a lack of information about foster children, inefficiencies regarding payments and poor out-of-hours support. Turnover was low when there was good support by link workers, higher than average allowances/ fees and training and support from other carers. The study concluded that 'a combination of allowances, training, support from other carers and from family placement workers seems to provide the key to support' (Sinclair et al. 2000: 5).

Implications for policy and practice

Recent research, especially the wide-ranging studies of Triseliotis et al. (2000) and Sinclair et al. (2000), allow us to take a wide view of the family placement scene while focusing on some key issues. Triseliotis and his colleagues, for example, concluded that the strengths of the foster care service could be attributed to the commitment of carers, the link worker system, how enquiries were dealt with, the process of selection, preparation and training, support groups, the fee-paying structure and the move within some agencies towards the integration of residential and fostering services. Significant associations were found between, on the one hand, finding the children difficult, expectations not having been met and thinking about giving up fostering and, on the other hand, the non-availability of the children's social worker and poor general support.

Before the recent national recruitment campaign, the shortage of public sector foster carers reached crisis point. Its apparent failure to attract anything like its target figure of a further 7000 approved foster carers will probably mean more carers will be over-stretched and possibly overwhelmed as they care for troubled and troubling children, including those outside their approval range. Meanwhile, more children are likely to be placed with family and friends or with foster carers in the independent and private sectors. Some local authorities and independent agencies are entering into formal agreements that will regulate placement numbers and costs, and the Care Standards Act will require all fostering agencies to be inspected. The real challenge will be to retain and develop all foster carers, whether they be relatives or strangers or in the public or independent sectors, by a combination of sensitive and sophisticated support methods.

PERMANENT SUBSTITUTE FAMILY PLACEMENT

KEY POINTS

- Although the factors that contribute to the success or failure of a placement are complex, age at placement has been found to be consistently important.
- Outcome measures most frequently used are placement longevity and the child's well-being and satisfaction.
- Placements with relatives or friends tend to be more successful overall.
- Although findings are mixed, few differences appear to emerge between adoption and 'permanent' foster care in terms of the respective outcomes for children. The child's choice and sound professional judgement remain the crucial elements associated with success.
- Evidence continues to accumulate that placement with siblings is a protective factor.
- Where successful efforts are made to maintain contact with birth families, the number of breakdowns tends to be lower.
- There is no evidence that trans-racial placements are less successful if measured by breakdown rate; there are frequent accounts from children, however, that suggest a strong sense of cultural loss.
- Delay in permanent placement, while important, is likely to be far more relevant for an infant than an older child, who may need more time to adjust to the change in circumstances.

When assessing 'what works' when placing children with permanent substitute families, one has to evaluate the characteristics of the child being placed, especially age at placement, which is a 'proxy' for other variables. It has been shown that the characteristics of the child requiring placement will have an impact on the nature of practice and on success. A 6-week-old baby will usually be placed before too much harm has been done. Teenagers are often 'on the move', even in 'ordinary families', and most studies of the placement of teenagers show quite high rates of breakdown. The larger the study cohort, the more these individual differences can be allowed for when considering the relationship between any one variable and an outcome. Thus from larger-scale research studies, we can determine whether, in most cases, a particular aspect of the service is associated with a successful outcome for a subgroup of children, such as emotionally disturbed 12-year-old boys or infants who have Down's Syndrome (for a discussion on controlling the impact of one variable on another, see the appendix by Sapsford in Fratter *et al.* 1991; Thoburn 1994). Increasingly, researchers confront this problem from the start by evaluating placements for particular groups. Recent examples include the Maudsley 'middle childhood' studies (Rushton *et al.* 1995, 2001; Quinton *et al.* 1998) and Neil's (2000) study of infants adopted under the age of 4. Three recent sources of summary information are the Department of Health (1999) research overview *Adoption Now: Messages from Research*, the British Agencies for Adoption and Fostering (BAAF) review of statistics (Ivaldi 2000) and the *Prime Minister's Review of Adoption* (Cabinet Office 2000). The Department of Health's annual statistics show that 5 per cent of the almost 60,000 children 'looked after' in England in 2000 were placed with new families prior to legal adoption. There are no national statistics on children placed with foster families with the intention of establishing a life-long relationship, although some indication of proportions is provided by Sinclair *et al.* (2000), who found that 23 per cent of foster placements were described as long-term.

What the research tells us

The research will be reviewed under two broad headings: (1) the decision-making process about legal status, type of family and continuing contact and (2) the different aspects of practice. There have been no randomized controlled trials of permanent substitute family placement in the UK or USA. Most research comprises a descriptive account of children placed. Some provide a detailed account of process and some also measure outcome after varying lengths of time. Some studies involve only adoptive placements with families not previously known to them, while others include children placed for permanence with relatives, with permanent foster families or with short-term foster families confirmed as their 'forever families'. The most robust studies involve 'natural experiments', in that larger numbers included in prospective longitudinal studies make it possible to control for variables when considering outcomes for different groups of children in different types of 'permanent' placements.

The most frequently used outcome measure is whether or not the placement was disrupted within a given period of time. For some recent studies that provide a detailed account of social work practice (e.g. Quinton *et al.* 1998; Schofield 2001), only an interim outcome measure is available, sometimes as little as 12 months after placement, although with both of the above the intention is that they will become longitudinal prospective studies. Outcome data are more reliable if the outcome measure is taken after a longer period, as in Thoburn and colleagues' (2000) study of children from an ethnic minority. However, these children were placed in the early 1980s when some aspects of practice were different. Other outcome measures used in smaller-scale studies involve a range of measures of well-being and satisfaction, most often of the adoptive parents or adult adoptees but sometimes also of younger adopted children and, less frequently, of birth parents. Here we concentrate on outcomes for the children.

The placement decision

The decision to place a child with a substitute family is jointly made by some or all of the parents, young people, social workers, local authority solicitors, team managers, 'looked after' reviews, adoption and/or permanence panels and courts. There are descriptive accounts of these processes but no research that relates different processes to long-term child outcomes. Three important recent UK studies that provide detailed descriptive data on decision-making processes are Lowe and Murch's (1999) survey of 115 adoption agencies placing children aged over 5 (including detailed postal survey responses from 226 adoptive families and some qualitative interviews), Neil's (2000) survey of a 10 per cent sample of English children adopted under the age of 4 years and Harwin *et al.* (2001) study of care plans for 100 consecutive care order cases. Harwin and Owen found that adoption plans were made for around a third of the children (all under 7 with an average age of less than 3 years). Attempts were made to implement these plans, but some had been changed to long-term foster care within a two year period. Long-term foster care was the plan for just over a fifth of the children aged between 5 and 15, with an average age of 10 years. Just over one in ten were placed with relatives on a long-term basis.

When age at placement (and, sometimes, other key variables) has been controlled for in larger-scale studies, long-term placement with relatives or friends has been found to be more successful for the full range of children than placement with families not previously known to the child (for an overview of earlier studies, see Sellick and Thoburn 1996; for a review of the North American literature, see Maluccio *et al.* 2000).

There are three types of permanent placement with non-relative foster parents. The most successful on a range of measures is the confirmation of an already existing 'temporary' foster placement as a permanent placement. When such placements are included in a sample of 'permanent placements', as in the

Lothian study (Borland *et al.* 1991) and several American studies (e.g. Festinger 1986; Barth and Berry 1988), the breakdown rate is lower.

In a review of the literature, Schofield *et al.* (2001) found limited information about outcomes for children placed as long-term foster children, even though, as several studies of looked after children make clear, this is by far the most common 'permanence option'. Surveys of adolescents with a range of problems (youth offenders, homelessness and teenage pregnancy) have found that children who were once in foster care are greatly over-represented. However, this mainly reflects the fact that a large proportion of young people are already experiencing difficulties, often involving homelessness and criminal behaviour, at the point of entering care. No large-scale longitudinal study has yet been completed in the UK of a cohort of foster placements made with the intention that the children will remain in care until at least 16 years of age. In the USA, a prospective longitudinal study of older children placed in the Casey long-term foster care programme (Pecora *et al.* 1998) found the same rate of placement breakdown (around 50 per cent) as that found by Thoburn (1991) for adoptive and permanent foster placements in the UK. Smaller-scale studies provide contradictory findings. The placement breakdown rates reported by Berridge and Cleaver (1987) for long-term placements are similar to those reported by Thoburn and by Pecora *et al.* Gibbons *et al.* (1995) concluded from their study of children abused when under the age of 5 and followed up eight years later, that the well-being of those placed for adoption was no better than those in foster care, even though those in foster care had been placed later than those with adoptive families. However, long-term foster children who were subsequently adopted, when interviewed by Triseliotis and Russell (1984) and Hill *et al.* (1989) in a series of Scottish studies, came down firmly in favour of adoption. On a range of measures, the adopted young people were doing better than those brought up by long-term foster parents, and both were doing better than children brought up mainly in residential care.

Reporting on the first stage of a longitudinal study of long-term foster placements, Schofield *et al.* (2000) found that these are predominantly older children with complex family relationships and often traumatic backgrounds. Smaller-scale studies of young people 'ageing out' of stable foster family care at 18 and remaining in close touch with their foster families (Thoburn *et al.* 2000) report satisfaction for young people and foster parents. The work of Stein (1997, this volume) suggests that most placements that last until adulthood are successful on a range of well-being measures. Sinclair and colleagues (2000) found that more than half of the 151 foster children who responded to their survey wished to remain with their present foster families until age 18 or beyond.

The third group for whom more reliable outcome data are available are children placed with families not previously known to them, with the clear intention that this will become a 'family for life'. These are often placed by specialist 'adoption and permanence' teams and placement practice differs little from adoption practice. Thoburn (1991) and Thoburn *et al.* (2000) found

that around 20 per cent of 1165 permanently placed children were permanently fostered; almost 30 per cent of these children were of minority ethnic
origin. When other variables were controlled for, they found no difference
in breakdown rates between those placed for adoption and those placed as
permanent foster children. When other variables are considered, including
satisfaction of the new parents and young people, findings vary and numbers
are small. Thoburn (1990) found that the adopted and the permanent foster
children were equally likely to have a 'sense of permanence', although some of
the children chose to be adopted in their late teens.

The safe conclusion is that adoption will work best for and is preferred by
some children, whereas it will be foster care for others. It is important for
practitioners to look closely at the results of qualitative studies to help them
to decide which is best. Interviews with adopters and adopted young people
in the above studies and in the study of Thomas and Beckford (1999) provide
helpful clues. Several writers have noted that there is a group of mainly older
children who would not allow themselves to be placed with substitute families
if they had to break close links with their families of origin; here, foster
placement rather than adoption is likely to be more appropriate.

The most reliable information on outcomes concerns adoptive placements.
Below the age of 11, the younger the child at placement, the more likely the
placement will be successful on all measures. The breakdown rate for children
placed when under 6 months of age is around 5 per cent. The hazard here is
that a proportion of teenagers and adults placed as babies in 'closed-model'
adoptive families develop emotional problems – in a small minority of cases of
a chronic nature – regarding identity (Howe and Feast 2000). However, there
are indications that once older than 6 months of age, the risks associated with
placement increase. For a cohort of children who were older or who had
special needs, Thoburn (1991) found an average breakdown rate of 22 per
cent for children placed at the age of 8, rising to around 50 per cent for those
placed at the age of 10 or 11 years, and then dropping slightly.

Only around 200 infants are 'voluntarily' relinquished in England each year
and even in these cases the situation may be complex. Neil (2000) found that
of 62 children placed when under the age of 12, only 23 (37 per cent) were
relinquished infants; 34 per cent were more complex cases but not contested
in court; 29 per cent were adopted from care against parental wishes.

There is little robust evidence on the type of family likely to be successful
for different groups of children needing permanent substitute placement. Apart
from a heightened risk found in some studies if parents have 'own grown'
children close in age to the child being placed, no other easily measurable
characteristics are associated with more or less successful outcomes. Successful families may be older or younger, single or with a partner (Owen 1999),
with or without children of their own. The studies describe a wide range of
motivations. What seems to be important is that self-directed motives such as
wanting to become a parent are combined with an element of altruism, mani-
festing itself in the ability of the parents to empathize, not only with the child
but also with his or her biography, and thus develop an understanding of the

problems in the birth family which led to the need for placement. This characteristic is linked with the ability to help a child retain a clear sense of identity and probably goes a long way towards explaining the finding of many studies that families who can facilitate post-placement birth family contact are less likely to experience placement breakdown (for discussions of this complex issue, see Thoburn 1991; Sellick and Thoburn 1996; Quinton 1998; Ryburn 1997; Neil 2000).

Neil (1999), Dance and Rushton (1999) and Rushton *et al.* (2001) have summarized the evidence on the importance of placing children with substitute families who can either look after sibling groups together or ensure that they continue to have comfortable contact with each other. Rushton *et al.* (2001) provide a descriptive account of the characteristics, pre-placement experience and first 12 months in their substitute families of 133 children in sibling groups, some placed together and some 'split' or 'splintered'. This is the first stage of a detailed and complex longitudinal study. At this stage, there can be only pointers to assist practice in making decisions about placing siblings together or separately, but there is nothing to date to contradict other studies that have indicated that being placed with a sibling will usually be a protective factor.

On the question of ethnicity, there is no statistically significant difference in placement breakdown rates for families when the child and new parents are of similar or different ethnic origin (Thoburn *et al.* 2000). However, this and other qualitative studies (Kirton 2000; Kirton *et al.* 2000) provide evidence that some young people consider that they have lost out by being placed transracially. When parents and children are visibly different, there are extra obstacles to overcome in adapting to adoptive family life.

To summarize these findings, when the outcome measure used is whether the placement did not break down within a period of five or more years, whatever the route to permanence chosen, age of the child at placement appears to be the key variable. Other variables significantly associated with placement breakdown include being emotionally or behaviourally disturbed or 'institutionalized' at the time of placement, and having been maltreated prior to placement (Thoburn 1991). Others identify being 'singled out' for rejection by the birth parents (Quinton *et al.* 1998) or having experienced multiple moves, as associated with breakdown or lower well-being, but the data on these are less robust. Having two black or Asian parents does not appear to be associated with placement breakdown, although Thoburn (1991) found that children of mixed-race parentage were more likely to have disrupted placements.

The evidence about practice

There is very little robust evidence to link outcomes for children with aspects of placement practice. Rushton *et al.* (2001) have made the most comprehensive study of practice with parents and children around the time of placement. When reviewing case histories a year after placement, they concluded:

'in the cases of positive outcome it was impossible to say whether it was the intervention itself, the efforts of the parents, the passage of time, or a combination of factors that made the difference' (p. 145). Most of the studies already cited provide 'service outcome' data in that they describe the types of services provided at the various stages. The study of Lowe and Murch (1999) is particularly useful and draws out some differences between practice in the voluntary agency and local authority sectors. Most of the smaller studies provide information on the satisfaction (mainly of adopters) with different aspects of the service. Thoburn *et al.* (2000) and Howe and Feast (2000) supplement the earlier literature summarized by Sellick and Thoburn (1996). Thomas and Beckford (1999) provide compelling evidence on the views of 41 recently adopted children (mostly aged between 8 and 12) about the whole adoption process. In reviewing the evidence for a 'Quality Protects Briefing' (Department of Health 2002), Thoburn summarizes the evidence for services to adoptive families, services to children and young people and services to birth parents. Many of the messages echo those already reported above for short-term placements. Perhaps the strongest message is that clear and accurate information has to be provided at all stages to birth parents, new parents and (in an age-appropriate way) children. Since continuing direct or indirect contact is now a feature of most permanent arrangements, the evidence provided by Neil (2000) is also relevant. She found that the why and the how of contact were not adequately covered in the recruitment and training of adopters.

For adopters, there is a general acceptance that the home study stage has to be rigorous but that an empathic attitude by the social worker is essential. The positive aspect of this is that, during the assessment and approval stage, a relationship of trust and mutual respect develops. There is a consistent message from qualitative studies that after placement the adoptive family prefers the worker who did the 'home study' to be the main support worker. A readily available 'sounding board', reliable advice, advocacy to ensure that appropriate education and other services are provided, and help to negotiate the most appropriate contact arrangements are the preferred mode of intervention in the early months after placement. Sometimes out-of-home placement in a respite foster family or boarding education are required to sustain parent–child relationships. The cogent argument of Hill *et al.* (1989) for the generous provision of financial assistance is supported by Gibbons *et al.* (1995) and Lowe and Murch (1999), who found that the stressful lives of some adoptive families were made worse by financial problems.

The message that comes through most loudly from the young people is the request to be allowed to settle in and be 'a normal member of the family'. Any therapy deemed necessary at these early stages has to be carefully negotiated with the young person. However, several studies report positive feedback from young people and their adoptive parents about the help provided by educational and clinical psychologists. Another strong message from most studies is that, although a small proportion would prefer not to, most would like to see such professionals more frequently than they do.

Discussion points on permanent family placement

There is a lack of fit between current concerns about the adoption process and the research evidence. Much attention is placed on 'delay' in reaching a decision that a child should be placed, proceeding to placement and then to adoption. 'Common sense' and theories of child development suggest that delay is likely to be associated with poorer outcomes. However, no empirical study has shown this to be the case. One of the problems for researchers, policy makers and practitioners is that there can be no single 'best practice' for permanent substitute family placement when the children themselves have such different needs. Average time-scales are meaningless. A delay of six months before placing a relinquished infant will take him or her past the age at which risks start to accumulate. On the other hand, to expect a traumatized 9-year-old to have 'cut her losses' on a mum and dad she still cares and worries about and move on to a new 'forever family' all within six months may compound the significant harm already suffered. Consumer studies provide evidence of adopters and some children greatly regretting the lost months or years before they came together as a family, but other new parents and young people, who only make their voices heard when the placement breaks down, say it was all done too quickly and their opinions and doubts were not heeded.

Despite the many published studies, robust research on outcomes is only beginning to unravel the complex biographies, relationships, feelings, attitudes, practices and events that contribute to the success or otherwise of permanent family placements. Each year more pieces of the puzzle are slotted in. We have given details here of some of the most recent British studies, which are also sources of rich information on new research from across the world. We have not, in the space available, tackled the issue of inter-country adoption, but refer the reader to the volume on research policy and practice edited by Selman (2000). In drawing together what we do know, we conclude that, when children of any age cannot go safely home or to relatives, it is more likely than not that their needs can be met and their well-being enhanced by being placed with a permanent substitute family. No category is unsuitable for permanent family placement but, for a minority of *individual* children, the nature of their attachments to the parents they cannot safely live with, or the damaging impact of trauma, separation and loss, will make the risks to themselves and to any available new family too high. Other older children will just decline the offer and prefer group living, a move to independence or to remain in 'temporary' care, hanging on to the hope that a miracle will happen to mend their shattered families.

Once the decision to look for a new family has been taken, a careful assessment and scrutiny of the research will take the worker some way towards deciding what sort of placement and what sort of practice will be most likely to succeed with that particular child. Guidance can be helpful, but rigid rules based on age or type of maltreatment are to be avoided. For some children, only adoption and for others only foster placement will be acceptable. For some, legal status is much less important than finding a family who can empathize with the child's earlier life and facilitate the appropriate form of contact with birth parents and siblings. In such circumstances, the outcome research would support looking concurrently for *either* an adoptive *or* a foster family, thus widening the pool of potential families and decreasing the delay caused by only starting to look for foster carers after months or even years have elapsed and no adopters have been found. Similarly, there appears to be merit in the 'concurrent placement' practice of recruiting adopters or permanent foster parents who will work with the parents and social workers to get the child safely back home, but provide a permanent family home if returning home proves not to be possible. There are descriptive but as yet no published outcome studies of this model of practice in the USA. In the UK, it is in its infancy and used almost entirely with very young children. Finally, on the question of age, although the numbers of children being adopted from care are rising, the numbers placed for adoption when over the age of 5 are falling. It would be unfortunate if the drive to place more children for adoption led to a focus on the youngest (and easiest to place) children at the expense of the majority of children who are over 5 when they start to be looked after. It may be that the needs of these children are being met in stable long-term or permanent foster families, but that particular gap in our knowledge is only starting to be filled.

CONCLUSION

The Quality Protects targets draw on the available evidence on family placement when they stress a child's need for stability and a sense of permanence, alongside his or her need to know about and value cultural and personal identity. 'Permanence' has been the watchword for family placement, repeated in all government policy documents and legislation since the 1975 Children Act. However, micro-policies and practice in individual cases have fallen short of making it a reality for too many children. A review of the evidence since the early 1980s, when serious attempts were first made to introduce permanence policies pioneered in the USA (see Thoburn 1999), indicates that many children have benefited, but that two major mistakes were made.

The first was to underestimate children's need for continuity and connection with the family and culture of origin. This has often led to unnecessarily prolonged contested court cases and all too often delayed the child's move to substitute families, since the most contentious issue is often not whether the 'significant harm' threshold has been crossed, but the nature of any continuing birth parent and sibling contact. The evidence that continuing birth family contact is in most cases a protective rather than a destabilizing factor is leading to contact arrangements being part of the package for more children being placed permanently with foster or adoptive families. If more families are recruited who recognize the value of appropriate contact, the reduced conflict should lead to more children being placed more quickly.

The second major mistake was to undervalue temporary foster care. No 'permanence policy' can be successful without a choice of skilled short- and intermediate-term foster carers. Their place is essential in safely holding the child for as long as needed in a skilled and loving family home. They also provide the healing environment necessary if the child who has been harmed is to have the best possible chance of settling back permanently with the birth family or moving to a substitute family. Research has also shown that a minority will themselves become the permanent substitute parents for children placed with them on a temporary basis. After the early neglect of the essential contribution of foster care to child welfare policy and practice, there are encouraging signs that research and practice are joining together in a concerted attempt to ensure that long- and short-term family placements maximize the life chances of the increasing numbers of children who need their skill, perseverance and love.

REFERENCES

Aldgate, J. and Bradley, M. (1999) *Supporting Families Through Short-term Fostering.* London: The Stationery Office.

Association of Directors of Social Services (1997) *The Foster Care Market: A National Perspective.* London: Association of Directors of Social Services.

Barth, R. and Berry, M. (1988) *Adoption and Disruption: Rates, Risks and Responses.* New York: Aldine de Gruyter.

Bebbington, A. and Miles, J. (1990) The supply of foster families for children in care, *British Journal of Social Work*, 20: 283–307.

Berridge, D. (1997) *Foster Care: A Research Review.* London: The Stationery Office.

Berridge, D. and Cleaver, H. (1987) *Foster Home Breakdown.* Oxford: Basil Blackwell.

Borland, M., O'Hara, G. and Triseliotis, J. (1991) Placement outcomes for children with special needs, *Adoption and Fostering*, 15(2): 18–28.

Butler, S. and Charles, M. (1999) The tangible and intangible rewards of fostering for carers, *Adoption and Fostering*, 23(3): 48–58.

Cabinet Office (2000) *Prime Minister's Review of Adoption.* London: Performance and Information Unit.

Dance, C. and Rushton, A. (1999) Sibling separation and contact in permanent placement, in A. Mullender (ed.) *We are Family: Sibling Relationships in Placement and Beyond.* London: British Agencies for Adoption and Fostering.

Department of Health (1995) *Looking after Children: Assessment and Action Records, Aged Ten to Fourteen Years/Aged Fifteen Years and Over.* London: HMSO.

Department of Health (1998) *Quality Protects: Transforming Children's Services.* London: Department of Health.

Department of Health (1999) *Adoption Now: Messages from Research.* Chichester: Wiley.

Department of Health (2000) *Children Looked After by Local Authorities: Year Ending 31 March 1999, England.* London: Department of Health.

Department of Health (2002) *Quality Protects Briefing: Adoption and Permanence for Looked After Children.* Dartington: Research in Practice.

Festinger, T. (1986) *Necessary Risk: A Study of Adoptions and Disrupted Adoptive Placements.* New York: Child Welfare League of America.

Fisher, T., Gibbs, I., Sinclair, I. and Wilson, K. (2000) Sharing the care: qualities sought of social workers by foster carers, *Child and Family Social Work*, 5(3): 225–33.

Fratter, J., Rowe, J., Sapsford, D. and Thoburn, J. (1991) *Permanent Family Placement: A Decade of Experience.* London: British Agencies for Adoption and Fostering.

Gibbons, J., Gallagher, B., Bell, C. and Gordon, D. (1995) *Development after Physical Abuse in Early Childhood.* London: HMSO.

Gilligan, R. (2000) Men as foster carers: a neglected resource?, *Adoption and Fostering*, 24(2): 63–9.

Harwin, J., Owen, M., Locke, R. and Forrester, D. (2001) *Making Care Orders Work: A Study of Care Plans and their Implementation.* London: The Stationery Office.

Hill, M., Lambert, L. and Triseliotis, J. (1989) *Achieving Adoption with Love and Money.* London: National Children's Bureau.

Howe, D. and Feast, J. (2000) *Adoption, Search and Reunion: The Long-term Experience of Adopted Adults.* London: The Children's Society.

Inch, L. (1999) Aspects of foster fathering, *Child and Adolescent Social Work*, 16(5): 393–412.

Ivaldi, G. (2000) *Surveying Adoption.* London: British Agencies for Adoption and Fostering.

Kirton, D. (2000) *'Race', Ethnicity and Adoption.* Buckingham: Open University Press.

Kirton, D. (2001) Love and money: payment and the fostering task, *Child and Family Social Work*, 6: 199–208.

Kirton, D., Feast, J. and Howe, D. (2000) Searching, reunion and transracial adoption, *Adoption and Fostering*, 24(3): 6–18.

Lord, J. (1998) *Working with Independent Fostering Agencies: Guidance for Local Authorities in England and Wales.* London: British Agencies for Adoption and Fostering.

Lowe, N. and Murch, M. (1999) *Supporting Adoption: Reframing the Approach.* London: British Agencies for Adoption and Fostering.

McCracken, S. and Reilly, I. (1998) The systematic family approach to foster care assessment, *Adoption and Fostering*, 23(3): 16–27.

Maluccio, A.N., Ainsworth, F. and Thoburn, J. (2000) *Child Welfare Outcome Research in the United States, United Kingdom, and Australia.* Washington, DC: CWLA Press.

Minnis, H., Devine, C. and Pelosi, T. (1999) Foster carers speak about training, *Adoption and Fostering*, 23(2): 42–7.

National Foster Care Association (1999a) *UK National Standards for Foster Care.* London: National Foster Care Association.

National Foster Care Association (1999b) *Code of Practice on the Recruitment, Assessment, Approval, Training, Management and Support of Foster Carers.* London: National Foster Care Association.

National Foster Care Association (2001) Recruitment campaign update, *Foster Care*, 104: 3.

Neil, E. (1999) The sibling relationships of adopted children and patterns of contact after adoption, in A. Mullender (ed.) *We are Family: Sibling Relationships in Placement and Beyond.* London: British Agencies for Adoption and Fostering.

Neil, E. (2000) The reasons why young people are placed for adoption: findings from a recently placed sample and a discussion of implications for subsequent identity development, *Child and Family Social Work*, 4(6): 303–16.

Newstone, S. (2000) Male foster carers: what do we mean by 'role models'?, *Adoption and Fostering*, 24(3): 36–47.

Nixon, S. (1997) The limits of support in foster care, *British Journal of Social Work*, 27: 913–30.

Nixon, S. (2000) Safe care, abuse and allegations of abuse in foster care, in G. Kelly and R. Gilligan (eds) *Issues in Foster Care: Policy, Practice and Research*. London: Jessica Kingsley.

Owen, M. (1999) Single adopters and sibling groups, in A. Mullender (ed.) *We are Family: Sibling Relationships in Placement and Beyond*. London: British Agencies for Adoption and Fostering.

Pecora, P.J., Le Prohn, N.C., Nollan, K., *et al.* (1998) *How are the Children Doing? Assessing Your Outcomes in Family Foster Care*. Seattle, WA: The Casey Family Program.

Pithouse, A. and Parry, O. (1997) Fostering in Wales: the All Wales Review, *Adoption and Fostering*, 21(2): 41–9.

Pithouse, A., Young, C. and Butler, I. (1994) *The All Wales Review: Local Authority Fostering Services*. Cardiff: The University of Wales.

Quinton, D. (1998) Contact with birth parents in adoption – a response to Ryburn, *Child and Family Law Quarterly*, 10(4): 349–61.

Quinton, D., Rushton, A., Dance, C. and Mayes, D. (1998) *Joining New Families: A Study of Adoption and Fostering in Middle Childhood*. Chichester: Wiley.

Rowe, J., Hundleby, M. and Garnett, L. (1989) *Child Care Now – A Survey of Placement Patterns*. London: British Agencies for Adoption and Fostering.

Rushton, A., Treseder, J. and Quinton, D. (1995) An eight-year prospective study of older boys placed in permanent substitute families, *Journal of Child Psychology and Psychiatry*, 36(4): 687–95.

Rushton, A., Dance, C., Quinton, D. and Mayes, D. (2001) *Siblings in Late Permanent Placements*. London: British Agencies for Adoption and Fostering.

Ryburn, M. (1997) In whose best interests? Post-adoption contact with the birth family, *Child and Family Law Quarterly*, 53: 53–70.

Schofield, G., Beek, M., Sargent, K. with Thoburn, J. (2000) *Growing Up in Foster Care*. London: British Agencies for Adoption and Fostering.

Schofield, G. (2001) Resilience and family placement: a lifespan perspective, *Adoption and Fostering*, 25(3): 6–19.

Sellick, C. (1992) *Supporting Short-Term Foster Carers*. Aldershot: Arena.

Sellick, C. (1999a) The role of social workers in supporting and developing the work of foster carers, in M. Hill (ed.) *Signposts in Fostering: Policy, Practice and Research Issues*. London: British Agencies for Adoption and Fostering.

Sellick, C. (1999b) Can child and family social work research really assist practice?, *Children Australia*, 24(4): 93–6.

Sellick, C. (1999c) Independent fostering agencies: providing high quality services to children and carers?, *Adoption and Fostering*, 24(1): 7–14.

Sellick, C. and Connolly, J. (2001) *National Survey of Independent Fostering Agencies*. Norwich: University of East Anglia, Centre for Research on the Child and Family.

Sellick, C. and Connolly, J. (2002) Independent fostering agencies uncovered: findings of a national survey, *Child and Family Social Work*, 7(2): 107–20.

Sellick, C. and Thoburn, J. (1996) *What Works in Family Placement?* Ilford: Barnardos.

Selman, P. (ed.) (2000) *Intercountry Adoption: Developments, Trends and Perspectives*. London: British Agencies for Adoption and Fostering.

Sinclair, I., Wilson, K. and Gibbs, I. (2000) *Supporting Foster Placements.* http://www.york.ac.uk/inst/swrdu/fosterplacements.

Stein, M. (1997) *What Works in Leaving Care.* Barkingside: Barnardos.

Stone, J. (1995) *Making Positive Moves: Developing Short-Term Fostering Services.* London: British Agencies for Adoption and Fostering.

Thoburn, J. (1990) *Success and Failure in Permanent Family Placement.* Aldershot: Gower/Avebury.

Thoburn, J. (1991) Permanent family placement and the Children Act 1989: implications for foster carers and social workers, *Adoption and Fostering*, 15(3): 15–20.

Thoburn, J. (1994) The use and abuse of research in child care proceedings, in M. Ryburn (ed.) *Contested Adoptions: Research, Law, Policy and Practice.* Aldershot: Arena.

Thoburn, J. (1999) Trends in foster care and adoption, in O. Stevenson (ed.) *Child Welfare in the UK.* Oxford: Blackwell.

Thoburn, J., Norford, L. and Rashid, S.P. (2000) *Permanent Family Placement for Children of Minority Ethnic Origin.* London: Jessica Kingsley.

Thomas, C. and Beckford, V. with Murch, M. and Lowe, N. (1999) *Adopted Children Speaking.* London: British Agencies for Adoption and Fostering.

Triseliotis, J. and Russell, J. (1984) *Hard to Place – The Outcome of Adoption and Residential Care.* Aldershot: Gower.

Triseliotis, J., Sellick, C. and Short, R. (1995) *Foster Care: Theory and Practice.* London: Batsford.

Triseliotis, J., Borland, M. and Hill, M. (2000) *Delivering Foster Care.* London: British Agencies for Adoption and Fostering.

Utting, W. (1997) *People Like Us: A Report on the Safety of Children Living Away from Home.* London: Department of Health.

Warren, D. (1997) *Foster Care in Crisis: A Call to Professionalise the Forgotten Service.* London: National Foster Care Association.

Waterhouse, S. (1997) *The Organisation of Fostering Services: A Study of the Arrangements for Delivery of Fostering Services in England.* London: National Foster Care Association.

Waterhouse, S. and Brocklesby, E. (1999) Placement choices for children – giving more priority to kinship placements, in R. Grieff (ed.) *Fostering Kinship: An International Perspective on Kinship Foster Care.* Aldershot: Ashgate.

2

SONIA JACKSON

Promoting stability and continuity in care away from home

KEY MESSAGES

- Stability of care experience should be a central aim of the whole care system.
- Continuity of care is one of the main objectives of Quality Protects and its promotion is a key performance indicator for local authorities.
- The average number of placements increased during the period 1995–2000. Ten or more moves are not uncommon.
- Continuity of placement should be the default position in decision making. A move in care is only justified by clear evidence that it will contribute to the child's present or future welfare.
- Children have been insufficiently involved in decisions regarding placement changes. Little is known about the issue of instability from the child's perspective.
- Lack of stability and continuity of care affects children's lives in several crucial dimensions:

  - educational performance;
  - physical health, notably chronic conditions;
  - relationships, especially the ability to retain long-term attachments;
  - emotional, behavioural and mental health.

- Placement breakdown is distressing and expensive. Investment in strategies that may reduce the number of breakdowns will save money as well as help children.
- Future research should focus on methods of increasing placement stability and continuity of care.

INTRODUCTION

Almost all studies of children in public care identify the instability and unpredictability of their lives as prime causes of poor outcomes. Yet, surprisingly, little research has focused on the issue of stability itself. The purpose of this chapter is to ask:

- What do we mean by stability? Can we move beyond defining it simply as avoidance of placement breakdown?
- What is the extent of stability and instability in the care system now?
- What are the main causes of instability in care?
- How does stability relate to other aspects of quality of care for separated children?
- How does instability affect children's well-being and development?
- Do we know what might help to promote and maintain greater stability for children?

Despite the large volume of research on child welfare and local authority care over the past 20 years, it is still hard to locate good quality research studies that seek to answer these questions, especially the last one. There is the additional problem that few studies are precisely replicated. Where findings are contradictory, we often cannot tell if this is due to differences in the population being studied or to policy change over time at national or local level. For example, since 1997 the policy context of child care has been transformed, but much of the literature has barely caught up with the changes brought about by the Children Act implemented in 1991 and the later legislation in Scotland and Northern Ireland (1995). Apart from two surveys carried out in the 1980s, for large-scale quantitative studies we have mostly to look to North America. But we then have to ask how far we can rely on findings from different times and other countries.

The small-scale and context-specific nature of much UK research also raises questions about how far findings can be generalized. As Quinton *et al.* (1998: 205) have pointed out: 'studies that provide new insights can too easily be treated as "breakthroughs"', forgetting that any particular piece of research tends to capitalize on chance and can produce seemingly important predictors that are not replicated in further research.

In the past, instability has generally been equated with placement breakdown. This chapter looks at the problem more broadly, considering what factors in the care system as a whole work for and against stability and how we might make the best use of research knowledge to increase stability for children and young people looked after by local authorities.

MOVEMENT WITHIN THE CARE SYSTEM

It is difficult to know if instability within care has increased because there is so little firm information on the subject, but almost all studies show a high rate of placement turnover, affecting around half of children who remain in care for any length of time. The most reliable information on placement movement before implementation of the Children Act 1989 comes from a survey of admissions to care, discharges and moves in six local authorities (Rowe *et al.* 1989). This only measured moves of children who had been in care for a year over a further 12 month period. Over half (57 per cent) of the cohort of 2010 children had no moves during the year, but 38 children had five or more moves over this short time, including six pre-schoolers. There were no reports of children having the high numbers of moves found by some studies in the 1990s (Jackson and Thomas 1999).

Packman and Hall (1998) compared children entering care in the same two cities before and after implementation of the Children Act in 1991 and found that the rate of placement change had doubled. Biehal *et al.* (1995) studied 74 young people leaving care in three contrasting areas. Only one in ten had remained in the same placement throughout their care career and 10 per cent had moved more than ten times. The young people who had many moves, categorized by Biehal *et al.* as 'unsettled', tended to continue the pattern of instability and frequent movement after care.

Berridge and Brodie (1998) compared the circumstances of 70 young people living in children's homes with the similar population in Berridge's (1985) earlier study. They found that children were much less likely to stay long in public care, almost half having been away from home for under a year. In adolescent homes, three-fifths of the residents had been present less than three months. The proportion of fostering breakdowns and moves within care was less than in the earlier study, but the average number of placements for adolescents, despite the short time they had been looked after, was 3.3 and a third had already lived in five or more different settings.

A questionnaire survey of over 2000 looked after children carried out by the Who Cares? Trust (Shaw 1998) reported that, among those in care for five years or more, only one in ten had experienced a single placement and nearly a quarter, irrespective of age, had been in 11 or more different placements. Despite the difficulty in comparing disparate samples, it is probable that these figures represent a real increase in the instability of care since the survey of Rowe *et al.* (1989). Department of Health statistics show a rise in the average number of placements from 2.9 to 3.5 over the five years 1995–2000 (Department of Health 2001).

Children who are not already in a well-functioning long-term foster home when they enter adolescence appear especially vulnerable to serial placement breakdown (Sinclair *et al.* 1995; Triseliotis *et al.* 1995), or what John Brown (1998) memorably called 'accommodation pinball'. But children who enter care at an early age cannot rely on a stable care experience either.

Research on the implementation of the Looking After Children (LAC) materials found a disturbingly high level of movement even among the 16 per cent of children who began to be looked after under the age of 1 (Ward and Skuse 1999). Many had already had four or five changes of carer in the course of their first year, almost always initiated by social workers or managers for administrative reasons. This finding is confirmed by Gilles Ivaldi's (2000) analysis of the 1998–99 adoption statistics for the British Agencies for Adoption and Fostering (BAAF). He found that 44 per cent of infants between the ages of 1 and 12 months had four or more changes of carer while awaiting placement for adoption.

Young people who are relatively unproblematic and have done well despite spending several years in care do not seem much more likely to have a stable care career. In a study of 'high achievers' – care leavers who had gone on to further or higher education – the average number of placement moves for boys was 3 and for girls 5.5 (Jackson and Martin 1998). Among the comparison group of care leavers who had not been educationally successful, the boys had had 5.7 moves on average and the girls 4.4. In both groups, there were several individuals who had experienced more than 20 moves. One young woman, on obtaining access to her case file, discovered that she had been moved 36 times during her 15 years in care.

SETTING TARGETS FOR STABILITY

Greater stability, especially in long-term care, was one of the objectives of Quality Protects, the comprehensive programme launched in 1998 with the aim of improving outcomes for looked after children (Department of Health 1998). The specific objective set under the government's National Priorities Guidance was to reduce to 16 per cent in all authorities by 2001 the number of children looked after continuously for a year who have three or more placements, although the Department of Health (2001) admits that the three placement indicator only gives a 'rough measure' of the stability of care that a child experiences.

Although there is a constant flow of children in and out of the care system (approximately 81,500 in England, excluding those looked after under a series of short-term placements), there are also many children who remain for longer periods. In the year 1999–2000, nearly half of local authorities failed to achieve the 16 per cent criterion, with very wide variations – the range was 2–40 per cent. Some of the differences may result from inconsistencies in reporting, but it is clear that, overall, many English local authorities are falling a long way short of the target, whereas others are achieving better stability for children they look after (Department of Health 2001) (no comparable figures are available for other parts of the UK).

The focus on stability of placement as a performance indicator has also resulted in more information becoming available about numbers of placement moves during children's care history. Looking at children in continuous out-of-home care for four years or more, 46 per cent had been in their current foster placement for at least two years, a figure that remained remarkably constant between 1997 and 1999. Again the range was wide; for example, in Barnet, 78 per cent of children had experienced a stable foster placement for at least two years, whereas the figure for Wokingham was 15 per cent. Thirty-seven per cent of children leaving care in 1999–2000 had only a single placement, but 1600 had ten or more; among these, we know from other evidence, there will be some who had many more moves, with 30–50 not uncommon and in exceptional cases rising into the hundreds (Walker 2001).

WHAT CAUSES INSTABILITY?

The aspect of instability that has attracted most attention is placement breakdown, usually caused by the refusal of foster carers or residential workers to continue to look after a child, less often by the child's request for a change of placement. Significantly, the latter reason hardly figures in the literature at all. Foster care breakdown has tended to be viewed from a rather narrow perspective. Researchers have been preoccupied with the characteristics of the children and their families of origin, or the match between children and carers. Much less attention has been paid to characteristics of the receiving families or to the process of placement ending. Who decides that a placement has 'broken down'? How does it seem to the child concerned and to what extent are they consulted about the desirability of a move?

Another neglected aspect of instability is the part played by the care system itself. Moves are often dictated by policy or management considerations and may have nothing to do with the needs or behaviour of children. The most obvious example is the widespread closure of residential homes that took place throughout the 1980s and 1990s (Cliffe and Berridge 1992; Berridge and Brodie 1998). Children in long-term care might find their home swept from under them several times in succession. Although they sometimes protested, their views carried very little weight set against the substantial financial savings achieved by the local authority. Instability may also be built into placement policy, for example by an inflexible division between temporary, intermediate and long-term care, by arbitrary cut-off points linked to chronological age rather than individual circumstances (Marsh and Peel 1999), or by misguided policies, such as the discouragement of adoption by existing foster parents (Schofield *et al.* 2000).

Major sources of instability are also to be found outside the care system. Beckett (2001) has drawn attention to the huge increase in court proceedings, from 2657 initiated in 1992 to 6728 in 1998. The resulting delays leave children spending long periods in temporary placements with no idea what the future holds. Beckett points out that, just when the child most needs a stable attachment figure, he or she is least likely to have one. The education system, too, plays its part in creating instability. Exclusion from school, for example, is strongly associated with placement breakdown, as discussed later.

STABILITY AND CONTINUITY

It is useful to break down the concept of stability into several different aspects, which interact with each other but can still be seen as distinct.

> **KEY POINTS**
>
> - We might define *stability of placement* to mean not only that the child remains in the same home, but that it is seen by all the people involved as a secure setting within which the child can grow up or remain as long as needed.
> - *Stability of relationships* means children being part of a network of family and social relationships that remain stable and continuous over time. This includes not just the household and kinship group, but relationships with important people in their lives, such as friends and their parents, teachers, social workers and other professionals.
> - *Stability of education* ideally means staying in the same school, only moving with the year group, and with opportunities for learning geared to the child's interests and aptitudes.
> - *Stability of health care* means receiving services based on a full knowledge of the child's history and a regard for his or her individual needs, continuously monitored by carers.
> - *Stability of community* implies both remaining in a familiar neighbourhood and continuing involvement in activities taking place in that community.
> - *Stability of personal identity* is a more elusive concept with several different components. It means children having a clear understanding of who they are, what they are called, how they fit into their wider family, a sense of self-esteem and self-efficacy, and a cultural reference group that they can recognize and identify with, especially if this differs from that of their carers.

Another way of looking at the multidimensional character of stability is to distinguish more clearly between stability of placement and these other aspects of stability, which might be better described as continuity. In most cases they will go together, but the advantage of disaggregating them is that it becomes easier to balance the aspiration of placement stability against other needs.

In general, placement stability should take precedence if there are no overwhelming arguments for a change. It sometimes seems that moves are initiated by hopes of finding an 'ideal' placement. In the climate of acute placement shortage that exists in most areas, this is likely to be unrealistic. Unsettling a child by suggesting a move, even when the current placement is unsatisfactory in some respects, may do more harm than good. However, an over-emphasis on placement stability could lead to a move being resisted even when it would be in the child's interest or when he or she clearly expresses the desire for a change with good reason.

This point is made strongly in a study by Hedy Cleaver (2000) of the effects of increased emphasis on family contact following the Children Act. She observes:

> Changes of placement are generally considered to have negative consequences for children. However, in many cases a single, well-planned placement move, particularly when children went to live with relatives, had a positive impact on the child's well-being. In most cases moves also benefited contact because they allowed contact arrangements to be renegotiated.
>
> (Cleaver 2000: 275)

However, many moves are not well-planned, if planned at all, and the views of children and young people are seldom adequately considered (Folman 1998; Thomas and O'Kane 1999).

Continuity is harder to measure than placement stability and just as hard to achieve. What little we know about it from research suggests that its importance is greatly underestimated by social workers, especially in relation to health and education, but also, for example, in maintaining links with previous carers and other people who matter to the child. Research has shown that most care leavers feel part of extensive family networks with an average of over 20 members (Marsh and Peel 1999). When they were asked to rate the significance of different people in their lives, only a quarter nominated their natural mother as 'key kin'. Yet social workers typically focused on contact with mother to the exclusion of other relationships, often without listening to what the children might have to say. In the study of Marsh and Peel, fewer than half of social worker nominations for 'key kin' coincided with those of the young people.

STABILITY IN DIFFERENT SETTINGS

Most children looked after away from home are in foster care (65 per cent), a trend that is unlikely to be reversed. But there are also 11 per cent 'placed at home', a similar number in family group homes and many more who pass through residential care at some time in their care career. There is increasing diversity, too, in types of placement, some of which appear to hold out greater prospects of stability than others.

Surveying different kinds of substitute care underlines the weakness of the evidence on what works in creating stability. In all but a handful of studies, information on stability is a by-product of the research and not its main focus. That can make comparing categories of care a misleading exercise, both because many children move from one to another and because the meaning of the category changes. What do today's small residential units have in common with the 60-bed homes of the past? Once foster parents were enjoined to treat foster children as if they were their own; now their job is more often to work towards the child's return home and avoid taking over the parental role. In addition, research studies use different time spans and different criteria for inclusion.

Nevertheless, with these reservations, it is possible to place the main types of placement on a continuum from most to least stable. The evidence is reviewed in detail by Jackson and Thomas (2001).

1 *Staying at home* or returning there quickly generally offers the best hope of stability, although not necessarily the best quality of care (Schofield *et al.* 2000). Many children only have one episode of care and then go back to their own families without ever needing to be looked after again. Remaining in one's own family tends to be the most stable form of placement, especially for teenagers. Interdisciplinary adolescent support teams have achieved considerable success in avoiding the need for accommodation (Biehal *et al.* 2000). One study estimated that only 9 per cent of adolescents referred for care need it for their own protection and the rest could be safely maintained at home (Brown 1998).

2 *Adoption* has been the subject of more research than any other form of placement. The findings are extremely positive, showing consistently that adoption offers by far the best hope of stability for children who cannot live with their own families (Triseliotis *et al.* 1997; Jackson and Thomas 2001). It is rare for placements to break down once the adoption order has been made (Lowe *et al.* 1999) and outcomes are usually much better than for children who remain in care. In Howe's study of 211 children, for example, only two placements broke down, even though 89 of the children were 'late-placed' and 69 were considered to have had a particularly poor start in life (Howe 1996, 1997). There has been a dramatic swing of public and professional opinion in favour of adoption since it was the subject of a Prime Minister's Review (Cabinet Office 2000), but the number adopted from care is still very small, with long intervals and sometimes several changes of carer between first placement and adoption (Ivaldi 2000). Continuity of care, even for babies and very young children, does not seem to be given high priority, suggesting an unawareness of attachment theory among social workers and their managers.

Age at placement is a significant factor, with all studies showing the proportion of failed placements increasing the older the child, but adoption continues to be substantially more stable than long-term fostering. Perhaps, more importantly, it creates a life-long relationship, with adoptive parents providing emotional and practical support into adulthood, just as birth parents do. With the move towards more open adoption, it becomes a possibility for children who want to retain some contact with their birth families. Earlier predictions about the numbers of looked after children potentially available for adoption may prove far too pessimistic (Parker 1999).

3 Several American studies have shown that *placement with relatives* or kinship care is the most stable form of foster placement, although once placed children are less likely to return to their parents (Hegar and Scannapieco 1999). Kinship care is extensively used in the USA but less so in the UK, with wide variations between local authorities.

4 *Specialist foster care* is usually provided for a limited period and has a good record of placements lasting as long as planned. One of the first projects to be set up, Pro-Teen in Kent, is run as a cooperative of foster families with professional support (Fenyo *et al.* 1989; Jackson and Thomas 2001). It is also one of the few to have been formally evaluated, although there are now many independent fostering agencies. They usually pay much higher rates than local authorities and provide more support and training for foster carers, but evidence of their effectiveness in achieving stability for children is as yet only anecdotal.

5 *Residential care* has been the subject of much research, with rather discouraging findings (Department of Health 1998). In contrast to many other European countries and Israel, where group living seems able to provide a therapeutic and educational refuge for disturbed children from abusive backgrounds, residential care in the UK is highly unstable and is often seen by social workers as a last resort. As Berridge and Brodie (1998) showed, the population of most residential homes is transient and children do not stay long enough to gain any sense of community. Residential education appears more able to provide stability, although usually at the cost of removing young people far from their families and neighbourhood (Gibbs and Sinclair 1998).

PROMOTING CONTINUITY

KEY POINTS

- Educational continuity is vital to children's futures. Discontinuities may have serious effects not just on children's academic attainments, but on other areas of children's lives.

- While acute health problems may be addressed, chronic or apparently less severe problems may be ignored due to the lack of a consistent oversight of children's health needs.
- Discontinuity of care fractures personal relationships, impairs the child's ability to form attachments and may have severe psychosocial consequences.
- Frequent moves may exacerbate the already high prevalence of emotional and behavioural problems from which many looked after children suffer.

Social workers have a very important role ensuring that, when a placement move is unavoidable, serious efforts are made to minimize ill-effects for the child in relation to the different aspects of stability previously outlined.

Education

Education is the aspect of children's lives where it is most essential to preserve continuity, in relationships with teachers and friends, attendance at lessons, keeping up with curriculum content, and ensuring understanding of important elements of each subject. There is much evidence of the failure of social services to give sufficient attention to these matters (Fletcher-Campbell and Hall 1990; Bullock *et al.* 1994; Fletcher-Campbell 1997; Jackson 2000; Jackson and Sachdev 2001). Moves in care nearly always involve changes of school, or such long and difficult journeys to avoid a transfer that the benefits of not changing are lost. Berridge and Cleaver (1987) noted that placements were more likely to break down when children had to move school as the result of a change. Farmer and Parker (1991) found that half the older children in their study had been in three or more placements, each involving a change of school, to which they partly attribute the poor attendance records of the young people after their return home. The relationship works both ways; doing well at school makes it more likely that the placement will be a success, and school problems are a significant cause of coming into care and of placement breakdown (Francis 2000).

Placements of children excluded from school are especially likely to fail. Both foster and residential carers find it difficult to occupy bored and restless young people who should be in school, and the children are at high risk of being drawn into offending or health-threatening behaviour (Brodie 2001).

Borland *et al.* (1998) point out the impact of frequent moves on school attainment, but add that this does not inevitably lead to educational failure. A minority of children do well at school despite typically unstable care careers. It is the emphasis on continuity of learning opportunities, which need to be highly individualized and subject-related, that appears to make the difference. This is particularly essential for teenagers. The loss of GCSE coursework during transitions and disruption of school attendance in the period before exams are frequently reported by young people. A study by Ray Evans (2000) found that changes of placement – back home, into 'independence' or into residential units – often occurred only a few months or even weeks before their exams. In his study, 38 per cent of year 11 children in care experienced at least one move within six months of sitting their GCSEs. This must at least partly account for their very low success rate; only 5 per cent achieve five good passes, compared with over 50 per cent for the age group as a whole (Jackson and Sachdev 2001).

Health

Placement change leads to serious shortcomings in health care unless detailed information is passed to the new carer. Research by the Looking After Children (LAC) team found that although acute illness was treated, chronic conditions were often overlooked and dental care was neglected (Ward 1995). A case-controlled study comparing looked after children with a matched sample of those living in their own families found that those in care were four times more likely to have changed general practitioners and usually had no-one with an overview of their health needs and history. Foster carers complained that social workers, with the exception of those who conscientiously completed the LAC assessment and action records, provided very inadequate information about the children's health, especially their emotional and behavioural difficulties (Jackson *et al.* 2000; Williams *et al.* 2001).

Relationships

Attachment theory would predict that a child who has experienced even one extended separation from a primary care-giver is at risk of psychological ill-effects. When this experience is repeated many times, the child is placed in a state of chronic insecurity and learns not to form attachments or relationships to avoid the pain of losing them. New carers then see the child as cold and unresponsive.

Most looked after children have experienced neglect and ill-treatment and are likely to display disorganized attachment patterns (Howe *et al.* 1999), with emotional reactions and behaviour that make them hard to look after and love (Cairns 1999). They badly need to feel secure and safe and to live with adults who are predictable and reliable. Further rejections within the care system can only confirm their sense of worthlessness and low self-esteem (Schofield *et al.* 2000).

Other relationships are also important and more could be done to preserve them. For example, an intensive study of children during the first two years of a planned long-term placement found that loss of contact with school friends and teachers as a result of placement changes was a cause of sadness and resentment for many (McAuley 1996). Maintaining links with relatives, friends and previous foster carers and social workers can be important sources of continuity.

Emotional and behavioural problems

All studies of children in public care report a very high level of emotional disturbance and behaviour difficulties (Jackson *et al.* 2000). This is usually attributed to their almost universal experience of abuse and neglect within their birth families. Minnis and Devine (2001), for example, found that this was the case for 93 per cent of their sample of 182 children. However, like previous researchers, they also found that the severity and frequency of mental health problems were significantly associated with the number of previous placements. It is probable that whatever problems children bring with them into their placements will be exacerbated by the unpredictability of their living arrangements, often spending months if not years in a state of uncertainty. Young people themselves describe how this undermines their sense of self-efficacy, making it not worth while to think ahead or have any plans for the future (Jackson and Martin 1998).

PROMOTING STABILITY AND CONTINUITY

Mysteriously, there have been very few well-designed research studies that focused explicitly on the question of stability and continuity over a child's care career. We have to glean what information we can from research that looked in other directions and only incidentally provides evidence on stability. Staff and Fein (1995) remark on this phenomenon in the USA, despite the huge literature on out-of-home care. They comment that the few studies that exist 'command our attention; they define the enormity of the phenomenon of placement change' (p. 380).

In their large-scale quantitative study, Staff and Fein (1995) showed that organizing placement moves occupies a high proportion of social work time, which might be better spent supporting existing placements or working with birth parents. The cost of instability is another neglected issue. An informal survey carried out by participants in a series of workshops that I directed found that the cost of a placement move, taking into account meetings, telephone calls, travel and staff time, varied between £2500 if the move was relatively straightforward to £20,000 in a more complex case. Managers from larger authorities estimated that they could save substantial sums by relatively modest improvements in placement stability. Perhaps if this were more widely understood, it would provide an additional incentive to meet the Quality Protects target.

As has been shown, the prospects for a child remaining in a stable living situation vary markedly between types of placement, but the possibilities for placement choice are restricted by many factors beyond the control of social workers or social services departments. Only a small proportion of children in the population (under 1 per cent in most areas) ever need to be looked after by local authorities, usually for quite short periods, but those who stay longer tend to come from highly disorganized families under acute stress.

This means that the ideal of partnership and of keeping children in contact with birth parents can sometimes in itself be a source of instability (Hill 2000). Repeated attempts to return children to parents who are unable to provide adequate care account for some of the many placement changes that have been recorded. Sometimes these attempts are dictated by courts against the judgement of social workers, who may know the families better. A study of 58 children under 12 years in long-term foster care paints a bleak picture of their home life. For these children, the majority of whom had suffered overt hostility and rejection by their parents, 'long periods of stability in the birth family without social services involvement appeared to be a recipe for extended exposure to rejecting parenting and emotional distress' (Schofield *et al.* 2000: 45).

Promoting stability by changes at policy and management levels

It should be assumed that a child will remain in the same placement unless there are very strong reasons for a move on grounds of their present or future welfare. But this, as I have tried to show, is only one aspect of stability. Continuity depends not only on the primary carer, but on social workers and other professionals in contact with the child. Children who are able to form a long-term relationship with one social worker often speak warmly of their support and friendship, but far more often they experience frequent changes of social workers, who rarely stay long enough to get to know them. Resisting the urge to reorganize, measures to increase social work job satisfaction and reduce stress, enabling workers to retain responsibility for individual children or sibling groups even if they change teams or offices, all are management decisions with important implications for continuity; likewise, keeping the same doctor, dentist, optician and staying in the same school when a placement change is unavoidable. Of course, all these have to be balanced against practical considerations and take account of the child's own wishes. But in the past, stability has carried little weight in comparison with adult convenience and cost factors.

A consistent finding from studies in several countries is that paying enhanced rates for foster placements increases their stability. There is a difficulty, however, that if such placements are reserved for children seen as particularly problematic, when their behaviour improves there may be pressure to move them to less expensive 'ordinary' foster placements. For this reason, it is helpful to have a clear policy that *not* moving is the default option, especially since the change is quite likely to be counter-productive. The quality of the relationship between children and their carers is both crucial and unpredictable. It may not have any relation to official categories but is so precious that it should override them, enabling a temporary placement to become long-term for instance. All policies need to be flexible and subject to professional judgement and children's own wishes. Another example is a policy that no child under 12 should be in residential care – desirable in itself, but it can lead to children experiencing repeated unsuccessful foster placements when they would be happier to remain in the children's home they know.

IMPROVING STABILITY IN FOSTER CARE

Long-term or 'permanent' foster care has not been seen as a desirable form of placement. Indeed, the classic American study of stability in care suggests that social workers use it as a device for 'stacking' cases and avoiding the need to make decisions (Stein *et al.* 1978). In reality, this is the type of placement in which many looked after children find themselves (Schofield *et al.* 2000). They often have very unstable care experiences, moving backwards and forwards between foster homes and residential care with no chance to settle anywhere.

A comprehensive review of the evidence relating to stability of placement (Jackson and Thomas 2001) identified several factors well supported by research as leading to greater stability in foster placement, some of which have already been mentioned:

KEY POINTS

Factors associated with greater stability in foster care

- Placement with relatives.
- Placement with siblings.
- Intensive social work support during the early stages of placement.
- Maintaining the child's social networks.
- Previous acquaintance with foster parents.
- Involving parents in planning the placement.
- Continuing contact with parents or other family members after placement.
- Regular school attendance and average or better attainment.
- Paying foster carers higher rates.

There were also some less strongly supported findings. Some studies found that children's participation in decision making reduced the risk of placement breakdown. A short period in residential care before a foster placement could be helpful. Other foster children in the family contributed to stability, whereas research going back to the early 1960s has found that placements are less successful when the foster parents have younger children of their own, or children who are close in age to the fostered child (Parker 1966; George 1970; Wedge and Mantle 1991). Relationships between birth children and foster siblings are an important and under-researched aspect of placement stability.

Some studies have suggested that placing children with older, more experienced foster carers leads to greater stability, but more recent research has questioned this. One intriguing finding from a study by Minnis and Devine (2001) in Scotland is that, contrary to previous reports, very experienced foster carers, defined as those who had looked after more than 30 children in the past, were ten times more likely to have placements break down than those who had previously looked after five or fewer. Minnis and Devine speculate that they might have had more difficult children placed with them or they might have been suffering from burnout. Another possible explanation is that these seasoned foster parents were less likely than newer foster carers to form a strong affectional bond with a child who is merely one of a procession passing through their home. When problems arise, they may have less emotional investment in hanging on to difficult and unrewarding children. Minnis and Devine (2001) also note that social workers appear reluctant to record anything negative about foster carers on the file, so that possibly unsatisfactory foster homes, having passed the initial assessment, continue to be used. Quinton *et al.* (1998) also judged placements with more experienced foster carers to be less stable, but they suggest that this may only be because they tend to have children of their own. Difficulties between birth and foster children are a common reason for carers to end a placement.

A very consistent finding is that children who have suffered severe abuse or neglect, in particular those who have been singled out for rejection or victimization by their parents, are more likely to be rejected again by their carers. Not surprisingly, they are also likely to have the most serious emotional and behavioural problems. But the children with the most severe problems are not necessarily those seen as most problematic by their carers. It is the care-givers' perceptions that count for most, not the objective level of difficulty.

Does training for foster carers help to make placements more stable?

In contrast to some other European countries, foster carers in the UK have usually had limited educational opportunities and not much preparation for the task of fostering (National Foster Care Association 1997). There is still a perception that it is a practical job that can be done by anyone who has run a household and brought up children. This takes no account of the incidence of emotional problems among looked after children and the strong association between such problems and placement breakdown. Various attempts have been made to help foster carers deal with difficulties more effectively. Two randomized controlled trials, one in Scotland and one in Wales, have measured the effects of training on children's behaviour. Although not strictly comparable, since they used different approaches to training and had slightly different aims, their findings were broadly in line with each other.

Minnis and Devine (2001) report on a study of 121 foster families with 182 children aged 5–16 from 17 Scottish local authorities. The families were randomly allocated to intervention and control groups. The children were all in mainstream fostering and not considered to have special needs, but Minnis (a psychiatrist) comments that nearly two-thirds met the threshold criteria for detailed psychiatric assessment. Foster carers who participated in the training enjoyed it very much and thought it had improved their ability to communicate with and care for the children. However, it did not significantly reduce the children's problems. Although there were some positive effects on all measured areas of the children's functioning, there were no statistically significant differences in outcome between the training and control groups.

The Welsh study (Pithouse *et al.* 2001) was rather different in that it specifically targeted children with 'challenging' behaviour and developed a training package designed to help foster carers to understand and deal with it. One hundred foster families took part in the study and retention was very good. The research findings were similar to those of the Scottish research. The foster carers (mainly mothers) who participated were extremely positive about the training, but objective measures of outcome found no significant differences between intervention and control groups. The researchers concluded that training can help carers feel more confident and competent in dealing with difficult behaviour, but changing underlying attitudes and assumptions is much more difficult. Foster carers with their own children found it particularly difficult to accept that 'ordinary' parenting might not work with foster children whose previous experience had been so traumatic.

One explanation for these disappointing results may be that the training and subsequent reinforcement and support was simply inadequate to make any real impact. Minnis and Devine (2001) contrast the three days training in their scheme with the intensive support provided in successful projects evaluated by Chamberlain *et al.* (1992). These projects included weekly two-hour group sessions, three to five hours weekly contact with project workers, individual meetings at least once a week, individual work with young people and, perhaps most importantly, a substantially increased fostering allowance.

The strongest predictor of success, or at least continuation, of placements is the commitment of the care-giver. This has been found to be more significant than any other single factor and may partly account for the very low breakdown rate in completed adoptions. To a lesser extent, it seems also to hold true for long-term fostering (Quinton *et al.* 1998; Schofield *et al.* 2000). With increasing shortages of placements for children who cannot live at home, the possibility of adoption or fostering has been extended to many categories of people who would previously have been excluded. Being unmarried, single, lesbian or gay no longer automatically rules out individuals who want to offer a child a home (McCann and Tasker 2000). There is no evidence that such placements are less successful. If anything, being placed with a single carer is associated with greater stability, perhaps because the child is not having to compete for attention with another adult (Owen 1999).

CONCLUSIONS

By making the number of placement changes a performance indicator in the performance assessment framework of social services and setting a clear target for improvement, the government has ensured that more attention will be paid to stability than in the past. There is consistent evidence that a high proportion of children in the care system experience unacceptable instability and that this has negative effects on their quality of life and developmental progress. On the other hand, there is only limited information from research on what leads to greater stability. In common with many other aspects of social work with children, the evidence on what doesn't work is stronger than that on what does.

It is quite clear that stability and continuity are of the greatest importance to children and young people who cannot live with their birth parents. They are the foundation for all other aspects of healthy development. At the same time, we also need to remember that remaining in the same placement is neither essential nor sufficient for good outcomes. Some moves are a change for the better and, as has been suggested, the negative effects could, to a certain extent, be offset by much closer attention to continuity in all other aspects of children's lives. However, this in no way justifies the multiple placement changes experienced by some children, which cannot be other than intensely damaging to them.

Even with our present state of knowledge, there is much that could be done by local authorities to create greater stability. First, there needs to be a clear understanding that providing a stable care experience for children and young people should be a central aim of the whole system, both for those who come into care for a short time and those who remain for long periods. This means examining all policies and procedures to ensure that there are no built-in causes of instability, some of which were discussed earlier. All plans for reorganization, decisions about recruitment and deployment of social workers, allocation of caseloads, location and staffing of residential units, payment and training of foster carers, and guidelines on placement choice should be considered in relation to their impact on stability for children.

At management level, the key is to make stability the default option, so that any proposed move has to have the strongest possible justification as contributing to the child's welfare, both immediately and in the longer term. Taking this position can often lead to more creative answers to problems for which a placement change seemed at first to be the obvious solution. Moves dictated by short-term financial considerations should in particular be avoided. Keeping the same social worker is an important source of continuity for looked after children and should always be given preference over administrative tidiness. First-line managers have a crucial role in directing attention to continuity in all aspects of children's lives. Several research studies have shown the Looking After Children materials to be a useful tool for this purpose if they are used effectively, but social workers will only treat them as an aid to practice rather than as a form-filling exercise if they are promoted and supported by management (Ward 1995; Jackson 1998). The LAC system also encourages cooperation with other services, of which education is particularly important in relation to stability (Rees 2001; Skuse and Evans 2001).

As most children are looked after in foster homes, reducing failure rates could significantly improve stability. The evidence on what makes for greater stability is fairly consistent; the problem is finding the resources to apply it. Choosing the right placement for the child, preparing the ground carefully, involving birth families and keeping them informed, providing intensive support to foster carers right from the beginning, anticipating difficulties rather than waiting for trouble to blow up, all of these have been shown to reduce the risk of breakdown. In practice, most new placements are made in an emergency, there is likely to be little choice, administrative requirements are pressing and, as soon as the children have a roof over their heads, the social worker must move on to the next case. Increasing the supply and retention of social workers is a matter for government, but different priorities in the management of workloads could also help to support foster placements more effectively.

Social workers should be making contingency plans for adoption of young children as soon as they begin to suspect that there may be a need for long-term care. The evidence is very strong that early adoption holds by far the best promise of stability. Adoption by foster parents also has a high success rate. However, the number of children adopted from care remains low and despite considerable political pressure is rising only very slowly. The opportunities offered by the move towards more open adoption have yet to be tested, but have the potential to unlock the possibility for more children and challenge the idea of what constitutes 'availability' (Jackson 2001).

I have suggested in this chapter that wider issues of stability have been confounded with the question of placement breakdown, the focus of most research, and yet in some ways this is the least researched question of all. Although we know quite a lot about what characteristics of children and, to a lesser extent, of foster families are likely to make placements more fragile, no recent studies have tracked the care careers of children with multiple placement changes and looked in detail at the cause of each move and how it might have been avoided. Hardly any research has looked at instability from the child's perspective.

There are many other gaps. We need to explore further how whole systems work to create or undermine stability. We need well-designed studies to compare local authorities with high and low levels of placement movement. Interventions and projects intended to promote stability should be realistically evaluated. Random allocation may be unacceptable on ethical grounds, but naturally occurring experiments could have much to tell us. We need research that focuses specifically on stability and looks at it over longer time spans. However, we do not need more research to recognize instability as a fundamental weakness of our present system of public care and one that needs to be vigorously tackled if we are to achieve better outcomes for children and young people looked after by local authorities.

ACKNOWLEDGEMENTS

Thanks to Nigel Thomas for permission to use material from our jointly authored books, *On the Move Again* and *What Works in Creating Stability for Looked After Children*. My thanks also to Diana McNeish and Barnardo's for commissioning this work, which focused my longstanding unease about the number of placement changes suffered by so many of the children I met through the Who Cares? Trust, Children in Wales and during research on other topics.

REFERENCES

Beckett, C. (2001) Critical commentary: the great care proceedings explosion, *British Journal of Social Work*, 31(3): 493–502.

Berridge, D. (1985) *Children's Homes*. Oxford: Blackwell.

Berridge, D. and Brodie, I. (1998) *Children's Homes Revisited*. London: Jessica Kingsley.

Berridge, D. and Cleaver, H. (1987) *Foster Home Breakdown*. Oxford: Blackwell.

Biehal, N., Clayden, J., Stein, M. and Wade, J. (1995) *Moving On: Young People and Leaving Care Schemes*. London: HMSO.

Biehal, N., Clayden, J., Stein, M. and Wade, J. (2000) *Home or Away? Supporting Young People and Families*. London: National Children's Bureau.

Borland, M., Pearson, C., Hill, M., Tisdall, K. and Bloomfield, I. (1998) *Education and Care Away from Home*. Edinburgh: Scottish Council for Research in Education.

Brodie, I. (2001) *Children's Homes and School Exclusion: Redefining the Problem*. London: Jessica Kingsley.

Brown, J. (1998) *Family and Adolescent Support Services: New Social Work Crisis, Support and Assessment Services for Adolescents and Their Families*, discussion paper, April. London: National Institute of Social Work.

Bullock, R., Little, M. and Millham, S. (1994) Children's return from state care to school, *Oxford Review of Education*, 20(3): 307–16.

Cabinet Office (2000) *Prime Minister's Review of Adoption*. London: Performance and Information Unit.

Cairns, K. (1999) *Surviving Paedophilia*. Stoke-on-Trent: Trentham Books.

Chamberlain, P., Moreland, S. and Reid, K. (1992) Enhanced services and stipends for foster parents: effects on retention rates and outcomes for children, *Child Welfare*, LXXII(5): 387–401.

Cleaver, H. (2000) *Fostering Family Contact*. London: Stationery Office.

Cliffe, D. and Berridge, D. (1992) *Closing Children's Homes*. London: National Children's Bureau.

Department of Health (1998) *Caring for Children Away from Home*. Chichester: Wiley.

Department of Health (2001) *Children Looked After by Local Authorities Year Ending March 31 2000*. London: Department of Health.

Evans, R. (2000) The educational attainments and progress of children in public care. Unpublished PhD thesis, Institute of Education, University of Warwick.

Farmer, E. and Parker, R. (1991) *Trials and Tribulations: A Study of Children Home on Trial*. London: HMSO.

Fenyo, A., Knapp, M. and Baines, B. (1989) Foster care breakdown: a study of a special teenage fostering scheme, in J. Hudson and B. Galaway (eds) *The State as Parent*. Dordrecht: Kluwer Academic.

Fletcher-Campbell, F. (1997) *The Education of Children Who are Looked-After*. Slough: National Foundation for Educational Research.

Fletcher-Campbell, F. and Hall, C. (1990) *Changing Schools, Changing People: The Education of Children in Care*. Slough: National Foundation for Educational Research.

Folman, R. (1998) I was tooken, *Adoption Quarterly*, 2(2): 7–35.

Francis, J. (2000) Investing in children's futures: enhancing the educational arrangements of 'looked after' children and young people, *Child and Family Social Work*, 5: 23–33.

George, V. (1970) *Foster Care: Theory and Practice*. London: Routledge & Kegan Paul.

Gibbs, I. and Sinclair, I. (1998) Private and local authority children's homes: a comparison, *Journal of Adolescence*, 21(5): 517–28.

Hegar, R.L. and Scannapieco, M. (eds) (1999) *Kinship Foster Care: Policy, Practice and Research*. New York: Oxford University Press.

Hill, M. (2000) Partnership reviewed: words of caution, words of encouragement, *Adoption and Fostering*, 24(3): 56–68.

Howe, D. (1996) Adopters' relationships with their adopted children from adolescence to early adulthood, *Adoption and Fostering*, 20: 35–43.

Howe, D. (1997) Parent reported problems in 211 adopted children: some risk and protective factors, *Child Psychology and Psychiatry*, 38(4): 401–11.

Howe, D., Brandon, M., Hinings, D. and Schofield, G. (1999) *Attachment Theory, Child Maltreatment and Family Support: A Practice and Assessment Model*. London: Macmillan.

Ivaldi, G. (2000) *Surveying Adoption: A Comprehensive Analysis of Local Authority Adoptions 1998–1999 (England)*. London: British Agencies for Adoption and Fostering.

Jackson, S. (1998) Looking after children: a new approach or just an exercise in form filling?, *British Journal of Social Work*, 28(1): 45–56.

Jackson, S. (2000) Raising the educational achievement of looked after children, in T. Cox (ed.) *Combating Educational Disadvantage: Meeting the Needs of Vulnerable Children*. London: Falmer Press.

Jackson, S. (2001) Sharp message, blunt practice, *Adoption Forum News*, 6 (June–August): 1.

Jackson, S. and Martin, P.Y. (1998) Surviving the care system: education and resilience, *Journal of Adolescence*, 21: 569–83.

Jackson, S. and Sachdev, D. (2001) *Better Education, Better Futures: Research, Practice and the Views of Young People in Public Care*. Ilford: Barnardo's.

Jackson, S. and Thomas, N. (1999) *On the Move Again?* Ilford: Barnardo's.

Jackson, S. and Thomas, N. (2001) *What Works in Creating Stability for Looked After Children*. Ilford: Barnardo's.

Jackson, S., Williams, J., Maddocks, A. *et al.* (2000) *The Health Needs and Health Care of School Age Children Looked After by Local Authorities*. Cardiff: Wales Office of Research and Development.

Lowe, N., Murch, M., Borkowski, M. *et al.* (1999) *Supporting Adoption: Reframing the Approach*. London: British Agencies for Adoption and Fostering.

Marsh, P. and Peel, M. (1999) *Leaving Care in Partnership: Family Involvement with Care Leavers*. London: Stationery Office.

McAuley, C. (1996) *Children in Long-term Foster Care: Emotional and Social Development*. Aldershot: Avebury.

McCann, D. and Tasker, F. (2000) Lesbian and gay parents as foster carers and adoptive parents, in A. Treacher and I. Katz (eds) *The Dynamics of Adoption: Social and Personal Perspectives*. London: Jessica Kingsley.

Minnis, H. and Devine, C. (2001) The effect of foster carer training on the emotional and behavioural functioning of looked after children, *Adoption and Fostering*, 25(1): 44–54.

National Foster Care Association (1997) *Crisis in Foster Care*. London: NFCA.

Owen, M. (1999) *Novices, Old Hands and Professionals: Adoption by Single People*. London: British Agencies for Adoption and Fostering.

Packman, J. and Hall, C. (1998) *From Care to Accommodation: Support, Protection and Control in Child Care*. London: Stationery Office.

Parker, R. (1966) *Decision in Child Care – A Study of Prediction in Fostering*. London: George Allen & Unwin.

Parker, R. (1999) *Adoption Now: Messages From Research*. Chichester: Wiley.

Pithouse, A., Hill-Tout, J. and Lowe, K. (2001) *Managing Challenging Behaviour in Foster Care: Developing Best Practice Through Training and Evaluation*. Unpublished report to the National Assembly for Wales.

Quinton, D., Rushton, A., Dance, C. and Mayes, D. (1998) *Joining New Families: A Study of Adoption and Fostering in Middle Childhood*. Chichester: Wiley.

Rees, J. (2001) Making residential care educational care, in S. Jackson (ed.) *Nobody Ever Told Us School Mattered: Raising the Educational Attainments of Children in Care*. London: British Agencies for Adoption and Fostering.

Rowe, J., Hundleby, M. and Garnett, L. (1989) *Child Care Now: A Survey of Placement Patterns*. London: British Agencies for Adoption and Fostering.

Schofield, G., Beek, M. and Sargent, K. with Thoburn, J. (2000) *Growing Up in Foster Care*. London: British Agencies for Adoption and Fostering.

Shaw, C. (1998) *Remember My Messages*. London: Who Cares? Trust.

Sinclair, R., Garnett, L. and Berridge, D. (1995) *Social Work and Assessment with Adolescents*. London: National Children's Bureau.

Skuse, T. and Evans, R. (2001) Directing social work attention to education: the role of the Looking After Children materials, in S. Jackson (ed.) *Nobody Ever Told Us School Mattered: Raising the Educational Attainments of Children in Care*. London: British Agencies for Adoption and Fostering.

Staff, I. and Fein, E. (1995) Stability and change: initial findings in a study of treatment of foster care placements, *Children and Youth Services Review*, 17(3): 379–89.

Stein, T., Gambrill, E. and Wiltse, K. (1978) *Children in Foster Homes: Achieving Continuity of Care*. New York: Praeger.

Thomas, N. and O'Kane, C. (1999) Children's participation in reviews and planning meetings when they are 'looked after' in middle childhood, *Child and Family Social Work*, 4(3): 221–30.

Triseliotis, J., Borland, M., Hill, M. and Lambert, L. (1995) *Teenagers and Social Work Services*. London: HMSO.

Triseliotis, J., Shireman, J. and Hundleby, M. (1997) *Adoption: Theory, Policy and Practice*. London: Cassell.

Walker, T. (2001) The place of education in a mixed economy of child care, in S. Jackson (ed.) *Nobody Ever Told Us School Mattered: Raising the Educational Attainments of Children in Care*. London: British Agencies for Adoption and Fostering.

Ward, H. (ed.) (1995) *Looking After Children: Research into Practice*. London: HMSO.

Ward, H. and Skuse, T. (1999) *Looking After Children: Transforming Data into Management Information*. Report for first year of data collection. Totnes: Dartington Social Research Unit.

Wedge, P. and Mantel, G. (1991) *Sibling Groups and Social Work*. Aldershot: Avebury.

Williams, J., Jackson, S., Maddocks, A. *et al.* (2001) Case-control study of the health of those looked after by local authorities, *Archives of Disease in Childhood*, 85(4): 280–5.

3

MIKE STEIN

Leaving care

KEY MESSAGES

- Many young people leaving care have to cope with the challenges and responsibilities of major changes in their lives at a far younger age and in a shorter time than other young people.
- The challenges include leaving foster or residential care and setting up home, leaving school and entering the world of work, or more likely being unemployed and surviving on benefits, and being young parents.
- Black, Asian and mixed-heritage young people leaving care may face additional problems due to isolation from their families and communities as well as racism.
- Young disabled people leaving care may experience abrupt and delayed transitions.
- Many care leavers are poorly prepared, having experienced movement and disruption while in care.
- Specialist leaving care services can contribute to positive outcomes for care leavers in helping them with accommodation, life skills, social networks and building self-esteem.
- Specialist services are most effective if they build upon a foundation of stability, family and carer links, continuity, a supportive environment for study and the opportunity for a gradual and planned transition from care.

- The discretionary leaving care provisions of the Children Act 1989 and the complex, inconsistent and generally discouraging wider social policy framework disadvantaged many care leavers.
- The Children (Leaving Care) Act 2000 introduces a new legal framework in England and Wales. New responsibilities include: needs assessment, pathway planning, providing personal advisers, keeping in touch and revised financial arrangements for 16- and 17-year-olds. These are intended to lead to improved outcomes for this highly vulnerable group of young people.

INTRODUCTION

This chapter reviews a wide range of research studies to explore four questions:

- What are the problems experienced by young people leaving care?
- What services are being provided to assist them?
- What are the outcomes of those services?
- What are the implications of these studies for policy and practice?

The research examined includes studies with quasi-experimental and non-experimental designs, studies of young people's views and their personal accounts, as well as surveys and cohort studies. The strengths and weaknesses of the research evidence will be discussed within the respective sections. The chapter draws largely on research completed during the last 25 years, including international research, and provides additional and updated material to an earlier review by the author (Stein 1997).

WHAT ARE THE PROBLEMS FACED BY CARE LEAVERS?

KEY POINTS

- Many young people leaving care are likely to have experienced multiple placements and a weakening of family and community ties, often contributing to identity problems.

- Young people leave care and live independently at a much earlier age than other young people leave home.
- Many care leavers have lower educational attainment, higher unemployment rates, more unstable career patterns and greater dependency on welfare benefits than other young people.
- Young women leaving care aged between 16 and 19 are more likely to be young mothers than other young women of that age group.
- Black, Asian and mixed-heritage young people may face additional problems due to lack of contact with their families and communities as well as experiencing racism.
- Young disabled people leaving care may experience abrupt or delayed transitions from care due to restricted housing and employment options and inadequate support.

Early research: 1960–90

From the mid-1970s, several small-scale surveys and qualitative studies have increased our awareness of the range of problems faced by young people leaving care and made connections between these difficulties and the quality of their pre-care and in-care experiences. These studies have highlighted the diversity of the care experience and have shown that care leavers are not a homogeneous group in terms of their pre-care experiences, their care histories, their needs and abilities, or their cultural and ethnic backgrounds. Children's 'in-care' experience may have been valued by them and helped them, but it may have also contributed to other problems. They were likely to have experienced further movement and disruption during their time in care. For those in longer-term care, there was a weakening of links with family, friends and neighbourhood and, for some of these young people, identity confusion stemming from incomplete information, separation and rejection. As Biehal *et al.* (1995: 4) noted: 'Young people often lacked a detailed knowledge of their past, a convincing narrative of who they were and why events had taken the course they had'.

These feelings and confusions were often amplified for black and mixed-heritage young people brought up in a predominantly 'white' care system, particularly if they became detached from their families and communities. These early British studies also documented their poor educational performance, their feelings of being stigmatized by care and their variable preparation for leaving care. And, upon leaving care, at between 16 and 18 years of age, loneliness, isolation, unemployment, poverty, movement, homelessness and 'drift' were likely to feature significantly in many of their lives (Godek 1976; Mulvey 1977; Kahan 1979; Triseliotis, 1980; Burgess, 1981; Stein and Ellis 1983; Lupton 1985; Morgan-Klein 1985; Stein and Maynard 1985; Stein and Carey 1986; First Key 1987; Randall 1988, 1989; Barnardo's 1989; Bonnerjea 1990).

As suggested earlier, this picture of needs was derived from small-scale qualitative research, in the main based on selected samples. Nor were any of the early British studies able to make comparisons with young people from the general population in any systematic way.

Early research studies from the USA, Canada and continental Europe were also limited in size and scope; at best, their findings were impressionistic (McCord *et al.* 1960; Van der Waals 1960; Meier 1965; Bohman and Sigvardsonnon 1980; Raychuba 1987). There was, however, one exception, Trudy Festinger's (1983) seminal study, *No One Ever Asked Us: A Postscript to Foster Care*.

Festinger (1983) followed up 349 young people who had been discharged from foster and residential group care in New York City in 1975. They had been in care for at least five years and were aged 22–25 when they were followed up. In contrast to all previous studies, comparisons were made with sameage adults in the population at large. This was achieved by using data from identical questions in two youth surveys, augmented by New York City census data.

There were two main differences between the care leavers and the comparison sample. First, those who had been in care completed less education and gained poorer qualifications. Second, they were less likely to marry or live with a partner. In other respects – perceptions of self and others, health, friendships, dependence on welfare, records of arrest, areas of living – the care leavers, as a whole group, were more alike than different to the comparison sample of 'non-care' young adults. However, there were significant differences between young people leaving foster care and those leaving residential group care. The former, who constituted 75 per cent of the sample, corresponded with the findings outlined, whereas those leaving residential care (25 per cent) were the most disadvantaged group in respect of education, employment, single parenthood, dependency on welfare and their personal satisfaction rating.

In contrast to Festinger's research, the early UK studies left unanswered the question of how the needs of care leavers differed from those of other young people, although they did provide some signposts for future research.

Recent research: 1990 onwards

More recent research has been able to build upon these early studies. Four studies in particular, two from England and two from the USA, have compared the experiences of care leavers with other young people using comparison samples and secondary data sources: analysis of the National Child Development Study data, census material, government information and contextual research findings (Biehal *et al.* 1992, 1995; Cheung and Heath 1994; Cook 1994; Iglehart 1994, 1995). These studies, taken together, indicate four main areas of contrast between care leavers and other young people.

Leaving home, leaving care and homelessness

Young people leave care to live independently at a much earlier age than other young people. Biehal *et al.* (1995), who used a quasi-experimental design, found that in both their survey (*n* = 183) and qualitative sample (*n* = 74), nearly two-thirds of the young people left care before they were 18 and just under a third did so at just 16. This contrasts with 87 per cent of a similar age group who were living at home, and another study which found that the median age of leaving home was 22 years for men and 20 years for women (Jones 1987). The main reasons for leaving care included placement break-down and the assumption by carers that they should move on having reached 16 or 17 years of age. Whereas the current trend for young people in the general population is for delayed household formation, care leavers have to make accelerated transitions and thus shoulder adult householder respons-ibilities at a much earlier age than other young people.

For many of these young people, their first two years out of care were marked by movement, with over half making two or more moves. Just over 20 per cent became homeless at some stage, a figure lower than some estimates, particularly those based on young adults in hostels who have been in care at some time in their lives (Randall 1988, 1989). These estimates vary between 30 and 59 per cent, depending on the type of care. This demonstrates the difference between follow-up and retrospective studies, but in both types of study care leavers would be over-represented compared with the youth popu-lation in general.

Education

Young people leaving care have lower educational attainment and post-16 participation rates in education than young people in the general population. In the 'Moving On' survey sample (Biehal *et al.* 1995), two-thirds had no qualifications at all, only 15 per cent had a GCSE (A–C grade) or its equival-ent and only one young person gained an A level pass. The qualitative sample revealed a similar pattern. Those who did gain some qualifications were over-whelmingly female (85 per cent) and from fostering backgrounds (70 per cent). The differences are striking in comparison with data from both national and participating local area school attainment tables. For the relevant year nationally and locally, 38 per cent and 30 per cent, respectively, attained five or more A–C GCSE passes. At A level, 25 per cent of boys and 29 per cent of girls attained at least one pass.

Again, whereas the trend is for increased attainment and participation edu-cation, the findings from 'Moving On' and earlier studies reveal a depressing consistency of young people with care backgrounds ill-equipped to enter an increasingly competitive labour market. These findings on educational attainment are also supported by other research studies from the UK, USA, Ireland, Canada and Australia (Festinger 1983; Raychuba 1987; Jackson 1988–89; Heath *et al.* 1989; Biehal *et al.* 1992; Aldgate *et al.* 1993; Cook 1994;

Stein 1994; Cashmore and Paxman 1996; Pinkerton and McCrea 1999; Stein *et al.* 2000).

Analysis of data from the National Child Development Study (NCDS), a cohort study of 17,000 children born between 3 and 9 March 1958, and followed up in 1965, 1969, 1974, 1981 and 1991, reveals lower educational attainment among cohort members who had experienced care than for those who had never been in care:

> Perhaps the most striking percentages are those for respondents with no qualifications. Of the people (aged 23) who had been in care 43 per cent had no qualifications compared with only 16 per cent of their peers who had never been in care. In a society in which qualifications are of major importance for success in the labour market, the educational disadvantage suffered by children in care hardly needs emphasising.
>
> (Cheung and Heath 1994: 365)

More specifically, when respondents who had been in care secured qualifications, they tended to be of a lower standard. Whereas two-thirds of their peers secured qualifications at O level or above, only one-third of the respondents who had been in care achieved an equivalent number of passes.

The NCDS data were also analysed to include divisions within the 'care' category. This pointed to two main conclusions. First, respondents who were only briefly in care were not disadvantaged in terms of educational attainment or subsequent educational or occupational status compared to non-care respondents. Second, the most disadvantaged group were those who came into care before 11 years of age and typically remained in care for about nine years. They not only had low educational attainment, but also had even lower occupational attainments than would have been expected given their qualifications.

The NCDS data were further analysed to consider the effects of social origin on the findings. Is it possible that children who have been in care come from particularly disadvantaged backgrounds, and that the findings simply indicate that poverty leads to a cycle of disadvantage? When controlling for social origin, however, this explanation was not supported. The study concluded that 'the legacy of care cannot be explained purely as a legacy of poverty' (Cheung and Heath 1994: 371).

The factors contributing to poor educational attainment have been less systematically researched. Hypotheses and speculation arising from earlier qualitative studies include damaging pre-care experiences, non-attendance, exclusion, emotional stress, low expectation of carers and teachers, the prioritization of welfare above educational concerns and disruption caused by placement moves (see Stein 1994). A study by the Audit Commission (1994) found that nearly half of the children of school age living in local authority children's homes were not attending school and over one-third were not receiving any formal education. The main reasons for their non-attendance at school were being excluded or refusing to attend.

Employment, careers and benefits

Closely connected to education, care leavers are more likely to be unemployed than other young people aged 16–19 in the population at large. In the study of Biehal *et al.* (1995), 36.5 per cent of the survey sample and 50 per cent of the qualitative sample were unemployed, compared to a mean of 19 per cent for other young people. In the follow-up sample, half of the young people were unemployed within a few months of leaving care and nearly two-thirds failed to establish a stable career pattern during the course of the research, facing periods of short-term casual work interspersed with episodes of training and unemployment.

Analysis of the NCDS data revealed that respondents in 1981 and 1991 who had been in care were much more likely to be unemployed, were more likely to be in semi- or unskilled manual work and were less likely to be in managerial work than their peers who had never been in care. Through statistical modelling of the data, Cheung and Heath (1994) suggested that respondents who had been in care in 1981 and 1991 fared less well than would have been expected:

> these results suggest that unqualified respondents who had been in care were more likely to be unemployed or, if employed, were more likely to be restricted to low skilled manual work than were the unqualified respondents who had never been in care. In this respect there does appear to be a continuing legacy of care. Respondents who had been in care suffered an additional penalty when they entered the labour market over and above the penalty that they suffered in the educational sphere.
>
> (Cheung and Heath 1994: 369)

A consistent finding from the UK research studies completed since the 1970s has been that the vast majority of care leavers live at or near the poverty line. They struggle to survive and to make ends meet, something which affects their whole life.

The 'Westat' study in the USA (Cook 1994), another quasi-experimental design, made systematic comparisons between its sample of care leavers (*n* = 1644) and two other groups: 18- to 24-year-olds in the general population and 18- to 24-year-olds living below the poverty level. Cook (1994: 217) concluded:

> In general, the status of discharged foster care youth is only adequate at best. With respect to education, early parenthood, and the use of public assistance, discharged foster care youth more closely resembled those 18–24 year olds living below the poverty level than they did the general 18–24 population.

Young parenthood

The fourth area of contrast between care leavers and other young people is in relation to early parenthood. In the study of Biehal *et al.* (1995), one-quarter of the young women in the survey sample and a half of young women in the follow-up sample were coping with early parenthood, being aged 16–19 years when their babies were born, a finding consistent with other research (e.g. Garnett 1992). These patterns contrast sharply with those for the population as a whole. In the same year, only 5 per cent of young women aged 15–19 had children and only 2.8 per cent were lone mothers at 19 years of age. The average age for maternity at that time was 26.5 years and recent research suggests that this age is increasing, indicating another difference in transitions to adulthood between care leavers and other young women (Kiernan and Wicks 1990).

However, despite re-occurring panics about teenage parenthood and lone mothers being seen as social problems, this is not inevitable. Research has also drawn attention to the social context in which mothering takes place, the financial dependence it entails and, where young mothers have sufficient support, especially from their mothers, their ability to cope and provide good-quality care for their children (Sharpe 1987; Phoenix 1991). There is also evidence from young mothers who had been in care of a feeling of maturity and status, thus contributing to achieving an adult identity. The gains for some included a renewal of family links and improved relationships with their mothers and their partners' families. Hutson (1997) found that young mothers in supported accommodation tended to experience less poverty and reduced social isolation.

Reasons for early parenthood are less well researched. Biehal et al. (1995) found that just over half of the parents said that their pregnancies were unplanned, nearly two-thirds of whom were aged 17 or younger. Disruption through movement in care, problems with truancy and the absence of a consistent carer capable of inspiring trust may mean they miss out on advice. As Biehal et al. (1995) remarked: 'safe sex requires an ability to communicate between partners and where young women have had poor chances for developing trust, confidence and a positive identity, relating to young men in a confident and assertive way can be difficult' (p. 132).

In addition to these four matters, a few studies have also contributed to our understanding of differences between black and white young care leavers, disabled young people and young people with health problems.

Differences between black and white young care leavers

Few studies have made significant comparisons between black and white young people leaving care or have concentrated solely on black youth. An early study that focused exclusively on black young people found that transcultural placements, or placements in predominantly white areas, could leave them confused about their cultural identity. A lack of cultural knowledge affected their confidence and self-esteem and was an additional burden at the time of leaving care (Black and In Care 1984; First Key 1987). More recently, Ince's (1998, 1999) qualitative work with ten black care leavers has also highlighted identity problems derived from a lack of contact with family and community, as well as the impact of racism and direct and indirect discrimination upon their lives after leaving care.

Consistent with other findings, by far the largest group of 'black' young people (using the term in the meaning of black/Asian/mixed heritage) in both the survey and qualitative samples of Biehal *et al.* (1995) were young people of mixed heritage (Bebbington and Miles 1989; Rowe *et al.* 1989; Garnett 1992). As a group they tended to enter substitute care earlier and stay longer than white young people (Barn 1993; Barn *et al.* 1997). However, apart from this factor, there were few differences between their care careers and those of white young people. After leaving care, they had similar housing and employment careers, although they were slightly more likely to make good educational progress after leaving care than white young people. Most of these young people had experienced racist harassment and abuse; some of the mixed-heritage young people felt that they were not accepted by black or white people.

Young people's definitions of their ethnic identity were often complex, varied and shifted over time. Their identification with a particular ethnic group was strongly related to young people's identification with, or rejection of, family members (Hall 1992; Tizard and Phoenix 1993; Owusu-Bempah 1994).

Young disabled people and young people with health problems

Twenty-three disabled young people and young people with health problems (13 per cent of the survey sample) were identified by Biehal *et al.* (1995). The largest group – over half – consisted of young people who had been classified as emotionally or behaviourally disturbed; four had severe learning disabilities, three had a physical disability and two had a mental health problem. Compared with other young people in the survey sample, they had fewer educational qualifications, were more likely to be unemployed and were over-represented among the homeless.

There has been little research into the experiences of young disabled people leaving care (Rabiee *et al.* 2001). A survey of young disabled people in the general population that included a comparison sample of non-disabled peers estimated that up to 40 per cent 'find great difficulty in attaining independence in adult life comparable to that of young people in the general population' (Hirst and Baldwin 1994: 110). The study showed that disabled young people were less likely than their non-disabled peers to be living independently of their parents and to be in paid employment; they were also more likely to be dependent on benefits or lower incomes, to have lower self-esteem and to have more restricted social lives (Hirst and Baldwin 1994). The literature has also highlighted the problems young disabled people face in accessing housing, moving away from parents, being involved in leisure activities and finding employment (Morris 1995, 1998, 1999).

The only recent study of the experiences of young disabled care leavers identified the problems they experience in their transitions to adulthood. Rabiee *et al.* (2001) gathered data on 131 young disabled people, including a qualitative sample of 28 young people. They found that, for many of these young people, there was a lack of planning, inadequate information and poor consultation with them. Their transitions from care could be abrupt or delayed by restricted housing and employment options and inadequate support after care.

Recent research has identified greater behavioural and emotional disturbances among young people referred to social services. Triseliotis *et al.* (1995) found that the behaviour of 90 per cent of young people was rated above the 'normal' cut-off point using an adaptation of the Rutter scale (thus allowing comparisons with the general population). In another study, over three-quarters of young people referred for assessment were thought by professionals to be displaying disturbed or disturbing behaviour (Sinclair *et al.* 1995). The most disturbed behaviour was to be found among those young people living in residential care. A recent study of young people who went missing from substitute care also found that those with emotional and behavioural difficulties were over-represented among those who went missing often and were at risk of detachment from safe adult networks (Wade *et al.* 1998).

The health needs of young people leaving care have also been largely neglected. However, recent research reported a high incidence of smoking, drug and alcohol use, high numbers of chronic physical conditions and of mental health problems, including self-harming and attempted suicides (Save the Children 1995; Saunders and Broad 1997).

The contribution of recent research studies

In addition to their similar results, what these studies contribute by drawing on comparative data, and what was lacking in earlier research, is an empirical underpinning to our assessment of need, an essential foundation for conceptual clarification and the planning of intervention. The analysis of the NCDS data is particularly pertinent, as it provides substantial evidence for a connection between the main areas of comparison by what is referred to as 'the legacy of care'. To avoid over-simplification, this legacy should perhaps be considered as deriving from a process linking reasons for being 'looked after', including pre-care experiences, with early interventions as well as subsequent care careers.

The evidence from these studies shows that young people leaving care have to cope with the challenges and responsibilities of major changes in their lives – leaving foster and residential care and setting up home, leaving school and entering the world of work (or, more likely, being unemployed and surviving on benefits) and being parents – at a far younger age than other young people. In short, they have compressed and accelerated transitions to adulthood.

WHAT SERVICES ARE BEING PROVIDED TO ASSIST CARE LEAVERS?

KEY POINTS

- Specialist leaving care schemes were developed from the mid-1980s to respond to the core needs of care leavers for help with accommodation, personal support, financial assistance and help with careers.
- Social Services authority-wide provision for care leavers may include specialist leaving care teams, general mainstream social work support and integrated services for a wider range of vulnerable young people.

The development of leaving care schemes

From the mid-1980s, partly in response to the growing awareness of the problems faced by young people, some voluntary organizations and local authorities pioneered specialist leaving care projects and schemes. Of 33 leaving care schemes surveyed in 1989, only one had been in existence in 1978 and most (82 per cent) had started in or after 1985 (Stone 1990). The introduction of specialist schemes and projects was seen by social services as a way of meeting their new legal responsibilities under the Children Act 1989. However, as has been observed:

> This was a rediscovery rather than an innovation for working boys' and working girls' hostels and designated after-care probation and children's officers were in existence between 1948 and 1971. It was after 1971 that the needs of care leavers were increasingly neglected in many authorities, until the rediscovery of specialist responses during the 1980's.
> (Stein 1999: 184)

Specialist schemes were developed to provide a focused response to the core needs of care leavers, for help with accommodation, social support, assistance with finance and help with careers.

The literature on leaving care services is, in the main, descriptive and suggests there are differences in terms of service delivery, philosophy and in the range and intensity of service. Earlier research made the distinction between specialist and non-specialist models of service delivery, as well as differences in philosophy between independence and inter-dependence models and linked programme content (Stein and Carey 1986).

The rationale of independence schemes is that young people should be trained to manage on their own from sixteen onwards through instruction in practical survival skills – domestic combat courses – and by coping with minimum support. In contrast, inter-dependence models see leaving care as a psycho-social transition, a high priority being placed on inter-personal skills, developing self-esteem and confidence and receiving ongoing support after a young person leaves care.

(Stein 1997: 28)

In their in-depth study of four leaving care schemes, Biehal *et al.* (1995) proposed a three-dimensional basis for classifying scheme distinctiveness:

1 How do schemes compare in their approaches to service delivery, in terms of perspective, methods of working and the extent to which their work is young person demand-led or social work planned?
2 How do schemes compare in terms of the nature of the providing agency, including its culture and organizational, management and staffing structures?
3 What contribution do schemes make to the development of leaving care policy within their local areas?

In the USA, there have been two main approaches to classifying scheme distinctiveness. First, whether, how and in what combination schemes provide *hard living skills* (for example, practical and functional competencies, such as employment, independence training, home management) and *soft living skills* (such as promotion of self-esteem or personal development). Second, the extent to which development of general life skills is aimed at *all* young people, or whether the focus is on specialist approaches for *vulnerable* young people.

The results of a 1999 English survey of best practice in leaving care (based on responses from 42 local authorities) suggest that, despite the diversity of service types, four main models of authority-wide provision are currently common (Stein and Wade 2000):

1 A *non-specialist service*, where responsibility for delivering a service rests primarily with field social workers, sometimes in collaboration with carers.
2 A *centrally organized specialist service*, consisting of a centrally organized team of workers providing an authority-wide service, primarily to care leavers.
3 A *dispersed specialist service*, where individual specialist leaving care workers are attached to area-based fieldwork teams.
4 A *centrally organized integrated service*: an emerging model that attempts to provide an integrated service for a wider range of vulnerable young people 'in need', such as homeless young people, young offenders and disabled young people. Integration is facilitated through a multi-agency management and staffing model.

WHAT ARE THE OUTCOMES OF LEAVING CARE SERVICES?

KEY POINTS

- Leaving care schemes can make a positive contribution to specific outcomes for care leavers.
- They work particularly well in respect of accommodation and life skills, including budgeting, negotiation and self-care skills and, to some extent, in furthering social networks, developing relationships and building self-esteem.

Attempts to evaluate the impact of scheme services on subsequent outcomes for young people are at an early stage in the leaving care field. The growing literature on outcomes acknowledges the complexity of the task, given the range of contextual and interpersonal factors that help to structure the life chances of young people (Knapp 1989; Parker *et al.* 1991; Cheetham *et al.* 1992; Ward 1995). In the past 20 years, no studies in this area have adopted an experimental design (Stein 1997) and very few longitudinal studies have used a quasi-experimental design to compare outcomes for young people in receipt of specialist services with those who are not (Cook 1994; Biehal *et al.* 1995). Cook's evaluation of independent living programmes in the USA found that such preparation programmes tended to have the most beneficial impact on a range of subsequent outcomes when a core group of skills were taught in combination and targeted towards specific goals.

The most comprehensive British study to date of different approaches to delivering leaving care services is that of Biehal *et al.* (1995). They evaluated four leaving care schemes situated in three local authorities and tracked a sample of 74 young people over their first 18–24 months of independent living. The sample was subdivided into a participating group of scheme users and a comparison group of young people not in receipt of scheme services. Biehal *et al.* identified considerable diversity in the organization of and approaches to delivering leaving care services. They suggested that there could be no single blueprint for schemes. Models of schemes and the shape of the services offered by them varied according to the geographical, policy and resource contexts within which they were embedded and the nature of the providing agency. However, all the schemes, with varying success, were working at several levels in an attempt to meet the core needs of care leavers: assisting their authorities to develop clear policies and access routes; developing a flexible range of resource options in cooperation with other agencies (especially in relation to accommodation, finance and careers); providing advice, information and consultancy services (including preparation and leaving care planning); and offering direct individual or group-based support to young people. However leaving care services are organized, these core functions are necessary if services are to be both effective and comprehensive.

The outcomes of scheme interventions were assessed across nine dimensions of young people's lives: accommodation, life skills, education, career paths, social networks, relationships, identity, drug use and offending. Two approaches to measuring outcomes were developed. First, comparisons of progress for those using or not using schemes were made for each dimension. However, schemes tended to work with young people who had more disadvantaged starting points. They were less likely to have positive family relationships, were more socially isolated and tended to have had less stable early housing careers. In recognition of this, a second approach was developed to assess young people's progress across these dimensions, taking account of their differential starting points. In relation to outcomes, the success of schemes was quite impressive, especially in the areas of accommodation and life skills. Although at the end of the study there had been no change for the comparison group, an increase was seen in the proportion of scheme users managing in good accommodation. Scheme users were also more likely to have improved their practical and budgeting skills and were more likely to have maintained their negotiating skills in the community. Schemes were less able to compensate for young people who had poor social networks and relationship skills; nor were they able to improve the career paths of young people, an area in which poor outcomes were the norm for both samples. Successful educational outcomes were closely linked to placement stability, more often achieved in foster care placements, combined with a supportive and encouraging environment for study. Without such stability and encouragement, post-16 employment and career outcomes were also likely to be very poor. Success in social networks and in having a positive self-image, although assisted by schemes, is also connected with young people having supportive links with family members or former carers. Stability, continuity and family and carer links are the foundation upon which specialist leaving care schemes must build if they are to be most effective.

WHAT ARE THE IMPLICATIONS FOR POLICY AND PRACTICE?

KEY POINTS

- Research, young peoples' voices, practitioners and campaigners have all contributed to policy changes.
- Research has highlighted the weakness of discretionary leaving care powers under the Children Act 1989, as well as the complex, inconsistent and discouraging wider social policy framework.

- The Children (Leaving Care) Act 2000 introduces new duties in terms of assessing and meeting needs, keeping in touch, the provision of personal advisers, pathway plans and new financial arrangements for 16- and 17-year-old care leavers.

Research and policy

Both the early British research and the more recent research discussed here have contributed to the development of leaving care policy. It is generally acknowledged that, despite their methodological limitations, the body of small-scale qualitative studies have contributed – alongside other activities by the small but powerful voices of young people belonging to 'in care' groups, by practitioners in statutory and voluntary agencies, by the campaigning activities of non-governmental organizations such as Barnardo's, Shelter and First Key – to the awakening of leaving care in the professional and political consciousness. An important outcome was new 'leaving care' duties and wider discretionary powers contained within the Children Act 1989 (Collins and Stein 1989; Stein 1991, 1993, 1999; Page and Clarke 1997).

Research carried out since the introduction of the Children Act 1989 (in October 1991) has highlighted the weaknesses of the permissive discretionary leaving care powers contained within the Act, as well as the complex, inconsistent and discouraging wider social policy framework, particularly in relation to benefits and housing (Lowe 1990; First Key 1992; Biehal *et al.* 1995; Save the Children 1995; Audit Commission 1996; Broad 1998; Biehal and Wade 1999). This has led to the development of national standards (First Key 1996) and the introduction of training materials (Frost and Stein 1995). In addition, as detailed above, Biehal *et al.* (1995) have identified the contribution of specialist leaving care schemes, combined with good-quality substitute care, to achieving positive outcomes for young people leaving care.

The Labour government elected in 1997, in its response to the Children's Safeguards Review (which followed the revelations of widespread abuse in children's homes) and in its plans to modernize children's services, committed itself to legislate for new and stronger duties to support care leavers. The proposed changes, detailed in the consultation document *Me, Survive, Out There?* (Department of Health 1999), were to build upon the Quality Protects Programme, National Priorities Guidance, the inspection of leaving care services and good practice guidance (Department of Health 1997, 1998a,b, 1999; Utting 1997). Wider government initiatives to combat social exclusion, including the introduction of the Connexions Service, and initiatives to tackle youth homelessness, under-achievement in education, training and employment, and teenage parenthood are also intended to impact upon care leavers.

The government also recommended 'Moving On' and 'What Works in Leaving Care?' (Biehal *et al.* 1995; Stein 1997) to all English local authorities to assist them in the development of specialist leaving care schemes, as well as identifying the contribution of research to the Children (Leaving Care) Act 2000, due to be implemented in October 2001. The Act introduces new duties in respect of assessing and meeting needs, personal advisers, pathway plans, keeping in touch and financial arrangements (Department of Health 2000).

Research and practice

Combining the research evidence discussed above with the findings from a survey of best practice carried out in 1999 (Stein and Wade 2000), core messages can be identified to inform best practice in leaving care services. These will be discussed in relation to the new responsibilities contained within the Children (Leaving Care) Act 2000 (implemented in October 2001).

Personal advisers

One of the main reasons why leaving care schemes were able to achieve successful outcomes was that young people had a key worker who could assist them in meeting their core needs – for accommodation, personal support, help with finances and careers – and who were committed to them and had the skills to engage and involve them. They could work with young people, not just for them (Biehal *et al.* 1995). The Children (Leaving Care) Act 2000 recognizes this by requiring local authorities to appoint personal advisers to provide advice and support, to play a core role in needs assessment and pathway planning, to coordinate services, to be informed about young people and to keep in touch with them.

Needs assessment and pathway planning

Local authorities are given new duties under the Act to assess the needs of young people with a view to determining what advice, assistance and support to provide, and to prepare a pathway plan based on the assessment, keeping the plan under regular review. The assessment, planning and review process prior to a young person leaving care is the foundation upon which good aftercare support can be built. Research and evaluations of best practice suggest that several elements are associated with smooth and well-planned transitions (Biehal *et al.* 1995; Stein and Wade 2000).

- It helps for planning to take place early – this should build upon the young person's existing care plan.
- The process must involve and empower the young person (Who Cares? Trust 1993; Stein 1997). The regulations require that the young person's wishes and feelings are taken into account and the guidance identifies the importance of scheduling meetings at convenient times, paying travel expenses and taking account of any disability (Department of Health 2000).

- All those with an interest in the support of the young person must be fully involved in the process, provided that this is consistent with the young person's wishes (Biehal *et al.* 1995; Stein and Wade 2000). In addition to the young person and their personal adviser, the regulations require that parents, carers, teachers, independent visitors and general practitioners should normally be involved, as well as anyone else whom the young person or local authority consider relevant. There is also strong evidence that where specialist leaving care schemes exist, they need to be integrated into this process at an early point (Biehal *et al.* 1995; Stein and Wade 2000).
- Research highlights the importance of holistic assessment and planning, recognizing the different dimensions to young people's lives (Clayden and Stein 1996). The regulations require the assessment to address health and development, education, employment and training, personal support from family and other relationships, financial needs, practical and other skills necessary for independent living, and young people's needs for care, support and accommodation. In addition, pathway plans require that contingency planning is undertaken.

Finally, there is evidence from evaluated practice that recording assessments and plans, and identifying those responsible for implementing plans, is very helpful to young people. This is a requirement for both needs assessments and pathway plans, and the young person must be provided with a copy of the pathway plan (Department of Health 2000).

Preparation for adult life: the practical and other skills necessary for independent living

Research and evaluation of best practice also contributes to specific areas of responsibility under the Act for needs assessment and pathway planning. Evaluations of good practice point to the importance of assessment to identify young people's needs and how they will be met, support and participation, involving discussion, negotiation and opportunities for risk taking, and the gradual learning of skills, in the context of a stable placement (Clayden and Stein 1996). Achieving such stability may present significant challenges to children's homes (Berridge 1985; Berridge and Brodie 1998; Sinclair and Gibbs 1998; Whitaker *et al.* 1998).

There is evidence to suggest that preparation should be holistic in approach, attaching equal importance to practical, emotional and interpersonal skills and responding to ethnic diversity (Ince 1999). Specialist leaving care schemes can assist carers with the development of skills training programmes and by offering intensive compensatory help at the aftercare stage (Biehal *et al.* 1995; Clayden and Stein 1996).

Disability and health

The neglect of disability and the health needs of young people leaving care in the research literature was referred to earlier (Stein and Wade 2000).

The available evidence points to the need for these areas to be given higher priority (Farmer and Pollock 1997; Saunders and Broad 1997; Berridge and Brodie 1998; Rabiee *et al.* 2001). The best practice survey suggests that health care may be assisted by a thorough health assessment and the maintenance of detailed health records while young people are looked after. This should provide a platform to promote a healthy lifestyle, ensure appropriate use of primary care services, provide access to specialist mental health and therapeutic services where necessary, and promote leisure services (Department of Health 1997; Stein and Wade 2000). Rabiee *et al.* (2001) argue for developments in monitoring, planning, supporting transitions, promoting involvement and training to improve policy and practice for young disabled people leaving care.

Education, training or employment

Improving the career chances of care leavers needs to build upon their educational progress while being looked after. Evidence suggests that placement stability, positive encouragement, proactive placement, school and education service links and compensatory assistance can be helpful to young people (Biehal *et al.* 1995; McParlin 1996). The assessment of skills and career planning can be assisted by being part of the leaving care planning and review process. There is also evidence that providing ongoing support for young people is essential to maintain motivation and to assist those wishing to return to learn. Also, inter-agency links can provide access to opportunities and to plan service developments, including links with careers, training agencies, further and higher education colleges, employers, benefits agencies and youth services (Smith 1994; Department of Health 1997). The collection of performance data by the Department of Health will assist this process (Department of Health 2001).

Financial needs

Maximizing young people's educational and career opportunities is the best way to protect young people against subsequent dependency on benefits and poverty; however, as already noted, the research evidence reveals high unemployment and low attainment and participation in education and training among care leavers. In addition, the discretionary and complex nature of the policy framework for financial assistance has resulted in major variations in the help young people receive.

Under the Children (Leaving Care) Act 2000, the local authority will become the sole agency responsible for providing financial assistance to 16- and 17-year-old care leavers (excluding disabled young people and lone parents). Personal advisers will still have a key role in accessing financial assistance for other care leavers, and research studies have shown the importance of providing clear accessible information to all parties, as well as developing formal links and protocols with relevant agencies (Biehal *et al.* 1995; First Key 1996; Department of Health 1997; Broad 1998).

Family and social relationships

Research findings suggest that, wherever it proves possible, young people's interests will be served best by efforts to maintain or create links with their families while they are being looked after (Millham *et al.* 1986; Marsh and Peel 1999). Even if relationships with parents have broken down, other members of a young person's extended family may be able to offer some support. There is evidence that contact with family members can contribute to a positive self-image, increase young people's sense of stability in foster placements and help preserve placements. Also, at a later stage, those lacking family support may have more difficulty creating new relationships (Biehal *et al.* 1995; Berridge 1996) and, as detailed earlier, black young people isolated from family and community may experience identity problems (Ince 1998).

Best practice will be assisted by assessing young people's sources of family, carer and informal support at the planning stage. This may include arrangements for young people to live close to supports, a continuing role for carers to support young people and the option for young people to remain with carers on a supported lodging basis (Fry 1992; Wade 1997). There is also evidence that specialist leaving care schemes can play an important role in helping young people form new networks and relationships (Biehal *et al.* 1995).

Keeping in touch with young people after they leave care, a new duty under the Act, will be assisted by well-planned transitions and clear support arrangements negotiated with the young person. They may benefit in particular from being aware of their entitlements to support and having a link person responsible for coordinating support and resources for them. Evaluations of specialist leaving care schemes by young people show their success in keeping in touch as a consequence of their presence, style of work and a social base that encourages young people's involvement.

Accommodation

Young people leaving care are a diverse group whose accommodation needs will vary accordingly. The Act requires local authorities to provide 'suitable' accommodation. There is substantial evidence that specialist leaving care services have been successful in developing a range of accommodation for young people leaving care, including supported lodgings, re-designating foster placements as supported lodgings, a range of provision offering accommodation and support (such as 'trainer' flats, supported hostels and floating support schemes), foyers and independent tenancies (Stein 1990; Stone 1990; Fry 1992; Anderson and Quilgars 1995; Wade 1997; Broad 1998; Biehal and Wade 1999).

There is evidence to suggest that, when planning to meet the needs of individual young people, positive outcomes will be assisted by: involving young people in planning and decision making; assessing needs and preparing young people; offering a choice in the type and location of accommodation; having a contingency plan; setting up a package of support to go with the accommodation; and having a clear financial plan (Hutson 1995).

Contingency plans

As indicated above, young people leaving care often have compressed and accelerated transitions to adulthood. It is not surprising that many experience difficulties and crises after leaving care. There is also evidence to indicate that few young people have the opportunity to return to care or sheltered provision and that they may experience difficulty in reconciling themselves to such a return (Biehal *et al.* 1995; Department of Health 1997).

Evidence of successful contingency arrangements include returning to successful foster care arrangements and specifically designated provision. Specialist leaving care schemes have been particularly effective in assisting young people through specialist worker support and access to a range of accommodation options. Their responsive approach also encourages young people to seek help when they are in difficulties (Biehal *et al.* 1995; Broad 1998).

CONCLUSION

From the mid-1970s, a body of small-scale surveys and qualitative research studies has increased our awareness of the range of problems faced by young people leaving care – their generally poor outcomes in education, employment, maintaining accommodation, sense of identity and self-esteem – and made connections with the quality of their experiences while in care. In addition to confirming their poor life chances, more recent research has illustrated that, compared with other young people, they have compressed and accelerated transitions to adulthood, and they have to cope with major changes in their lives at a far younger age and in far less time.

A few research studies evaluating the effectiveness of interventions have highlighted the positive contribution specialist leaving care schemes can make to both specific and general outcomes for care leavers. But the research has indicated that good-quality substitute care needs to be built upon to achieve positive outcomes. Stability, continuity and family and carer links are the essential foundations of effective interventions by specialist schemes. Research evidence indicating variations in the resourcing, range and quality of leaving care services has contributed to the strengthening of the legal and policy framework. Best practice guidance has also been informed by research and evaluation.

Finally, there is growing recognition that meeting the needs of this highly vulnerable group of young people requires a comprehensive strategy that addresses the resourcing of services and the wider social policy context, including an understanding of the dynamics of social exclusion, as well as more focused substitute care, leaving, aftercare policy and practice responses.

REFERENCES

Aldgate, J., Heath, A., Colton, M. and Simm, M. (1993) Social work and the education of children in foster care, *Adoption and Fostering*, 17(3): 25–34.

Anderson, I. and Quilgars, D. (1995) *Foyers for Young People: Evaluation of a Pilot Initiative.* York: University of York, Centre for Housing Policy.

Audit Commission (1994) *Seen but Not Heard.* London: Audit Commission.

Audit Commission (1996) *Misspent Youth: Young People and Crime.* London: Audit Commission.

Barn, R. (1993) *Black Children in the Public Care System.* London: Batsford.

Barn, R., Sinclair, R. and Ferdinand, D. (1997) *Acting on Principle: An Examination of Race and Ethnicity in Social Services Provision to Children and Families.* London: British Agencies for Adoption and Fostering.

Barnardo's (1989) *I Can't Go Back to Mum and Dad.* Ilford: Barnardo's.

Bebbington, A. and Miles, J. (1989) The background of children who enter local authority care, *British Journal of Social Work*, 19(5): 349–68.

Berridge, D. (1985) *Children's Homes.* Oxford: Blackwell.

Berridge, D. (1996) *Foster Care: A Research Review.* London: HMSO.

Berridge, D. and Brody, I. (1998) *Children's Homes Revisited.* London: Jessica Kingsley.

Biehal, N. and Wade, J. (1999) 'I thought it would be easier': the early housing careers of young people leaving care, in J. Rugg (ed.) *Young People, Housing and Social Policy.* London: Routledge.

Biehal, N., Clayden, J., Stein, M. and Wade, J. (1992) *Prepared for Living? A Survey of Young People Leaving the Care of Three Local Authorities.* London: National Children's Bureau.

Biehal, N., Clayden, J., Stein, M. and Wade, J. (1995) *Moving On: Young People and Leaving Care Schemes.* London: HMSO.

Black and In Care (1984) *Black and in Care Conference Report.* London: Children's Legal Centre.

Bohman, M. and Sigvardsonnon, S. (1980) Negative social heritage, *Adoption and Fostering*, 3: 25–34.

Bonnerjea, L. (1990) *Leaving Care in London.* London: London Boroughs Children's Regional Planning Committee.

Broad, B. (1998) *Young People Leaving Care: Life After the Children Act 1989.* London: Jessica Kingsley.

Burgess, C. (1981) *In Care and Into Work.* London: Tavistock.

Cashmore, J. and Paxman, M. (1996) *Wards Leaving Care: A Longitudinal Study.* Sydney: New South Wales Department of Community Services.

Cheetham, J., Fuller, R., Petch, A. and McIvor, G. (1992) *Evaluating Social Work Effectiveness.* Buckingham: Open University Press.

Cheung, Y. and Heath, A. (1994) After care: the education and occupation of adults who have been in care, *Oxford Review of Education*, 20(3): 361–74.

Clayden, J. and Stein, M. (1996) Self care skills and becoming adult, in *Looking After Children, Good Parenting Good Outcomes, Reader.* London: HMSO.

Collins, S. and Stein, M. (1989) Users fight back: collectives in social work, in C. Rojeck, G. Peacock and S. Collins (eds) *The Haunt of Misery.* London: Routledge.

Cook, R. (1994) Are we helping foster care youth prepare for their future?, *Children and Youth Services Review*, 16(3/4): 213–29.

Department of Health (1997) *When Leaving Home is also Leaving Care: An Inspection of Services for Young People Leaving Care.* London: Social Services Inspectorate.

Department of Health (1998a) *Quality Protects: Framework for Action*. London: Department of Health.

Department of Health (1998b) *Modernising Health and Social Services: National Priorities Guidance 1999/00–2001/02*. London: Department of Health.

Department of Health (1999) *Me, Survive, Out There? New Arrangements for Young People Living In and Leaving Care*. London: Department of Health.

Department of Health (2000) *Children (Leaving Care) Act 2000, Draft Regulations and Guidance: Consultation Document*. London: Department of Health.

Department of Health (2001) *Children Act Report 2000*. London: Department of Health.

Farmer, E. and Pollock, S. (1997) *Substitute Care for Sexually Abused and Abusing Children: Report to the Department of Health*. Bristol: School for Policy Studies, University of Bristol.

Festinger, T. (1983) *No One Ever Asked Us: A Postscript to Foster Care*. New York: Columbia University Press.

First Key (1987) *A Study of Black Young People Leaving Care*. Leeds: First Key.

First Key (1992) *A Survey of Local Authority Provision for Young People Leaving Care*. Leeds: First Key.

First Key (1996) *Standards in Leaving Care*. Leeds: First Key.

Frost, N. and Stein, M. (1995) *Working with Young People Leaving Care*. London: HMSO.

Fry, E. (1992) *After Care: Making the Most of Foster Care*. London: National Foster Care Association.

Garnett, L. (1992) *Leaving Care and After*. London: National Children's Bureau.

Godek, S. (1976) *Leaving Care*. Ilford: Barnardo's.

Hall, S. (1992) The question of cultural identity, in S. Hall, D. Held and T. McGrew (eds) *Modernity and its Futures*. Cambridge: Polity Press.

Heath, A., Colton, M. and Aldgate, J. (1989) The educational progress of children in and out of foster care, *British Journal of Social Work*, 19: 447–60.

Hirst, M. and Baldwin, S. (1994) *Unequal Opportunities: Growing Up Disabled*. London: HMSO.

Hutson, S. (1995) *Care Leavers and Young Homeless People in Wales: The Exchange of Good Practice*. Swansea: The University of Wales.

Hutson, S. (1997) *Supported Housing: The Experience of Young Care Leavers*. Ilford: Barnardo's.

Iglehart, A. (1994) Adolescents in foster care: predicting readiness for independent living, *Children and Youth Services Review*, 16(3/4): 159–68.

Iglehart, A. (1995) Readiness for independence: comparison of foster care, kinship care, and non foster care adolescents, *Children and Youth Services Review*, 17: 417–31.

Ince, L. (1998) *Making it Alone: A Study of the Care Experiences of Young Black People*. London: British Agencies for Adoption and Fostering.

Ince, L. (1999) Preparing Black young people for leaving care, in R. Barn (ed.) *Working with Black Children and Adolescents in Need*. London: British Agencies for Adoption and Fostering.

Jackson, S. (1988–89) Residential care and education, *Children and Society*, 4: 335–50.

Jones, G. (1987) Leaving the parental home: an analysis of early housing careers, *Journal of Social Policy*, 16(1): 49–74.

Kahan, B. (1979) *Growing Up in Care*. Oxford: Blackwell.

Kiernan, K. and Wicks, M. (1990) *Family Change and Future Policy.* York: Joseph Rowntree Foundation/Family Policy Studies Centre.

Knapp, M. (1989) *Measuring Child Care Outcomes,* PSSRU Discussion Paper 630. Canterbury: University of Kent.

Lowe, K. (1990) *Teenagers in Foster Care.* London: National Foster Care Association.

Lupton, C. (1985) *Moving Out.* Portsmouth: Portsmouth Polytechnic.

Marsh, P. and Peel, M. (1999) *Leaving Care in Partnership: Family Involvement with Care Leavers.* London: The Stationery Office.

McCord, J., McCord, W. and Thurber, E. (1960) The effects of foster home placement in the prevention of adult anti-social behaviour, *Social Services Review,* 34: 415–19.

McParlin, P. (1996) *The Education of Young People Looked After.* Leeds: First Key.

Meier, E. (1965) Current circumstances in former foster children, *Child Welfare,* 44: 196–206.

Millham, S., Bullock, R., Hosie, K. and Haak, M. (1986) *Lost in Care.* Aldershot: Gower.

Morgan-Klein, B. (1985) *Where Am I Going To Stay?* Edinburgh: Scottish Council for Single Homeless.

Morris, J. (1995) *Going Missing? A Research and Policy Review of Disabled Children and Young People Living Away from Their Families.* London: Who Cares? Trust.

Morris, J. (1998) *Still Missing? The Experiences of Disabled Children and Young People Living Away from Their Families.* London: Who Cares? Trust.

Morris, J. (1999) *Move On Up: Supporting Young Disabled People in Their Transition to Adulthood.* Ilford: Barnardo's.

Mulvey, T. (1977) After care – who cares? *Concern,* 26: 8–9.

Owusu-Bempah, J. (1994) Race, self-identity and social work, *British Journal of Social Work,* 24: 123–36.

Page, R. and Clarke, G. (eds) (1977) *Who Cares?* London: National Children's Bureau.

Parker, R., Ward, H., Jackson, S., Aldgate, J. and Wedge, P. (eds) (1991) *Assessing Outcomes in Child Care.* London: HMSO.

Phoenix, A. (1991) *Young Mothers.* Cambridge: Polity Press.

Pinkerton, J. and McCrea, J. (1999) *Meeting the Challenge? Young People Leaving Care in Northern Ireland.* Aldershot: Ashgate.

Rabiee, P., Priestley, M. and Knowles, J. (2001) *Whatever Next? Young Disabled People Leaving Care.* Leeds: First Key.

Randall, G. (1988) *No Way Home.* London: Centrepoint.

Randall, G. (1989) *Homeless and Hungry.* London: Centrepoint.

Raychuba, B. (1987) *Report on the Special Needs of Youth in the Care of the Child Welfare System.* Toronto, Ontario: National Youth in Care Network.

Rowe, J., Hundleby, M. and Garnett, L. (1989) *Child Care Now.* London: Batsford/British Agencies for Adoption and Fostering.

Saunders, L. and Broad, B. (1997) *The Health Needs of Young People Leaving Care.* Leicester: de Montfort University.

Save the Children (1995) *You're On Your Own: Young People's Research on Leaving Care.* London: Save the Children.

Sharpe, S. (1987) *Falling for Love: Teenage Mothers Talk.* London: Virago.

Sinclair, I. and Gibbs, I. (1998) *Children's Homes: A Study in Diversity.* Chichester: Wiley.

Sinclair, R., Garnett, L. and Berridge, D. (1995) *Social Work and Assessment with Adolescents.* London: National Children's Bureau.

Smith, C. (ed.) (1994) *Partnership in Action: Developing Effective Aftercare Projects.* Westerham: The Royal Philanthropic Society.

Stein, M. (1990) *Living Out of Care*. Ilford: Barnardo's.

Stein, M. (1991) *Leaving Care and the 1989 Children Act: The Agenda*. Leeds: First Key.

Stein, M. (1993) Protest in care, in B. Jordan and N. Panton (eds) *The Political Dimensions of Social Work*. Oxford: Blackwell.

Stein, M. (1994) Leaving care, education and career trajectories, *Oxford Review of Education*, 20(3): 349–60.

Stein, M. (1997) *What Works in Leaving Care?* Ilford: Barnardo's.

Stein, M. (1999) Leaving care: reflections and challenges, in O. Stevenson (ed.) *Child Welfare in the UK*. Oxford: Blackwell.

Stein, M. and Carey, K. (1986) *Leaving Care*. Oxford: Blackwell.

Stein, M. and Ellis, S. (1983) *Gizza Say*. London: National Association of Young People in Care.

Stein, M. and Maynard, C. (1985) *I've Never Been So Lonely*. London: National Association of Young People in Care.

Stein, M. and Wade, J. (2000) *Helping Care Leavers: Problems and Strategic Responses*. London: Department of Health.

Stein, M., Pinkerton, J. and Kelleher, J. (2000) Young people leaving care in England, Northern Ireland, and Ireland, *European Journal of Social Work*, 3(3): 235–46.

Stone, M. (1990) *Young People Leaving Care*. Redhill: The Royal Philanthropic Society.

Tizard, B. and Phoenix, A. (1993) *Black, White or Mixed Race?* London: Routledge.

Triseliotis, J. (1980) Growing up in foster care, in J. Triseliotis (ed.) *New Developments in Foster Care and Adoption*. London: Routledge & Kegan Paul.

Triseliotis, J., Borland, M., Hill, M. and Lambert, L. (1995) *Teenagers and Social Work Services*. London: HMSO.

Utting, W. (1997) *People Like Us: The Report of the Review of the Safeguards for Children Living Away from Home*. London: Department of Health/The Welsh Office.

Van der Waals, R. (1960) Former foster children reflect on their childhood, *Children*, 7: 29–33.

Wade, J. (1997) Developing leaving care services: tapping the potential of foster carers, *Adoption and Fostering*, 21(3): 40–9.

Wade, J. and Biehal, N. with Clayden, J. and Stein, M. (1998) *Going Missing: Young People Absent from Care*. Chichester: Wiley.

Ward, H. (1995) *Looking After Children: Research into Practice*. London: HMSO.

Whitaker, D., Archer, L. and Hicks, L. (1998) *Working in Children's Homes: Challenges and Complexities*. Chichester: Wiley.

Who Cares? Trust (1993) *Not Just a Name: The Views of Young People in Foster and Residential Care*. London: National Consumer Council.

4

DAVID BERRIDGE

Residential care

KEY MESSAGES

- Ascertaining 'what works' in children's residential care is complex. Research evidence remains limited, although areas of agreement have been identified in recent studies (see below).
- Residential homes vary considerably and some manage to be positive environments in which to live.
- Residents are a highly challenging group with complex long-standing problems. We should be realistic in our approach to what can be achieved, particularly as most stays are very short.
- Young people's assessments of residential care are often positive. However, any gains that occur during residence are often not sustained after leaving.
- Bullying and exploitation between peers are frequently problems. Relationships with peers in residential homes are probably more influential than relationships with adults.
- Homes should have better links with services for children in need, including education and health. Specialist therapeutic help for children is scarce.
- The most successful homes are small, demonstrate effective leadership, have clearly defined roles and staff consensus.
- We know insufficient about the particular attributes and skills of effective residential managers and staff.

INTRODUCTION

The question 'what works in residential care for children and families?' is deceptively straightforward. Unlike some of the more established disciplines, such as mathematics, physics and medicine, which have been accumulating a knowledge base over centuries, the social sciences are more recent and our understanding is correspondingly less developed. Furthermore, social work services for children and families have emerged in their current form only over the past 50 years, and so to ask at this stage 'what works?' might appear presumptuous. Explaining, for example, why an apple falls from a tree or a rainbow has colours are undoubtedly complicated, yet the intricacies and unpredictability of human behaviour pose greater complexity.

Yet as we see, in this and other chapters, several relevant research studies have been undertaken in children's residential care and other fields. We need to learn from them messages about what is and is not effective and seek to apply them to social policies and social work practice. The government has emphasized this 'evidence-based' approach as part of its modernizing agenda (Department of Health 2000a). Although few child welfare researchers would dissent from this general view, there is much epistemological and conceptual debate about the meaning of the terms 'what works?', 'effective' and, indeed, even what constitutes 'evidence'. This is discussed in the Introduction to this volume. Some may dismiss these nuances as harmless academic distractions. In fact, the debates have profound implications for social work services in the current political context. They relate, for example, to 'Quality Protects' (Department of Health 2000c) and other 'targets', the overall level of professional autonomy and individual discretion, the nature of regulatory frameworks, joint reviews and 'best value', and the role, function and indeed plausibility of a body such as the Social Care Institute for Excellence, which is charged with establishing, developing and disseminating the social work knowledge base (Department of Health 2000a).

Much of this debate about 'what works?' focuses on research methodologies and, in particular, the extent to which social scientists should emulate natural scientists in their approaches (positivism). Newman and Roberts (1997) have articulated this view; for example, they have argued for the greater use in social work research of experimental and quasi-experimental designs to evaluate the effects of social work interventions with children and families (see also Macdonald, this volume). In particular, randomized controlled trials are advocated ('it is necessary to recognise the primacy of the randomized controlled trial'; Newman and Roberts 1997: 287), in which service users are randomly allocated to two groups, one of which receives a service or treatment while the other does not. Those on a waiting list are sometimes used for the latter. Any differences in results are attributed to the intervention.

The subject of randomized controlled trials is controversial in academic debates between child welfare researchers; some have argued that this is an unduly narrow or even unfeasible approach. Broader evaluation methods have been urged in children's health services (McGuire *et al.* 1997) as well as social care (Lewis 1998). Smith's (2000) critique of positivism argues that some proponents of an evidence-based approach misconceive the nature of the social sciences. Politicians and bureaucrats seek a law-like certainty which will remain elusive. Smith asserts that we need to give greater attention in evaluative research to *context* and *process*:

> the experimental method of positivism, which, hypnotised by method to the point where theory is forgotten, has rarely managed to tell us anything helpful about the questions that matter: what is it about this programme that works for whom in what specifiable conditions and given what contextual features?
>
> (Smith 2000: 3)

Sinclair (2000), while sympathetic to a quantitative approach, highlights certain pitfalls of evaluative social work research (see also Fook 2000). He raises a fundamental point about outcome measures used by researchers:

> the criteria set may be too ambitious and out of all proportion to the scale of the intervention. As a very rough rule of thumb, social work interventions seem capable of improving mood, morale and satisfaction with service. They have great difficulty in changing the ways people behave – eg whether they engage in delinquency or suicide attempts. This is particularly so if the people concerned have not asked for the service . . . By concentrating on ambitious and inappropriate targets, social work research may have given social work an undesirably bad name. Judged against over-ambitious and inappropriate criteria it is set up to fail.
>
> (Sinclair 2000: 4)

Useful work clarifying the concept and measurement of outcomes in children's services has been undertaken by Parker and colleagues (1991), which acted as a forerunner to the *Looking After Children* materials (Department of Health 1995b). This asked, for example, for whom is something considered to be an outcome? (There are public, service, professional, family and child outcomes.) Should we be concerned with specific or general outcomes and when are outcomes assumed to occur?

I return later to some of these theoretical and methodological considerations. However, the main implication here is that posing the question 'what works?' is more problematic than it may initially appear. Consequently, in this chapter a more pluralistic, inclusive approach is favoured to what constitutes evidence about what works than some others may have adopted.

Clearly defined boundaries are essential in social research; therefore, the focus here is on children's homes rather than other forms of residence, such as boarding schools, residential special schools, young offender institutions, secure treatment facilities and homes specifically for disabled children, which raise particular issues. The discussion is also restricted to the UK. Research from other countries can be informative, but findings from elsewhere are not automatically transferable here.

Children's homes have recently had a very chequered history. Social workers, wider professionals and the general public alike have seen residential care as something to be avoided wherever possible. A stigma remains associated with living in public care, especially residence, and family placements have been preferred for younger children and those needing long-term care. The costs of children's homes, estimated in the mid-1990s at half a billion pounds annually, have also discouraged their use (Sinclair and Gibbs 1998). Over the past 20 years, the number of young people resident on any one day in England has plunged from some 20,000 to nearer 6000, which is a small proportion of the 58,000 or so total looked after and the estimated 380,000 children in need (Berridge 1985; Department of Health 2000b, 2001). A major factor associated with this unpopularity has been the series of scandals that have been reported concerning the physical and sexual abuse of residents, stretching back over 30 years (Utting 1991, 1997). As a consequence, most residents today are adolescents, who stay weeks or months rather than years. They tend to come from very troubled backgrounds, having experienced inconsistent parenting, neglect and abuse and schooling difficulties, as well as having presented behavioural problems at home and in the community. Social skills and self-esteem are often poor. As a group, they are more problematic than their predecessors and pose a significant challenge for staff looking after them (Berridge and Brodie 1998). In response to criticisms, government has set targets for children looked after, including placement stability, educational achievements, school attendance, proportions in family placements, final warnings, convictions and adoption rate (Department of Health 2000c).

RESEARCH REVIEWS

KEY POINTS

- Taking into account limitations in conceptualization and research methodology, early studies provided a quite positive portrayal of residential care.
- Early studies also indicated that the way homes were organized made a significant difference to the young person's experience.
- While descriptions of young people's experience of residential care are common, less attention has been given to detailed interventions – what it is that staff actually do.
- A range of options for looked after children is indicated; no single form of care can accommodate the needs of all children.

Two reviews of the research have been undertaken which provide useful background for this chapter. One needs, of course, to be cautious in interpreting research findings that are some years old. The first review was by Parker (1988), undertaken as part of the Barclay Committee (1982) review of social work. This considered residential settings in general and there was little material specifically on children's homes. Previous research had mainly focused on services for young offenders and had used outcome measures such as offending rates and absconding/going missing. Parker (1988) drew four general conclusions from this early body of research:

1 Different regimes had a differential effect on children's behaviour.
2 The regimes that achieved the 'best' results were 'child-oriented' rather than 'institution-oriented'.
3 The role of heads played a central part in influencing the regime.
4 Maintaining changes in children's behaviour on departure was difficult.

Parker also commented on the quality and nature of the evidence, pointing out that there was a lack of large-scale and national studies, residential care was seldom contrasted with its main alternatives and assessments of outcome were limited.

The second review followed five years later and was undertaken by the Dartington Social Research Unit (Bullock *et al.* 1993). Reviewing some 60 studies, the authors found that most children in residential care at the time were likely to be older adolescents, experiencing and presenting significant difficulties. Despite the overall decline in numbers, residential care was still widely used: 80 per cent of young people separated from their families for long periods experienced residence at some stage. Many children questioned claimed they preferred residential care to its main alternative, fostering, 'because it is less restrictive and minimises conflict with family loyalties, so preserving trust and confidence' (Bullock *et al.* 1993: 16). Surprisingly perhaps, in view of more recent concerns, the review's authors concluded that residential care 'confers educational benefits and offers children stability in an otherwise disrupted life' (p. 17). However, there was said to be a risk of poor outcomes, especially as 'secondary problems' could be generated by the residential experience itself, such as going missing/running away, and behavioural control within the institution, which could override the personal and family problems responsible for separation in the first place. Thus, the researchers maintained that subsequent delinquent behaviour, for example, was seldom reduced by residential placement. Indeed, they concluded that, 'In the context of a child's wider care career, the residential experience may be of only marginal relevance; major effects on behaviour are seldom to be expected' (p. 16).

Commenting on the nature of the research, the Dartington team described a growing interest in the use and effects of residential care, but far less detailed work on the interventions themselves. Limited attention had been paid to evaluating the quality of care offered to children. Long-term outcome studies have been based on earlier models of residential care and their results may no longer be valid. Research was recommended into the residential experiences of specific groups, such as girls, abuse victims and short-stay cases.

FOLLOW-UP STUDIES

It is of interest to explore how children who have experienced residential care and other family support services develop in later life. This is naturally complex, as many other factors intervene over the years, and positive or negative outcomes cannot simply be attributed to residence itself. Nonetheless, research, although now rather dated, has attempted long-term follow-ups involving residential populations. Triseliotis and Russell (1984), for example, contrasted two groups of men and women in their early to mid-20s, one group who had grown up in adoptive homes ($n = 44$) and the other who had grown up in residential care ($n = 40$). Both groups were considered 'hard to place'. The adopted children had moved into their new homes aged between 2 and 8 years, while the residential population had lived an average of 11 years in their children's homes. Generally, as one would expect, those who had been adopted had fared better than the residential group. The former spoke more positively about their upbringing. They also demonstrated better physical and mental health and more favourable personal, social and economic circumstances. However, the authors urged caution in interpreting these findings. It was possible to trace only about half of each group in the follow-up and this sample loss may have introduced a source of bias. Furthermore, there were important contrasts in the backgrounds of the two groups and simple comparisons of the differences in outcomes were unjustified; variables other than category of placement might well have been influential (see also Quinton and Rutter 1984a,b).

FOSTER AND RESIDENTIAL CARE COMPARED

When Parker wrote in 1988 that research had seldom contrasted residential care with its main alternatives, three investigations were underway. The first was a detailed observational and statistical study by Colton (1988), comparing 12 children's homes with 12 specialist foster homes, catering mostly for teenagers. The two samples of service users had many similarities, although the care careers of the foster children were longer; most of the residential group had been separated from their families during adolescence. The specialist foster homes compared favourably with the residential settings in many respects. In general, they were concluded to be significantly more *child-oriented* in the management of everyday events. Children had stronger community contacts, there were better physical amenities in the homes and techniques of control were more child-centred. Adults interacted more with the young people, were more likely to initiate that contact and were relatively more approving than disapproving in their behaviour. Foster children were more positive than the residential group in their perception of the placements.

However, there were no statistically significant differences in children's progress during the course of their stay between the two placement categories regarding, for example, running away, offending, displays of physical violence and aggression, having a negative effect on peers living with them, problems in relationships with carers, offending, educational performance or behaviour at school. Indeed, the children's homes were reported to be reasonably successful during the placement regarding school performance, attendance and behaviour, as well as in curbing offending and in improving general behaviour.

A rather different approach was adopted by Rowe and colleagues (1989) in their major study of placement patterns. Based on six local authorities, they amassed information on over 5800 children and 10,000 placements. Patterns of outcome were established by asking social workers the extent to which placements lasted as long as planned, whether they lasted as long as needed, and an estimation of the extent to which placement aims were met. Overall, 53 per cent of foster placements were deemed to be 'successful' on a combination of these criteria, 27 per cent 'mixed' and 20 per cent unsuccessful. Comparative figures for residential care were 46 per cent, 38 per cent and 16 per cent. It is important to note, however, that foster and residential care did not always have the same aims. Taking account of age, the difference in success rates disappeared for placements ending during adolescence.

A third study used comparative data from Rowe and colleagues' (1989) research and examined the decision in 1986 of one county, Warwickshire, to close the last of its own children's homes (Cliffe with Berridge 1991). Two hundred and fifteen children over 5 years of age were followed for 15 months. Most were placed in foster care and for 60 per cent of them there was no choice in venue – they went where there was a vacancy. Minority ethnic children were usually placed with white families due to the lack of an appropriate range of carers. In line with Rowe and colleagues' research, most placements in the county were found to be satisfactory or better than satisfactory. But there was more placement instability in Warwickshire than in the national study. Furthermore, using Rowe and colleagues' composite measure of success, Warwickshire came out worse than any of their six authorities, both regarding placements generally and foster care specifically, for young children and adolescents alike.

In 1994, I concluded that, with the current level of theorization and methodologies, most children were seen to benefit from their time in residential and foster care. Moreover, once age factors and differences in aims were taken into account, these and other studies indicated that both services were broadly equally effective in meeting their objectives. This view was in contrast to popular opinion. However, a note of caution was required:

This does not . . . mean that the two services are interchangeable or substitutes but that they should be seen as *complementary*. Residential environments are not suitable for children to grow-up in over long periods: younger children, especially, require more intimate care and greater daily continuity and predictability than residential settings can usually provide. Foster care, therefore, has clear potential advantages in these areas.

(Berridge 1994: 147)

Residential care was found to be used extensively for all groups, but in particular for adolescents in specific circumstances and in the short or medium term. These young people usually had families of their own, but for a variety of reasons either could not or did not want to live with them permanently.

YOUNG PEOPLE'S VIEWS

KEY POINTS

- Few studies of young people's views are representative of all looked after children and the same applies to professionals' views.
- Significant minorities of young people feel they have made progress in residential settings.
- Young people value staff who are practical, reliable, respectful and approachable. Most children report positive encounters with staff.
- Relationships with peers are the most frequently cited source of unhappiness. Appeals to staff for help are rarely reported as achieving a satisfactory resolution.

I have already alluded to young people's own views about services and this is a dimension that should not be ignored in seeking to understand 'what works' in residential care. Children's perspectives are now more likely to be taken into account by service providers, reinforced by legislation such as the Children Act 1989 and the United Nations Convention of the Rights of the Child, ratified by the UK in 1991. Although important, children's perspectives should not necessarily outweigh other considerations (Hill 1999). Nonetheless, a new paradigm in the sociology of childhood encourages us to consider children's *competencies* rather than deficits and leads us to explore their views of the world as social actors (Sandbaek 1999; see also Gilligan 2000). In relation to child welfare specifically, however, young people's expressed views may not always be representative of wider opinion, as responses to postal questionnaires or magazine surveys can be low, while those who volunteer to participate in national or local initiatives may have particular characteristics or attitudes. The same, of course, applies to adults.

The complexities in evaluating the outcomes of residential interventions were evident in a detailed study of the functioning of a therapeutic community (Little 1995). It interweaved an academic analysis with the diary reflections of a young woman resident for 20 months in her teenage years. The account revealed the ups and downs of residential life, including suicide attempts, as she confronted a range of personal problems and anxieties, including disclosure of earlier sexual abuse. She emerged with a successful educational record and greater insight into her background and difficulties, although she was socially and emotionally fragile and would have considerable challenges to face in adulthood. She spoke positively of the therapeutic community, especially the persistence of staff and the continuity it provided, their willingness to see beyond her behavioural challenges to the underlying problems, and those individuals with whom she forged deep personal relationships, giving her life meaning as well as self-belief. This was made possible by staff working an average of 75 hours a week (five days a week), with no shifts and only eight weeks holiday a year; as one interviewee expressed it, a lifestyle rather than a job.

This highly individualized experience would have been unavailable to respondents to the Who Cares? Trust (1993) survey of looked after young people's opinions. The exercise suffered from some of the disadvantages outlined earlier, being based on 600 replies to the 20,000 questionnaires distributed. Boys and minority ethnic groups were under-represented. Reference was made to the negative effect that living in a children's home could have on education, particularly the tendency to get into trouble, peer group pressure, uncertainty and low expectations of school attendance and achievement. Intimidation from other residents was another serious problem, which was rarely resolved by reporting it to staff. The inevitabilities of institutional life could outbalance the positive outcomes; some respondents spoke warmly of the friendship and support from staff, while simultaneously feeling empty, lonely and unhappy.

An empirical study of social work services for teenagers focused on 116 young people aged 13–17 years (Triseliotis *et al.* 1995). By interviewing young people, parents and social workers, contrasts were made between residential and foster care, living at home and supervision. Young people's initial attitude towards residential placement was usually one of passive acceptance. Eighty per cent of residents reported that they were getting on well with their key-worker and most had positive experiences to report of the children's home. Almost half, on the other hand, mentioned difficulties with other residents. Parents spoke approvingly about their contacts with children's homes and appreciated the efforts of staff to befriend young people and communicate with them, as well as exercise effective control. Reflecting on these placements a year later, young people's responses to the possible benefits of placements were as shown in Table 4.1. Overall, significant minorities identified improvements associated with residential placement. Interestingly, residential schools were rated more positively than these children's homes.

Table 4.1   Percentages of children and social workers attributing benefits to residential placements

Benefit	Children	Social workers
Improved school performance	41	40
Improved behaviour	48	37
Changed attitudes/point of view	41	30
Aided maturity/independence	17	26
Provided activities	34	23
Helped get a job	21	28

Source: Triseliotis *et al.* (1995).

The characteristics shown by the adults that young people related well to, and were likely to cooperate with, can be summarized as follows:

- informal in approach, easy to talk to;
- respect young people, listen to what they say, try to understand and not lecture them;
- be frank and sometimes challenging, rather than 'pushy' and 'nagging';
- are available, punctual and reliable;
- keep confidences;
- do practical things to help;
- keep their promises.

SERVICES FOR MINORITY ETHNIC GROUPS

KEY POINTS

- Local authority policies concerning services for minority ethnic groups are often inadequate.
- Little research has been conducted into the residential care experience of minority ethnic young people.
- There is no firm evidence that minority ethnic children spend a disproportionate time in residential care compared with white children.

There have been no major research studies of residential care for children from minority ethnic groups. An inspection of eight local authorities by the Social Services Inspectorate (2000) concluded that there was little evidence that anti-racist and equal opportunity policies had been implemented. Only two of the eight authorities provided specialist training on anti-racism and anti-discriminatory practice; the same number had good mechanisms in place for consulting community groups and minority populations. Practice concerning recruiting and developing black and Asian staff was variable. Families seeking support often had difficulty accessing the departments, particularly if their first language was not English. Workers' understanding of the circumstances of minority ethnic families varied considerably. Child and family assessments were often inadequate. Findings consistent with these were reported in a case study of services specifically for South Asian families (Qureshi *et al.* 2000).

The main study of services for minority ethnic children and families was carried out by Barn *et al.* (1997). Based in three authorities, they explored the experiences of 196 children, including interviews with 18 of the children themselves, together with interviews with some birth parents, social workers, foster and residential carers. Nearly half the children were white and almost one in six was of mixed parentage. They were of all ages but most were adolescents. Although there have been concerns about minority ethnic children languishing in residential care and being unable to find family placements, this did not apply to the authorities in this study; only 15 per cent were living in residence at the time of the research. Reservations were expressed in all three authorities about the extent to which residential placements could meet the cultural needs of minority children. In one, there were few black children in residence and an interviewee referred to the racist behaviour of some peers and staff inaction, together with a lack of staff awareness about food and hair care. In the second authority, residential care was held in low esteem, which some black residential workers saw as racist, despite examples of good practice mentioned by the researchers, for example in relation to young people's identity. The third authority had no residential care of its own and some children, therefore, were placed in private and voluntary provision in rural areas some distance from the borough. Some residents experienced living with an all-white staff in an all-white area.

EDUCATION

KEY POINTS

- The educational performance of young people in residential care is very poor. Most of this deficit may be related to their family experiences and upbringing. Children in foster care frequently also have low educational attainment.
- Young people's experiences can be hampered by low expectations, poor home–school liaison and lack of educational continuity.
- Greater emphasis on the value of education in social work planning and care settings should result in improved educational outcomes, including in post-school careers.

Doubts about the effectiveness of the care system often hinge on the poor educational achievements of care leavers; it has frequently been reported that up to 70 per cent of care leavers at 16 years of age have no educational qualifications (Jackson and Sachdev 2001). Although there is cause for concern, we should be cautious to avoid misinterpretation. Young people will seldom have grown up in foster or residential care and so earlier experiences will have a lasting influence. Official statistics report that of the 6800 care leavers in England aged 16 years and over during the year ending 31 March 2000, a quarter had been looked after for under six months and half less than two years (Department of Health 2001, table 15). This would have allowed limited time to reverse early failings. The link between social disadvantage and educational underachievement is well recognized (Brodie 2001). Indeed, attendance and behavioural problems at school may be a contributory factor to admission to accommodation, a cause rather than an effect. In one recent study, the proportion of children's homes' residents for whom education was considered to be 'a major problem' leading to the decision to accommodate was 59 per cent (Berridge and Brodie 1998).

A useful overview of the literature on the education of children in need was provided by Sinclair (1998). Building on Jackson's (1987) original work, Sinclair suggested five explanations for the poor educational performance of looked after children: pre-care experience, broken schooling, low expectations, low self-esteem and lack of continuity of care-giver. Sinclair stressed the significance of children's family upbringing, particularly where there has been trauma and neglect. A longitudinal study of the education of children in foster care found that those living in long-term foster homes that were felt to be stable and rewarding still did not make good progress (Heath *et al.* 1989, 1994). Those who entered care because of abuse or neglect did significantly worse than others.

Young people in the care system who have done well educationally have needed to be persistent. The presence of a role-model or mentor can be important to help fight the system. Interestingly, a number were enthusiastic and early readers, which suggests this should be encouraged more widely (Jackson and Sachdev 2001). Gilligan (2000) highlighted the importance of school success in bolstering children's resilience. He advocated greater interest from social workers and care-givers in all aspects of school life. Close links and dialogue with the school need to be maintained. Continuity in schooling is important both academically and socially; a change in placement should not necessarily mean a change in school. Adults should convey high but not unreasonable expectations about the child's achievements. Additional measures such as extra tutoring or homework clubs can also help. School should not have to wait until emotional problems are resolved; education itself may offer a route of escape for some (Aldgate 1990). In addition and in relation to children's homes specifically, proper attention should be paid to education in care planning and record keeping. Roles need to be clarified and residential staff could be more educationally stimulating, for example in offering to play games with children, watch informative television programmes and visit places of educational interest. Furthermore, there is much more discussion of school than college and the potential contribution of further education merits closer scrutiny (Berridge *et al.* 1997).

CARING FOR CHILDREN AWAY FROM HOME

KEY POINTS

- High-quality care has been associated with small homes with an effective leadership, with clearly defined roles and staff consensus.
- These factors have been associated with fewer children going missing/running away.
- Sustaining improvements after residents leave is difficult.
- Young people with traumatic pre-care experiences get insufficient specialist therapeutic help.
- Homes need to be fully integrated into the health, education and social welfare provision available in the wider community.

The final part of the discussion on 'what works' in children's residential care focuses on 12 studies published in the late 1990s, funded mostly as part of a Department of Health research initiative. Summaries and common themes are featured in the government publication *Caring for Children Away from Home* (Department of Health 1998).

Surprisingly, perhaps, in view of recent history, little specific attention was given in the research programme to issues of child abuse and child protection. An exception was Farmer and Pollocks' (1998) study of sexually abused and abusing children in substitute care. Based in two authorities, this study covered 250 case files, together with intensive interviews with 38 children over 10 years of age and a slightly smaller sample of care-givers and social workers. Placements of the 38 children who were interviewed were roughly evenly divided between residential and foster care. Many young people displayed highly sexualized behaviour in placements, yet staff lacked theory and practice ideas on which to base work with them. Few of the sexually abused children had been offered specialist therapeutic help to address the abuse and related issues.

The risk of abusive behaviour by young people, both inside and outside the placement, was less where there was 'high caregiver engagement':

> there were either regular keywork sessions or the caregiver made him or herself available for the child, there was a committed relationship of trust and acceptance, there was an extended view of the caring role in which the caregiver defined his or her role in terms of the individual child's emotional and material needs and there was a general concern for the child's long-term welfare.
>
> (Farmer and Pollock 1998: 178)

The greatest improvement in behaviour was seen when young people had been able to explore their experiences and feelings in a specialist therapeutic setting *and* with a caregiver in their placement. Although only 21 young people were living in residential care, 67 per cent were judged to have experienced high or medium caregiver engagement and 71 per cent were felt to be safe from sexual risks. Nevertheless, three-quarters had sexually abused others during their placement; for two-thirds it was felt that the child's sexual behaviour was poorly managed and over 70 per cent had outstanding needs that were not met. Only 39 per cent of young people themselves responded that they were 'very satisfied' with the residential placements. Recommendations from the study included: a need for greater consideration at the time of placement of the combination of needs and problems of the whole resident group; complete information should be given to caregivers about children's backgrounds; there should be enhanced opportunities for children to communicate their problems and worries; and practice ideas should be developed alongside improved training, consultancy and support for caregivers in this complex and stressful area.

Another study that was part of this research initiative looked at risk to children from a different angle – those who go missing from residential and foster homes (Wade and Biehal 1998). This consisted of mapping the patterns of going missing in four authorities as well as a more detailed qualitative study in two of them. The latter involved 36 young people, their carers and social workers. The findings revealed that there was wide diversity in the proportions of young people going missing from children's homes each year, ranging from 25 to 71 per cent. Some went to families or friends, others slept rough. Reasons for absence were linked both to their individual histories as well as care experiences. Contributory factors within children's homes included the influence of peers, such as bullying and intimidation, feeling insecure or unsettled in placements and 'a general lack of confidence and sense of disempowerment among residential staff' (Wade and Biehal 1998: 197). Strong leadership from heads of homes was singled out as particularly important in limiting this behaviour, linked to staff consensus, high morale and clear expectations for young people's behaviour. An early response to the problem of going missing is necessary before a pattern is established. Each placement needs to maintain good records. More generally, local authorities need to have developed policies on going missing and to have communicated these to caregivers. Effective liaison with school and police is considered important.

One of the most significant studies to illustrate what works in children's homes is that of Sinclair and Gibbs (1998). Its scale was larger than the other studies reported here, spanning a national sample of 48 homes and 223 of their residents. A range of quantitative and qualitative methods was used, including several postal questionnaires. Sinclair and Gibbs' main findings included the following. Residents' assessments of homes depended on whether they had wanted to be looked after, if the home was a reasonable place in which to live, whether they felt there was a purpose in being there, if they moved on at an appropriate time and their experiences since leaving. There was a preference for residential rather than foster care. Young people favoured homes in which they were not bullied, sexually intimidated or led into trouble, where other residents were friendly, where staff listened and the home's organization and rules were reasonable. Most parents welcomed the young person's spell in care and felt that it helped settle them down as well as improve family relationships.

Sinclair and Gibbs (1998) assessed outcomes for children in several ways. The existence of orderly homes with a positive resident culture was found to be unrelated to the previous delinquency and disturbance of residents, staffing ratios, the proportion of professionally qualified staff or whether the head of home was trained. Instead, successful homes had the following characteristics:

- They are small.
- The head of home feels that its roles are clear, mutually compatible, and not disturbed by frequent reorganisation and that he/she is then given adequate autonomy to get on with the job.
- The staff are agreed about how the home should run and are not at odds with each other.

(Sinclair and Gibbs 1998: 217)

However, change in residents' adjustment was usually quite minor and was often reversed on transfer to a new environment. These general findings were confirmed by another study, which found that the variables most strongly associated independently with the quality of care in children's homes were:

- the head of home being able to specify a clear theoretical or therapeutic orientation, or at least methods of work for the home;
- for homes to have a clear sense of their objectives and be able to keep to them;
- staffing stability (Berridge and Brodie 1998).

Summarizing the main themes to emerge from the 12 studies as a whole, the 'Green Book' (Department of Health 1998) reiterated that residents in children's homes were a particularly challenging group. We may need to be realistic about what can be achieved, especially as so many of their problems still defy our understanding. It reinforced the value of small homes, run by individuals who have a clear idea of what is trying to be achieved. Most importantly, perhaps, there is a need for children's homes to be better integrated into the wider continuum of services for children in need, including closer relationships with health and education professionals, schools, neighbourhoods and families.

CONCLUSION

The research evidence

Before attempting to identify some common themes, I first need to reflect on the nature of the evidence and return to my opening remarks. Readers should be reminded that the extent of empirical research on residential care is still very limited and we have barely begun to scratch the surface of some highly complex problems. Services evolve and earlier findings may no longer be applicable. At this stage, our conceptual tools remain restricted. It is only within the past decade that we have developed a more sophisticated theoretical understanding of the nature of child care 'outcomes' and how they can be assessed. Unlike the natural sciences, studies are seldom replicated and specific findings tend not to be reconsidered in detail. An exception was in relation to recent studies of children's homes, where research teams collaborated during the course of their work and similar findings emerged independently using different research methods. The current Department of Health approach to research programmes, whatever its advantages, means that major studies are unlikely to be revisited, as attention moves between service areas; for example, social work decisions (Department of Health 1985), child protection (Department of Health 1995a), teenagers (Department of Health 1996), residential care (Department of Health 1998), adoption (Department of Health 1999), family support and foster care. Proposals for research that may appear similar in focus can be discouraged, as there is a preference to cover a wide spectrum of topics and satisfy competing interests.

Few of the studies discussed had large sample sizes and there has been only one genuinely national study. There have been no randomized controlled trials and observational studies have been few. Little interest has been shown in services for minority ethnic groups and researchers tend not to adjust their methods, for example by 'oversampling', to provide sub-groups of an adequate size to enable comment. Not much is known about specific populations, such as residential care for girls or services for African-Caribbean teenage boys.

Depending on one's perspective, however, some of these methodological points may be unimportant. There are convincing arguments, outlined at the beginning of this chapter, that social work research is fundamentally different from the natural sciences and the chimera of positivism is misguided, although seductive in an age besotted with the certainty of audit, inspection, targets and task forces. An aspirin taken in Luton or New York has a similar effect, but a stay in a children's home will be a quite different experience. The nature of generalizations produced in social research are unlike those in the natural sciences. All this has important implications for 'evidence-based practice' – the balance between sharing complex findings with practitioners or telling them what they should be doing – and the status of research findings alongside received professional wisdom and reflective practice experience.

Over a short period, research has begun to lay a useful base to inform policy makers and practitioners in children's residential care and related fields. We have some good, systematic, descriptive data about residential services provided, users' characteristics and associated problems. Conceptualizations have been developed; for example, researchers have differentiated between various organizational forms of children's homes and different social patterns of children going missing. Qualitative studies use these to begin to make connections and theorize. A number of the studies reviewed have attempted to 'triangulate' (that is, cross-check) their data. Thus, interviews have often been held with young people, carers, birth parents and social workers, which highlight similarities and differences in perspectives and enable overall judgements to be formed. It is encouraging that many studies have canvassed young people's views. There is much consensus in findings across studies and the conclusions from research frequently resonate with accepted good practice. Results sometimes emerge that are unexpected or challenge the orthodoxy; for example, the findings that what otherwise appear to be good homes do not necessarily produce the best longer-term results, and the quality of care and young people's outcomes are unrelated to staffing levels and the extent of professional qualifications. These need careful explanation and dissemination as they are complex issues; there could be indirect associations and the factors involved (such as training) may be important for other reasons. Overall, therefore, adopting a pluralistic and inclusive stance, research has made a valuable contribution to understanding and hopefully improving children's residential care.

What works?

With these comments in mind, what can we deduce from the research evidence about what works in residential care for children and families and what are the implications for policy and practice? Four themes can be identified.

First, studies have indicated that children's homes vary considerably and some manage to become positive environments in which to live. It is, therefore, possible to offer high-quality care. However, we do not know how successful homes are at meeting the particular needs of children from minority ethnic groups. Residents generally seem to prefer children's homes over foster care, as they allow a negotiation of birth family relationships and roles. Once differences in aims and populations are taken into account, social workers have rated the two services about equally. An authority that discontinued its own residential care did not find a noticeable improvement in its results. A major problem with residential care is the threat of bullying and intimidation from other residents, which is a difficult problem to resolve. Relationships between peers are probably as important, if not more so, than those between young people and staff. Social networks and supports need to be strengthened during residence, not narrowed and weakened or become more delinquent. Whatever gains may be achieved during the period of residence, most researchers agree that these are unlikely to persist in the longer term. We would be unlikely to expect otherwise given the relatively brief stay of most residents and, therefore, need to be more realistic about what current approaches to residential care are likely to accomplish. The best we can aim for is a period of stability and safety, a decline in the extent and rate of deterioration, young people's satisfaction, the opportunity to communicate and discuss problems with concerned adults, and engagement with other supports and services. The following points appear to affect the likelihood of these. Whether they make any difference in the longer term depends on other events in young people's lives and what happens next.

A second theme concerns the relationship between children's homes and other services for children in need. Studies depict homes as professionally isolated, with too few drawing on specialist services, for example from health and education colleagues. The study of sexually abused and abusing children showed disconcertingly how most had not been offered specialist therapeutic help. Improvements were found to be most significant where children were communicating with caregivers *and* had received specialist help. In addition, schooling experiences are particularly important for the residential population, as successful educational achievement has been linked with resilience and social mobility. Most looked after children do poorly at school, largely because of early experiences, although the care system offers inadequate compensations and peer influences can be undermining. Social workers and residential staff need to be more involved in school life, educational matters should be more central to social work planning, continuity in schooling is important and there needs to be an expectation of children's potential.

A third cluster of points relate to the organizational features of successful homes. Although many researchers refer to the need for regimes to be 'child-centred', varying levels of social and psychological interaction with young people have been reported. Improvements in the behaviour of young people who had been sexually abused or who abused others depend in part on the amount of 'caregiver engagement'. Improved staffing ratios and professional qualifications are not in themselves the main determinants of effective homes. Instead, it has been agreed that homes should be small, heads should have a firm sense of the home's purpose and should be able to stick to it, there needs to be agreement among staff and there should be clear expectations of young people's behaviour.

The final and perhaps most important theme concerns the personal attributes and skills of social workers and residential staff working with children. Heads of homes are a key group. Previous research has pinpointed the crucial roles of school heads and probation hostel wardens (Sinclair 1975; Rutter *et al.* 1979). In the field of foster care, we sometimes talk of the 'chemistry' between carers and individual children, which can make for a successful placement, sometimes against the odds. Recent research has sought to explain this using attachment theory (Schofield *et al.* 2000). Several of the studies reviewed here explained successful residential care according to the quality of the interaction between young people and adults. Terms used included empathy, approachability, persistence, a willingness to listen and reliability. We know little about how to recognize these qualities on recruitment, how to reinforce them via training and supervision, and how they interact with the other variables discussed here. The challenge for researchers is how we can encourage these qualities and otherwise help develop evidence-based social work that enables staff to draw on appropriate research messages in their decision making and everyday work with children and families.

REFERENCES

Aldgate, J. (1990) Foster children at school: success or failure?, *Adoption and Fostering*, 14(4): 38–49.

Barclay Committee (1982) *Social Workers: Their Roles and Tasks*. London: Bedford Square Press/NCVO.

Barn, R., Sinclair, R. and Ferdinand, D. (1997) *Acting on Principle: An Examination of Race and Ethnicity in Social Services Provision for Children and Families*. London: British Agencies for Adoption and Fostering.

Berridge, D. (1985) *Children's Homes*. Oxford: Blackwell.

Berridge, D. (1994) Foster and residential care reassessed: a research perspective, *Children and Society*, 8(2): 132–50.

Berridge, D. and Brodie, I. (1998) *Children's Homes Revisited*. London: Jessica Kingsley.

Berridge, D., Brodie, I., Ayre, P. *et al.* (1997) *Hello: Is Anybody Listening? The Education of Young People in Residential Care*. Warwick: Social Care Association and the University of Warwick.

Brodie, I. (2001) *Children's Homes and School Exclusion: Redefining the Problem*. London: Jessica Kingsley.

Bullock, R., Little, M. and Millham, S. (1993) *Residential Care for Children: A Review of the Research*. London: HMSO.

Cliffe, D. with Berridge, D. (1991) *Closing Children's Homes: An End to Residential Childcare?* London: National Children's Bureau.

Colton, M. (1988) *Dimensions of Substitute Care: A Comparative Study of Foster and Residential Care Practice*. Aldershot: Avebury.

Department of Health (1985) *Social Work Decisions in Child Care: Research Findings and Their Implications*. London: HMSO.

Department of Health (1995a) *Child Protection: Messages from Research*. Chichester: Wiley.

Department of Health (1995b) *Looking After Children: Good Parenting – Good Outcomes*. London: Department of Health.

Department of Health (1996) *Focus on Teenagers: Research into Practice*. London: Department of Health.

Department of Health (1998) *Caring for Children Away from Home: Messages from Research*. Chichester: Wiley.

Department of Health (1999) *Adoption Now: Messages from Research*. Chichester: Wiley.

Department of Health (2000a) *A Quality Strategy for Social Care*. London: Department of Health.

Department of Health (2000b) *Children in Need in England*. London: Department of Health.

Department of Health (2000c) *Social Services Performance in 1999–2000*. London: Department of Health.

Department of Health (2001) *Children Looked After by Local Authorities, Year Ending March 2000, England*. London: Department of Health.

Farmer, E. and Pollock, S. (1998) *Sexually Abused and Abusing Children in Substitute Care*. Chichester: Wiley.

Fook, J. (2000) Theorising from frontline practice: towards an inclusive approach for social work research. Paper presented to the ESRC-funded seminar series *Theorising Social Work Research*, University of Luton, 11 July. http://www.nisw.org.uk/tswr/fook.

Gilligan, R. (2000) Adversity, resilience and young people, *Children and Society*, 14: 37–47.

Heath, A., Colton, M. and Aldgate, J. (1989) The education of children in and out of care, *British Journal of Social Work*, 19: 447–60.

Heath, A., Colton, M. and Aldgate, J. (1994) Failure to escape: a longitudinal study of foster children's educational attainment, *British Journal of Social Work*, 24(3): 241–60.

Hill, M. (1999) What's the problem? Who can help? The perspectives of children and young people on their well-being and on helping professionals, *Journal of Social Work Practice*, 13(2): 135–45.

Jackson, S. (1987) *The Education of Children in Care*. Bristol: University of Bristol, School of Applied Social Studies.

Jackson, S. and Sachdev, D. (2001) *Better Education, Better Futures: Research, Practice and the Views of Young People in Public Care*. Ilford: Barnardo's.

Lewis, J. (1998) Building an evidence-based approach to social interventions. *Children and Society*, 12: 136–40.

Little, M. with Kelly, S. (1995) *A Life Without Problems? The Achievements of a Therapeutic Community*. Aldershot: Arena.

McGuire, J., Stein, A. and Rosenberg, W. (1997) Evidence-based medicine and child mental health services, *Children and Society*, 11: 89–96.

Newman, T. and Roberts, H. (1997) Assessing social work effectiveness in child care practice: the contribution of randomized controlled trials, *Child Care, Health and Development*, 23(4): 287–96.

Parker, R. (1988) Children, in I. Sinclair (ed.) *Residential Care: The Research Reviewed*. London: HMSO.

Parker, R., Ward, H., Jackson, S., Aldgate, J. and Wedge, P. (eds) (1991) *Assessing Outcomes in Child Care*. London: HMSO.

Quinton, D. and Rutter, M. (1984a) Parents with children in care. 1. Current circumstances and parenting, *Journal of Child Psychology and Psychiatry*, 25(2): 211–29.

Quinton, D. and Rutter, M. (1984b) Parents with children in care – intergenerational continuities, *Journal of Child Psychology and Psychiatry*, 25(2): 231–50.

Qureshi, T., Berridge, D. and Wenman, H. (2000) *Where to Turn? Family Support for South Asian Communities – A Case Study*. London: National Children's Bureau.

Rowe, J., Hundleby, M. and Garnett, L. (1989) *Child Care Now: A Survey of Placement Patterns*. London: British Agencies for Adoption and Fostering.

Rutter, M., Maughan, B., Mortimore, P., Ouston, J. with Smith, A. (1979) *Fifteen Thousand Hours: Secondary Schools and their Effects on Children*. London: Open Books.

Sandbaek, M. (1999) Children with problems: focusing on everyday life, *Children and Society*, 13(2): 106–18.

Schofield, G., Beek, M. and Sargent, K. with Thoburn, J. (2000) *Growing Up in Foster Care*. London: British Agencies for Adoption and Fostering.

Sinclair, I. (1975) The influence of wardens and matrons on probation hostels, in J. Tizard, I. Sinclair and R. Clarke (eds) *Varieties of Residential Experience*. London: Routledge.

Sinclair, I. (2000) Methods and measurement in evaluative social work. Paper presented to the ESRC-funded seminar series *Theorising Social Work Research*, University of Luton, 11 July. http://www.nisw.org.uk/tswr/sinclair.

Sinclair, I. and Gibbs, I. (1998) *Children's Homes: A Study in Diversity*. Chichester: Wiley.

Sinclair, R. (1998) *The Education of Children in Need*. Totnes: Research in Practice/ Dartington Social Research Unit.

Smith, D. (2000) What works as evidence for practice? The methodological repertoire in an applied discipline. Paper presented to the ESRC-funded seminar series *Theorising Social Work Research*, University of Wales Cardiff, 27 April. http://www.nisw.org.uk/ tswr/smith.

Social Services Inspectorate (2000) *Excellence Not Excuses: Inspection of Services for Ethnic Minority Children and Families*. London: Department of Health.

Triseliotis, J. and Russell, J. (1984) *Hard to Place: The Outcome of Adoption and Residential Care*. London: Heinemann.

Triseliotis, J., Borland, M., Hill, M. and Lambert, L. (1995) *Teenagers and the Social Work Services*. London: HMSO.

Utting, W. (1991) *Children in the Public Care*. London: HMSO.

Utting, W. (1997) *People Like Us*. London: The Stationery Office.

Wade, J. and Biehal, N. with Clayden, J. and Stein, M. (1998) *Going Missing: Young People Absent from Care*. Chichester: Wiley.

Who Cares? Trust (1993) *Not Just a Name: The Views of Young People in Foster and Residential Care*. London: National Consumer Council.

PART 2

Preventing the social exclusion of children and young people

Tackling social exclusion in general, and the social exclusion of children and young people in particular, has been at the top of the policy agenda in recent years. A plethora of national, regional and local initiatives have emerged aimed at regenerating communities, reducing child poverty and addressing the exclusion of specific groups. But as far as understanding what works is concerned, we are better at talking the talk than walking the walk. While we now know quite a lot about the causes and consequences of social exclusion, we are still only beginning to develop the learning for what to do about it.

This part of the book considers some of the measures important to preventing social exclusion through an exploration of:

- children and young people's involvement in decision making;
- community-based interventions for young offenders;
- inclusive education;
- promoting the inclusion of disabled young people;
- community development with children and young people.

As the authors of these chapters make clear, we have some way to go in understanding which of our interventions are actually *effective* in promoting social inclusion. What can we do that might actually make a difference? The political prizes for improving educational outcomes and decreasing crime are considerable. The human costs of failing to promote inclusion in all the areas described here cannot be calculated. The authors all point to the need to understand what works in the process of implementation as well the interventions themselves. Even the most effective intervention will not work if we don't understand how to deliver it. What unites these chapters is the authors' assessment that process and context matter. This has implications for systematic reviews that bring together work from very different methodological traditions. The authors also share a view that the current state of evaluative research in these areas is insufficiently robust to enable us to claim a strong evidence base for the effectiveness or otherwise of interventions, although juvenile justice and education are better served than some of the other areas authors have tackled. In particular, politicians or pundits who prefer 'short sharp shock' treatment for young offenders may like to read of the relative lack of success of 'scared straight' programmes. In the summer of 2001, David Walker asked in both *The Guardian* and a Radio 4 *Analysis* programme whether we would ever know enough about whether all that money spent on crime and prison and a range of other interventions actually works. These chapters indicate that while we may not have a complete answer, there is a greater appetite for finding out than has sometimes been the case in the social sciences.

REFERENCE

Walker, D. (2001) Information gap, *The Guardian*, 26 July, p. 12 and 'Unreliable Evidence', Radio 4, 26 July.

5

GARY CRAIG

Community development with children

KEY MESSAGES

- Community development is increasingly being promoted energetically across the world but it is understood in different ways in different cultures.
- The language of community development and empowerment often masks different values and practices.
- It is important to distinguish between community development with communities in general and work targeted specifically at particular groups, including children.
- There is a wide range of practice of community development with children, in differing contexts and policy areas and using differing methods.
- The development of evaluative tools for this work is at an early stage and needs to involve children in the creation of appropriate measures.
- There are tensions between approaches focusing on children's rights and those focusing on children's needs.
- Empowering children challenges the power of adults and work with children needs to be set within an emancipatory framework.

INTRODUCTION: COMMUNITY DEVELOPMENT – TENSIONS AND CONTRADICTIONS FOR WORK WITH CHILDREN

This chapter reviews reported experience of community development with children and ways in which the effectiveness of that work might be assessed. Children and young people traditionally, almost as a matter of course, have been excluded from adult policy debate, being regarded as ill-equipped to contribute effectively. However, as the reviewed evidence shows, this need not be the case and there are many examples worldwide of the ways in which, using the techniques of community development, children and young people can make effective and appropriate contributions to policy issues that affect their lives. Although this evidence covers a range of contexts and children of mixed backgrounds and experience, much of it focuses on ways in which children and young people from more deprived backgrounds can become important policy actors in their own right.

A REVIVAL IN THE FORTUNES OF COMMUNITY DEVELOPMENT

The growth of this work has coincided with a more general revival of interest in community development. The language of 'community involvement' and 'participation' is again common coinage in political and policy circles, with the 1997 New Labour government locating a central plank of its policy approach to combating deprivation in the 'New Deal for Communities' (Social Exclusion Unit 1998). Although community development has long been associated with attempts to address poverty and deprivation, 'community', as one commentator once so aptly put it, has yet again become a 'spray-on additive', one which frequently obscures as much as it clarifies issues and processes under discussion. Hoggett (1997: 3) observes, 'nowhere is the idea of community more ubiquitous than in contemporary social and public policy'. This widespread usage, however, conceals widely differing meanings and political orientations. Frazer (1998: 8) suggests there is a danger that the fact that 'community has become the dominant political idea of the centre left ... will obscure the need for serious social analysis'. Consequently, it is important to clarify what is meant by the notions of community and community development.

Community development takes as a key tenet the importance of working with people starting with their own perceptions of their needs and then organizing with them to meet those needs in appropriate ways. In the context of this chapter, this raises several key ethical and methodological issues, both for children in general and for children with disability or impairment in particular, who are doubly impeded from fully participating in society. Some of these issues are addressed elsewhere in this book.

In discussing working with children, how far is it possible to work with children as independent actors in their own right, separate from the adults who have kinship, caring and/or legal responsibilities for them? Because of the contemporary legal frameworks defining the state of 'childhood' (albeit differently within particular cultures), children can never be seen as entirely autonomous. Childhood is now widely recognized not as a fixed concept, but as a social and political construct. It is not possible to review this issue here (although I do so in detail elsewhere; see Craig 2000), but the boundaries of the answer to this rather basic question are important in defining what is appropriate, possible and permissible in working with children. It is important to note the strong current of thinking that increasingly defines the child as a semi-independent actor with social and political rights, and provides a policy and political framework for working with children. This framework legitimizes the development of work with children but, at the same time, spells out the competing political and legal issues to be considered and clarified in the course of such work. Social research has incidentally made a useful contribution to exploring the ethical and methodological questions to be addressed in working with children. Research findings have much to offer practitioners and, to a large extent, have led where practice is following.

The practice of community development as a professional occupational form has evolved within the UK over the past 50 years, subject to a number of influences, identified in historical reviews of its growth (Thomas 1983; Craig 1989; Popple 1995). Although these reviews differ, sometimes considerably, in their political analysis and in the conclusions that the authors reach, they have in common the understanding that community development is both a way of working, a practice (or more precisely a *praxis*, a form of social action), which attempts effectively to unite theory and practice (Sayer 1986; *Community Development Journal* 1998) with a set of techniques and methods, and a broader philosophical approach to working with people.

This broader view of the community development approach to working with people is critical to understanding its contemporary importance, because it recognizes that it is possible for the principles of community development to inform work with people in a variety of policy settings (such as housing, education, planning, urban regeneration and health) or to influence other professions and social movements (Thomas 1995). For example, community development principles have informed a significant body of work attempting to give greater control over, and participation in, the work of social services to their consumers (Croft and Beresford 1993) and, increasingly, within primary health initiatives (Jones 1999).

At the same time, those working within communities have increasingly recognized the importance of approaches built as much on *difference* and *diversity* as on common interests and goals. Early sociological discussions about the meaning of 'community' identified the term (from a multiplicity of definitions) as not only referring to a set of social relations within a defined geographical area (community as *place*), but also, or alternatively, as 'a sense of belonging to a group' (Stacey 1969: 135) (community as *identity*) (Hillery

1955; Bell and Newby 1971). The Community Development Project (whose origins, ironically, lay in the changing legislative and policy framework for children and young people (Community Development Project 1977, 1978), working within neighbourhoods and using a strong class analysis, was rightly criticized for the underdeveloped gender dimension in its analysis. In the last 20 years, both community development practice and theory have been informed by an understanding of the importance of incorporating the dimensions of gender, race, disability and sexuality, for example (Flynn *et al.* 1986; Jacobs and Popple 1994). This has led to different strands of practice, for example so-called 'separatist work' with specific population groups, such as members of minority ethnic communities or people with disabilities, or work which has a specific rural focus (Henderson 1999) as opposed to the urban settings in which most community development work had previously taken place. One important issue emerging from practice has been the recognition that conflict is as likely to be a motive or context for organizing (Hoggett 1997) as is the consensus often associated with the romantic 'myth' of community. Increasingly, across the world, community development practice has had to develop quite explicitly in situations of (at times, extreme) conflict (*Community Development Journal* 1998). These insights are highly relevant to work with children.

Community development practice was undermined during the 1980s and 1990s in the UK by a combination of a centralizing national state and considerable fiscal and political pressure on the capacity of publicly controlled institutions to support it, leading in some commentators' views to it now being at something of a 'crossroads' (Miller and Ahmad 1997). Ironically, at the same time, its salience outside the UK apparently has become correspondingly greater, as argued elsewhere (Craig 1998: 4). The Brundtland Commission (World Commission on Environment and Development 1987) observed that one of the main prerequisites of sustainable development is 'securing effective citizens' participation', and the Human Development Report (United Nations Development Project 1993) commented that, in the face of current challenges for development, 'people's participation is becoming the central issue of our time'. Even the World Bank, better known for its fiscal conservatism than for its social and political risk taking, has argued that community participation can be a means for ensuring that 'projects reach the poorest in the most efficient and cost-effective way'.

LANGUAGE AND IDEOLOGY

This interest in community development outside the UK has been important in offering a framework for some imaginative work with children and young people, which is now increasingly mirrored within the UK. However, the apparent enthusiasm for community development and community participation reflects continuing political and ideological confusion about the goals of community development, this time on a global scale. In what follows, community development is taken to be a way of working with people, which starts with the needs and aspirations of groups of disadvantaged people in poor and deprived communities (whether socially or geographically defined). It seeks to articulate and organize politically (in the broadest sense) around these needs and aspirations, placing them at the front rather than at the end of political and policy debate. It strives to give ordinary people a voice for expressing and acting on their needs and desires and, through the process of participating in this approach to social change, offers people (again often the most powerless and deprived) support for their empowerment.

Empowerment is another of the terms associated with community development, which has become part of the common political lexicon but equally open to the charge of meaning everything and nothing. Here, the term 'empowerment' is taken to mean the creation of sustainable structures, processes and mechanisms, over which communities have increasing control, and which themselves have a measurable impact on public and social policy affecting those communities: this definition incorporates both outcome and process goals. These definitions have been used as a yardstick against which potential evidence has been assessed.

One important distinction is between community development work targeted at adults, but which claims to bring indirect benefits to children, and work directly with children themselves. This is an important distinction, because community development strategies are being turned to again as a potential panacea for dealing with a range of social issues such as the 'youth problem'. There is some evidence in recent literature of the indirect benefits that children derive from community development (Alexander 1992; Barr et al. 1995; Henderson 1995; and see below) and much basic community development work with adults – such as work with residents campaigning for better housing or clean water – brings fairly obvious benefits to children and adults alike. Much of this work is premised partly, however, on the assumption that it will bring benefits to children by a form of 'trickle-down' process. For example, community development-oriented public health, housing or employment programmes to reduce smoking, address dampness or disrepair, or improve labour market skills, should, it is claimed, impact on children in terms of health gains or improvements in their self-esteem. However, very little attention has been paid to evaluating the extent to which these assumptions are valid and, indeed, the 'trickle-down' theory of economic and social development is now thoroughly discredited within social development literature (Craig and Mayo 1995). It is important that these claims should be the focus of careful evaluative work.

Community development is, as we have noted, a highly complex organic process, in which it is not always possible to trace a definitive causal line between 'input' and 'outcome'. Most of the discussion in this chapter examines the impact of community development with children, but it has often been tentatively suggested that being part of a community and, therefore, also being involved in community development, has a beneficial impact on the life and well-being of the child, even when children do not form the direct focus of the intervention. Gaffikin and Morrissey (1994), in a review of one of the major UK interventions forming part of the European Third Poverty Programme (Geddes 1997), draw some cautious conclusions on the effects of the Brownlow Community Trust on the lives of the residents, including children, of Brownlow, Northern Ireland. They focus on tangible outputs, from which assumptions about lasting value are drawn. These outputs include the establishment of a women's centre and activities focusing on family support, a health centre users' group, crèche facilities and child play facilities, and the raising of awareness on policies as they affect young people.

The model employed within this programme has subsequently been applied to Barnardo's Anti-Poverty Strategy; Traynor *et al.* (1998) suggest that such an approach is promising in affecting the lives of children, but that it is too early to assert that the change will be sustained. Much early effort in this strategy went into the development of an infrastructure, without which long-term outcomes were unlikely to be achieved. Apart from these and other isolated examples, little reference is made in the literature to the impacts of an impoverished community on the child or of the impact of an improved or sound community on the child. One notable exception to date is Henderson (1997), who notes in a discussion of general community development work with children that:

> Other projects do not necessarily aim at children and young people but nevertheless involve and benefit them. A post-war council estate included a street where the houses had not been modernised like those in the surrounding streets. Part of the problem was the fact that kitchens and bathrooms were not properly separated, a situation which was seen as basic to the whole family's health.
>
> (Henderson 1997: 171)

What also remains largely untested, and this discussion is intended to advance the debate, is the extent to which community development *directly with* children offers benefits to the children themselves.

COMMUNITY DEVELOPMENT WITH CHILDREN: THE RESEARCH EVIDENCE

As much community development literature and practice now acknowledges, the distinction between 'developed' and 'developing' countries is often a misleading and unhelpful one (Craig and Mayo 1995). The processes impacting on local communities, resulting in poverty and deprivation, social and economic dislocation, are increasingly global in their origins and similar in their effects in disparate national contexts. Despite important local differences – in terms of social, economic, cultural and political contexts and differing understandings of the meaning of childhood in different countries – the local impacts and analyses of these global processes, and community responses to them, are increasingly following parallel paths.

Community development in the 'developed' world is increasingly recognizing the nature of these connections and how much it has to learn from the insights and practice of those in the 'developing' world: this was, for example, the critical insight which led Oxfam, the UK-based development aid non-governmental organization, to develop an anti-poverty programme within the UK, in parallel with its extensive work in other countries, and which has informed the cross-country comparative thinking within organizations such as Save the Children. The need for these connections is increasingly reflected in practice and the evidence drawn on here correspondingly comes from a very wide range of contexts from both the 'North' and the 'South'.

THE RELEVANCE OF SOCIAL RESEARCH

Social research has offered considerable methodological and ethical insights into working with children; it also demonstrates that there are few policy areas now where research has not sought their views. Social research and community development share common values, in particular the importance of listening carefully to what people have to say, the need to synthesize and analyse a range of data (both qualitative and quantitative) and the overriding importance of respect for the views of those with whom the professional is working. Research is, however, not the same thing as community development, although it is not uncommon that community development workers find that they need to draw on research findings to inform their activities. It is, in part, the process of moving across the threshold from research into action alongside individuals and community groups that differentiates the community development worker from the researcher. This raises further important issues about the capacity of children to be the subjects of community development work, not least because initiatives arising from community development work take these subjects into the world of political and social action, a world largely controlled and shaped by adults. The crucial question for those concerned with community development with children is, therefore, to what extent can groups of children, defined geographically or on the basis of some common interest, organize to change their world?

REVIEWING THE LITERATURE

Given the relatively recent development of a general awareness of children's rights, and the growing understanding of the need to offer children means to having a voice of their own, it is not surprising to find that the literature on community development with children is itself relatively recent and relatively sparse – although growing rapidly – much of it in the form not of books or

journal articles, but published in 'grey' sources such as magazines, house journals and monographs. In reading this literature, as suggested above, a clear
interpretation of the use of language remains crucial to understanding what is
happening: the boundaries between manipulation, consulting young people
(Kealy 1993) and full-blown community development with children are often
ill-defined, even within given cultural circumstances.

Although the following accounts demonstrate the encouragingly wide range
of actions in which children and young people have been helped to promote
their own interests in policy development, it is important to remember that
this work operates against a context of many structural inhibitors to effective
child or young person participation, such as dominant rural and urban planning
trends, or generalist community approaches that do not recognize the need for
children to have a separate voice.

General political and social arguments in favour of the participation of children and young people, particularly within a 'Northern' context, are explored
in Lansdown (1995), Goodman (1997), Treseder (1997), Wellard *et al.* (1997)
and New Economics Foundation (1998). Most of these also provide a range
of case studies, including pictures of a variety of structures and mechanisms
developed at local levels. Willow (1997) classifies initiatives into six approaches:
corporate strategies to promote participation, permanent structures and mechanisms, long-term projects, time-limited projects, national initiatives and European developments.

It is perhaps hardly surprising that the main focus of accounts of policy
development work with children within the UK and other 'Northern' countries is in relation to regeneration; such work is frequently associated with
policy issues, such as the environment, play and leisure with which children
can apparently engage more easily. Henderson (1995) provides several detailed
examples, organized into policy themes (such as environment, education,
care and protection, and the neighbourhood), describing case studies such as
work with children over traffic-calming measures, planning play provision
and the involvement of children in neighbourhood action. French experience
is cited where local children's councils have become an accepted part of civic
life in more than 700 towns. Willow (1997) reviews both the experience
of French children's councils and German children's parliaments. Reviews
of regeneration work are also provided by: Fitzpatrick *et al.* (1998), who
note that the intensity of support required for working with children is much
greater than that required for working with adults; Save the Children (1998),
which aimed to involve young people and children aged 9–25 years in forming
mechanisms for their inclusion in the seven-year regeneration programme in
Leeds; and Robinson (1997) in a review of Salford's regeneration strategy,
premised on the involvement of local communities, including children and
young people. Cannan and Warren (1997), covering experience in France,
Germany and the UK, unusually include case studies of the ways in which it
is possible to integrate both a child protection and a community development approach to working with children, providing illustrations of work
such as involvement in a Festival on the Rights of the Child and attempts

to encourage the participation of children within long-term neighbourhood work.

Adams and Ingham (1998) provide accounts of children's involvement in wider environmental issues and programmes, drawing on a range of local projects. These include case studies under six major headings: Local Agenda 21 groups; research; local plans; urban regeneration; art, design and the environment; and school grounds (see also Davis and Jones 1996 on play provision; and Nieuwenhuys 1997 on Dutch experience in relation to the built environment). Hart *et al.* (1997) provide a comprehensive review of experience of children's participation in environmental issues, drawing largely on experience from 'Southern' settings, such as Ecuador, Brazil, Nicaragua and the Philippines. The scope of 'the environment' and planning is widely defined, covering such issues as conservation, monitoring of school grounds, the conditions of working children and health hazards. Hart *et al.* (1997), defining childhood up to the age of 14 years, attempt to identify ways in which the experience they report could be used within differing cultures. The focus on environmental issues arises because, as they note, 'people's relationship to nature is the greatest issue facing the world at the turn of the century . . . [and] . . . the planning, design, monitoring and management of the physical environment is an ideal domain for the practice of children's participation; it seems to be clearer for children to see and understand than many social problems' (p. 3). This is perhaps the case because children can approach the environment in an holistic fashion, not subject to departmental or functional boundaries. In incorporating a community development approach to working with children on environmental issues, the authors challenge the increasingly discredited idea that development is essentially about growth (Korten 1990), arguing that an appropriate response to the over-exploitation of the world's resources requires a strategy that links the local to the global, an approach to which children can contribute strongly.

Pearce (1998) reviews the experience of involving children in the life of museums, especially from the USA. He demonstrates that by involving young people and older children as volunteers and through consultative exercises, 'the target age-groups of a children's museum could acquire both the right to influence and the means of influencing the organisation and the governance of the institution' (p. 115).

A growing body of writing nevertheless reports the involvement of children and young people in more 'difficult' policy areas, or with more 'hard-to-reach' groups. These reports include: work on health (de Groot 1996), which provides examples such as young people's health forums, in large housing estates and small markets towns, and working with young people with learning disabilities; anti-poverty work (Wilkinson 2000), which reviews ways in which children and young people have been involved in the development of strategic anti-poverty initiatives; residential care (Ward 1995), evaluating the development of regular community meetings within a residential care home; and housing and homelessness among 'at risk' American children and young people (Good 1992). A study of community safety in France and England

(Pearce 1995), exploring the link between bullying within schools and violence outside it, shows the value of comparative study. Students from East London, visiting French counterparts, came to appreciate the ways in which older youths took responsibility, including managing a school radio station, becoming involved in school management tasks and school–community relations. The English students developed in their own school ideas for working with local immigrant communities, a school safety committee and a mentoring scheme.

Work with the most excluded street children is described by West (1997), who analysed participatory research undertaken by street children in Bangladesh to establish a policy framework for change. Other examples of work with profoundly deprived children include Dallape and Gilbert's (1994) study of street children in Kenya and a similar study by Munene and Nambi (1996) in Uganda. Ennew (1994) includes short case studies of the Metro Manila Street Children's Conference in the Philippines, children's responses to a research project in India, campaigning around health issues near a waste tip in Peru and an investigation by children (with the help of adults) into the deaths of working children in India.

Another more sensitive policy area in which children and young people have effectively been engaged is race relations. For example, Treppte (1993) describes a community developmental approach to working with Turkish mothers and children in a German town. Similar community-focused approaches to pre-school children have been reported from the Netherlands (Kieneker and Maas 1997) and, drawing on the example of the *Head Start* programme of the US 1960s War on Poverty, from Ireland (Kellaghan and Greaney 1993). In the field of disability, Children in Scotland (1998) describe work to promote the involvement of children with special needs in Scotland. Russell (1998) and Beecher (1998) have analysed the work of the Council for Disabled Children and other agencies promoting the views of disabled children, including minority ethnic disabled children; McIvor (1995) provides examples of ways in which disabled Moroccan children have been encouraged to challenge their dependent status and others' oppressive perceptions of them.

A UNESCO-funded study (MOST, undated) includes accounts of work in eight countries, including Argentina and India, covering such disparate activities as dialoguing with local government representatives, planning resettlement from squatter camps, the creation of a young person's radio station and the use of modelling techniques as a way of designing safe play environments involving children as young as 3–4 years (see also Miller 1997). Johnson *et al.* (1998) review case study material from many countries, including instances of children faced with crisis, war or exploitation, within a number of settings (including school, the labour market, public services, the neighbourhood and in cultural activities). Save the Children (1995) provides brief accounts of children's participation, including an example of education and organization by village health workers who are children themselves, a children's parliament in India and children's involvement in participatory research in Kampuchea.

LESSONS FROM THE LITERATURE

Defining the characteristics of effective policy development work with children is an urgent political task. Although there is, on the one hand, growing concern about the ways of involving children and young people as a prelude to effective citizenship, increasingly young people have been driven further from participating in the life of their societies both indirectly and directly by the impact of government policy, not least in the UK (Craig 1991; Coles and Craig 1999); in many countries, children are predominantly seen only as units of labour. The literature reviewed briefly above suggests that there are few policy arenas, contexts or approaches where the involvement of children and young people in decision making is not possible or appropriate. This review encompasses work with children in war zones, with children who are profoundly disabled and with those whose entire life has been spent on the streets, disengaged from any of the normal trappings of citizenship. The scope of this work and the literature will doubtless continue to develop. Similarly, the techniques for engaging with children and young people, incorporating a range of innovative means of promoting such work – for example, the use of video and film, drama, narrative, fictionalized accounts and tape and, for very young children, through play – will expand.

This review of the literature draws on others' accounts of work, accounts which may be partial or limited and which might not have been written with wider evaluative goals in mind. It is, therefore, inappropriate to attempt to evaluate the range of work described here in detail. From these accounts, more general accounts of community development, analyses of the boundaries of childhood and the increasingly wide literature on the evaluation of qualitative social policy and community development interventions (Feuerstein 1986; Craig 1988; Harding 1991; Breitenbach and Erskine 1994; Barr et al. 1995, 1996a,b; Carley 1995; McKendrick et al. 1996; Connell and Kubisch 1998; Sanderson et al. 1998; Alcock et al. 1999), it is nonetheless possible both to draw out some general lessons from the literature and to provide a framework against which future policy development work with children might be assessed.

The literature suggests that it is possible for children and young people to have an effect on the policy process. Bringing young people together and supporting them with adequate resources has enabled their views to be elicited on policies and services, which have been adapted to suit their needs better. Children can be helped to become organized, to undertake research and to collate findings to present to policy actors. The literature reports many different types of structures, some of them developed specifically by children and young people themselves, through which this process of policy influence has been conducted. However, much work remains to be done.

FUTURE RESEARCH AGENDAS

An area worthy of exploration is the nature of the relationship between programmes that are developed for all members of a community and those developed specifically for children and young people. As with the marginalization of black and minority ethnic groups in, for example, regeneration programmes (Alcock *et al.* 1998) or within voluntary sector development work (Craig *et al.* 1999), there remains a real danger that children's interests may be marginalized within general community programmes. We still know relatively little about involving children effectively within community life, but the evidence reviewed above and from the general community work literature suggests it is better to explore this separately from work with adults.

Future work should also explore the appropriate balance between seeing the child as a person with needs and a person with rights. At present, and driven by the language and practice of the UK Children Acts and similar legislation elsewhere, there tends to be an overemphasis on children's needs – for protection and care – rather than seeing them as political actors, with a desire to become involved in discussions that affect them. The evidence suggests that, despite several barriers – cultural, political, attitudinal and resource barriers – the democratic participation of children and young people can function well, albeit still largely within paradigms shaped by adult expectations. Such participation needs to be linked to the overall context in which the child lives; otherwise it cannot succeed. Most children and young people do not feel constrained by the increasing 'compartmentalism' of policy and ideas with which adults are familiar. This participation needs to be seen not only as an end but also as a means, of helping children and young people explore ways in which they can most effectively express their ideas and needs. The task for those working with children and young people is a particularly difficult one, since it requires them effectively to empower children in ways that may be challenging to adult ideas and power, and to take social and political risks in a context of physical and emotional safety.

A MODEL OF BEST PRACTICE

Exploring the characteristics of effective community development work with children connects this discussion to the wider discussion of the evaluation of policy interventions. Again, it is not possible to review these debates in depth here (but see Alcock *et al.* 1999; Craig 2000). Although the language and practice of evaluation has developed considerably in the past 15 years in particular, and has challenged the dominant obsession of quantitative 'value-for-money' approaches of governments as largely irrelevant to the complex, multisectoral and qualitative approaches characteristic of community development, very little of this evaluative practice has yet found its way into the arena of work with children. A review of the evaluation literature (Craig 2000) highlights a number of key elements as the most important building blocks for the evaluation of community development. These building blocks could, in general, equally be applied in relation to community development work with children. The key elements are:

- the importance of *qualitative* indicators, used in a way that complements quantitative ones;
- the need to observe *process* goals as well as output and outcome goals;
- the stress on *participation* (which is not tokenistic) in all stages of programmes; and
- the importance of *sustainability* in thinking about empowerment.

To this list of basic criteria should be added a particular concern in relation to work with children: that it should attempt to meet the competing goals of being, on the one hand, *age-appropriate* (a consideration that runs the risk of being shaped entirely by adult views of what is appropriate, particularly given the continuing emphasis on child protection work) and, perhaps contradictorily, *liberating* rather than controlling. It is, incidentally, an important research task to determine whether the criteria developed by children match this, unavoidably, very adult formulation.

It was shown above that there are inevitable contradictions and tensions in working with children within what is essentially an adult-driven framework. These tensions are apparent when assessing the extent of participation. For example, Arnstein's (1969) famous ladder of participation has been adapted by others to apply specifically to the issue of participation by children. Wellard *et al.* (1997), drawing on Hart (1992), suggest that the eight rungs might be: manipulation, decoration, tokenism, assigned but informed, consulted and informed, adult initiated, child/young person initiated, and equal partnership. The highest level of participation in their view is where 'children and young people come up with the ideas for a project, they set it up and then involve adults as equal partners in taking decisions and implementing them' (p. 10). This view, however, still incorporates an understanding of children as inevitably dependent to some extent on the participation of adults in their lives. This tension is also apparent when involving children in evaluation where the goals of evaluation are not shaped by children themselves.

A long time-scale will be required to see through effective evaluations of human service programmes, in particular long-term interventions such as community development work, which should work at a pace determined by the capacity and the needs of those who are the intended beneficiaries of the programme. Unfortunately, it remains the case that most public policy interventions funding community development still expect it to produce results within a relatively short time, 'results' that are frequently in the form of relatively meaningless quantitative outputs rather than qualitative long-term outcomes. Where the subjects of community development work are children, long time-scales may be even more important.

The issue of sustainability is also critical to all community development work, to ensure that the mode of work encourages local communities to take control of initiatives as community development resources are withdrawn. The definition of empowerment outlined earlier involves the creation of structures, processes and mechanisms contributing to the goals of community development work with children beyond the initial impetus that helped establish them. Given the domination of most structures by adults, it is hardly surprising that the evaluation of community development work with children has to be seen as a long-term process (perhaps ending only as children cease being children). In this vein, Ennew (1994) suggests that evaluation should be an integral part of project work, a process of continuous learning in which the range of evaluative questions asked in work with children might be open to frequent review and revision. One tension apparent here is that children's interests change as they grow up through 'youth-hood' into adulthood and that time-scales in work with children may sometimes have to be limited. There are also tensions derived from particular cultural contexts, for example in social development work in the 'South', where the drive for participation may be overridden by the imperatives of meeting basic needs, such as ensuring the supply of adequate drinking water or food.

Those promoting the development of policy with children and young people, and its evaluation, also have to accept that the outcome of such work may not only be that the aims or methods of certain interventions are challenged, but that the challenge extends also to the organizational context within which such interventions are made: local input to evaluation may have knock-on effects in terms of local power structures. Put most simply, effective work with children may challenge the power of adults.

Notwithstanding the relative lack of proper evaluation in most cases, there is an enormous potential for consulting and encouraging the participation of children and the potential benefits that it can bring, not least of all in ensuring that children become active and participating citizens as they grow into adulthood. Children cannot, and in general should not, be treated as 'little adults': their intellectual and emotional sophistication and understanding of the adult world is limited by the very fact that they are partly or even largely dependent on others for the maintenance of their lives. Adults, however, have often been guilty of over-exaggerating the extent of that dependence, particularly perhaps in relation to children's ability to think critically.

Many of the lessons – and techniques – of research and community development are relevant, when used appropriately and sensitively, in working with children and the role of adults should be to liberate their abilities and creativity, within a negotiated framework of rights and responsibilities. The boundary of this framework will continue to be a subject of discussion and a source of tension, not least between children and young people and adults themselves, and the power of adults and the boundary between childhood and adulthood will continue to be tested through this process. Adults cannot, of course, absolve themselves from their legal and other responsibilities for the overall direction of children's lives and community development with children will always have to be seen within this overarching framework of responsibility. Similarly, governments need to ensure that their frameworks for legislation and policy do not, directly or indirectly, create obstacles to involving children and young people in important policy arenas. Despite all these caveats, there is much more that can be done to encourage children to take control of important aspects of their lives or of policies affecting them.

The benefits of this will be seen in their increasing engagement as they grow to adulthood.

CONCLUSIONS: WHAT WORKS AND WHAT IS THERE STILL TO LEARN IN COMMUNITY DEVELOPMENT WITH CHILDREN?

What works, then, in community development with children? The literature referred to in this chapter is, perhaps, surprisingly large and illustrates a growing range of work to engage the participation of children and young people in a very wide spectrum of settings and from many different cultural contexts. The sophistication with which the effectiveness of this work is evaluated remains, however, relatively crude.

The complex social, political and legal context for work with children has been developing rapidly in the past few years and, taken together with the relatively recent emergence of theoretical and political challenges to dominant evaluative currents, it would perhaps have been more surprising if there had been a strong body of evaluative outcomes. This clearly remains a major task for the next few years. Much of the literature exhorts the reader to accept that community development work with children is a 'good thing': politically, socially, educationally and developmentally. However, this is not enough. It has to be seen to work, to bring the benefits for children claimed of it and to do so as a result of the interventions described. We can also observe that the more general literature on community development generally fails to address the issue of its impacts on children. A review of the community development literature, both radical and more pluralistic, suggests that the relationship between community work in general and the lives of children is under-represented. Although it is reasonable to assume that a healthy community will be of advantage to the child, it has not been considered important to make this explicit or, with a few exceptions, to explain the relationship in depth. This task remains for those writing about community development.

At present, therefore, we cannot be sure of what works, except in a relatively few instances, although there is fairly convincing evidence from across the world that direct engagement with children in a community development context is possible and brings benefits to them. The extent to which those benefits can be attributed directly to the nature of that engagement remains to be tested in most cases. The evaluative literature, however, now provides more than adequate tools to make progress on this front. The literature on work with children also now provides a wide range of examples to test approaches in different contexts. More work also needs to be done in exploring more fully the boundaries of childhood and the appropriateness of differing interventions to work with children or young people of differing ages in these various cultural contexts. This is an area where research *with* children (as opposed to research *on* children) has offered and can continue to offer much. Some of the interventions described have in fact attempted to engage with children through a variety of methods: one useful further advance would be for the value of these different approaches to be assessed separately.

In facilitating this developing understanding, what might be encouraged is the development of more good-quality, critical but accessible literature. Until recently, the choice for those searching the literature had been between formal texts that had to meet certain perceived publishing standards (and, therefore, became increasingly inaccessible to a mass audience) or the 'grey literature' of project reports and monographs, much of which has never formally been published and has been difficult to access. Virtually all of this literature, of course, is more or less totally inaccessible (for reasons of cost or style) to the subjects of the writing, the children themselves. It is an important task for the future to engage children and young people in the process of disseminating the findings of their own work, using a variety of age-appropriate means. Most of all, it is important to build effective evaluative work into the growing body of direct work with children and young people, work that seeks the views of the subjects themselves as to 'what works'.

REFERENCES

Adams, E. and Ingham, S. (1998) *Changing Places: Children's Participation in Environmental Planning*. London: Children's Society/Planning Aid.

Alcock, P., Craig, G., Lawless, P., Pearson, S. and Robinson, D. (1998) *Inclusive Regeneration*. London: Department of Environment, Transport and the Regions.

Alcock, P., Barnes, C., Craig, G., Harvey, A. and Pearson, S. (1999) *What Counts, What Works?* London: Improvement and Development Agency.

Alexander, E. (1992) *From Store Cupboard to Family Room: How Parents Pushed Open the Doors of a Scottish Nursery School*. The Hague: Bernard van Leer Foundation.

Arnstein, S. (1969) A ladder of citizen participation, *Journal of the American Institute of Planners*, 35(4): 216–24.

Barr, A., Drysdale, J., Purcell, R. and Ross, C. (1995) *Strong Communities: Effective Government. The Role of Community Work*, Vol. 1. Glasgow: Scottish Community Development Centre.

Barr, A., Hashagen, S. and Purcell, R. (1996a) *Measuring Community Development in Northern Ireland: A Handbook for Practitioners*. Glasgow: Scottish Community Development Centre.

Barr, A., Hashagen, S. and Purcell, R. (1996b) *Monitoring and Evaluation of Community Development in Northern Ireland*. Glasgow: Scottish Community Development Centre.

Beecher, W. (1998) *Having a Say! Disabled Children and Effective Partnership in Decision-making, Section II: Practice Initiatives and Selected Annotated References*. London: Council for Disabled Children.

Bell, C. and Newby, H. (1971) *Community Studies*. London: George Allen & Unwin.

Breitenbach, E. and Erskine, A. (1994) *Partnership in Pilton*. Glasgow: University of Glasgow.

Cannan, C. and Warren, C. (eds) (1997) *Social Action with Children and Families: A Community Development Approach to Child and Family Welfare*. London: Routledge.

Carley, M. (1995) *A Community Participation Strategy in Urban Regeneration*. Edinburgh: Scottish Homes.

Children in Scotland (1998) *Onwards and Upwards: Enabling the Participation of Children with Special Needs*. Edinburgh: Children in Scotland.

Coles, R. and Craig, G. (1999) Young people and the growth of begging, in H. Dean (ed.) *Begging in the UK*. Bristol: Policy Press.

Community Development Journal (1998) Managing communities in conflict, *Community Development Journal*, 33(2) (special issue).

Community Development Project (1977) *Gilding the Ghetto*. London: Community Development Project Information and Intelligence Unit.

Community Development Project (1978) *The Costs of Industrial Change*. London: Community Development Project Information and Intelligence Unit.

Connell, J. and Kubisch, A. (eds) (1998) *Evaluating Comprehensive Community Initiatives*. Washington, DC: Aspen Institute.

Craig, G. (1988) Community work and the state, *Community Development Journal*, 24(1): 3–18.

Craig, G. (1989) *Questions of Value*. London: Law Centres Federation.

Craig, G. (1991) *Fit for Nothing?* London: Children's Society.

Craig, G. (1998) Community development in a global context, *Community Development Journal*, 33(1): 2–17.

Craig, G. (2000) *What Works? Community Development with Children*. Ilford: Barnardo's.

Craig, G. and Mayo, M. (1995) *Community Empowerment: A Reader in Participation and Development*. London: Zed Books.

Craig, G., Szanto, C., Taylor, M. and Wilkinson, M. (1999) *Developing Local Compacts*. York: Joseph Rowntree Foundation/York Publishing Services.

Croft, S. and Beresford, P. (1993) *Getting Involved*. London: Open Services Project.

Dallape, F. and Gilbert, C. (1994) *Children's Participation in Action-research*. Harare, Zimbabwe: ENDA.

Davis, A. and Jones, L. (1996) The children's enclosure, *Town and Country Planning*, September, pp. 233–5.

de Groot, R. (1996) Today and tomorrow, giving young people a voice, *Community Health Action*, 38: 12–15.

Ennew, J. (1994) *Street and Working Children: A Guide to Planning*, Development Manual 4. London: Save the Children.

Feuerstein, M.-T. (1986) *Partners in Evaluation: Evaluating Development and Community Programmes with Participants*. London: Macmillan/TALC.

Fitzpatrick, S., Hastings, A. and Kintrea, K. (1998) *Including Young People in Regeneration: A Lot to Learn?* Bristol: Policy Press.

Flynn, P., Johnson, C., Liberman, S. and Armstrong, H. (1986) *You're Learning all the Time: Women, Education and Community Work*. Nottingham: Spokesman.

Frazer, E. (1998) Community politics, *Citizen*, summer, pp. 8–9.

Gaffikin, F. and Morrissey, M. (1994) *Brownlow Community Trust Evaluation Report: Europe's Third Poverty Programme in Northern Ireland (1989–1994)*. Brownlow: Brownlow Community Trust.

Geddes, M. (1997) *Partnership Against Poverty and Exclusion*. Bristol: Policy Press.

Good, A.L. (1992) Alternatives for girls: a community development model for homeless and high-risk girls and young women, *Children and Youth Services Review*, 14: 237–52.

Goodman, H. (1997) *Encouraging Child and Youth Participation in Community Development*, Unpublished report to the Calouste Gulbenkian Foundation, London.

Harding, P. (1991) Qualitative indicators and the project framework, *Community Development Journal*, 26(4): 294–305 (special issue on Evaluation of Social Development Projects).

Hart, R. (1992) *Children's Participation: From Tokenism to Citizenship*, Innocenti Essays No. 4. Florence: UNICEF.

Hart, R. with Espinosa, M.F., Iltus, S. and Lorenzo, R. (1997) *Children's Participation: The Theory and Practice of Involving Young Citizens in Community Development and Environmental Care*. New York and London: UNICEF/Earthscan.

Henderson, P. (ed.) (1995) *Children and Communities*. London: Pluto Press/Community Development Foundation.

Henderson, P. (1997) Community development and children, in C. Cannan and C. Warren (eds) *Social Action with Children and Families: A Community Development Approach to Child and Family Welfare*. London: Routledge.

Henderson, P. (1999) Community work with children, in M. Hill (ed.) *Effective Ways of Working with Children and Their Families*. London: Jessica Kingsley.

Hillery, G. (1955) Definitions of community: areas of agreement, *Rural Sociology*, 20.

Hoggett, P. (ed.) (1997) *Contested Communities: Experiences, Struggles, Policies*. Bristol: Policy Press.

Jacobs, S. and Popple, K. (eds) (1994) *Community Work in the 1990s*. Nottingham: Spokesman.

Johnson, V., Ivan-Smith, E., Gordon, G., Pridmore, P. and Scott, P. with Ennew, J. and Chambers, R. (1998) *Stepping Forward: Children and Young People's Participation in the Development Process*. London: Intermediate Technology.

Jones, J. (1999) *Private Pain and Public Issues: A Community Development Approach to Health*. Edinburgh: Community Learning Scotland.

Kealy, L. (1993) *Consulting with Young People on Sealand Manor, Clywd*. Caerphilly: Wales Youth Agency and Wales Youth Forum.

Kellaghan, T. and Greaney, B.J. (1993) *The Educational Development of Students Following Participation in a Pre-school Programme in a Disadvantaged Area in Ireland*. The Hague: Bernard van Leer Foundation.

Kieneker, N. and Maas, J. (1997) *Samenspel – Mothers Speaking*. The Hague: Bernard van Leer Foundation.

Korten, D. (1990) *Getting to the 21st Century: Voluntary Action and the Global Agenda*. West Hartford, CT: Kumarian Press.

Lansdown, G. (1995) *Taking Part: Children's Participation in Decision-making*. London: Institute of Public Policy Research.

McIvor, C. (1995) Children and disability: rights and participation, in Save the Children (ed.) *In Our Own Words: Disability and Integration in Morocco*. London: Save the Children.

McKendrick, J., Lawson, N. and Robson, B. (1996) *Barnardo's Anti-Poverty Strategy: A Framework for Evaluation*. Manchester: University of Manchester.

Miller, C. and Ahmad, Y. (1997) Community development at the cross-roads: a way forward, *Policy and Politics*, 25(3): 269–84.

Miller, J. (1997) *Never Too Young: How Young Children Can Take Responsibility and Make Decisions*. London: National Early Years Network/Save the Children.

MOST (undated) *Growing Up in Cities: A Project to Involve Young People in Evaluating and Improving Their Urban Environments*, Project summary available from Barry Percy-Smith, Centre for Children and Youth, Nene College of Higher Education, Northampton.

Munene, J.C. and Nambi, J. (1996) Understanding and helping street children in Uganda, *Community Development Journal*, 31(4): 343–50.

New Economics Foundation (1998) *Participation Works! 21 Techniques of Community Participation for the 21st Century*. London: New Economics Foundation.

Nieuwenhuys, O. (1997) Spaces for children of the urban poor: experiences with participatory action-research, *Environment and Urbanisation*, 9(1): 233–49.

Pearce, J. (1995) French lessons: young people, comparative research and community safety, *Social Work in Europe*, 3(1): 32–6.

Pearce, J. (1998) *Centres for Curiosity and Imagination: When is a Museum not a Museum?* London: Calouste Gulbenkian Foundation.

Popple, K. (1995) *Analysing Community Work: Its Theory and Practice*. Buckingham: Open University Press.

Robinson, A. (1997) Can do on consultation, *Youth Action*, 60 (spring): 18–19.

Russell, P. (1998) *Having a Say! Disabled Children and Effective Partnership in Decision-making*, Section I: *The Report*. London: Council for Disabled Children.

Sanderson, I., Bovaird, T., Davis, P., Martin, S. and Foreman, A. (1998) *Made to Measure: Evaluation in Practice in Local Government*. London: Local Government Management Board.

Save the Children (1995) *Towards a Children's Agenda: New Challenges for Social Development*. London: Save the Children.

Save the Children (1998) *Leeds Single Regeneration Budget*, Phase 3. Leeds: Save the Children.

Sayer, J. (1986) Ideology: the bridge between theory and practice, *Community Development Journal*, 21(4): 294–303.

Social Exclusion Unit (1998) *Bringing Britain Together: A National Strategy for Neighbourhood Renewal*. London: Social Exclusion Unit, Cabinet Office.

Stacey, M. (1969) The myth of community studies, *British Journal of Sociology*, 20(2): 134–47.

Thomas, D. (1983) *The Making of Community Work*. London: George Allen & Unwin.

Thomas, D. (1995) *Community Development at Work: A Case of Obscurity in Accomplishment*. London: Community Development Foundation.

Traynor, T., Smith, K. and Hughes, M. (1998) *Still Challenging Disadvantage: First Report on the Evaluation of Barnardo's Anti-Poverty Strategy*. Ilford: Barnardo's.

Treppte, C. (1993) *Multicultural Approaches in Education: A German Experience*. The Hague: Bernard van Leer Foundation.

Treseder, P. (1997) *Empowering Children and Young People*. London: Children's Rights Office/Save the Children.

United Nations Development Project (1993) *Human Development Report*. Oxford: Oxford University Press.

Ward, A. (1995) Establishing community meetings in a children's home, *Groupwork*, 8(1): 67–78.

Wellard, S., Tearse, M. and West, A. (1997) *All Together Now: Community Participation for Children and Young People*. London: Save the Children.

West, A. (1997) *A Street Children's Research Project*. Dhaka, Bangladesh: Save the Children.

Wilkinson, M. (2000) *Involving Young People in Action Against Poverty: The Work of YAPP*. London: The Children's Society.

Willow, C. (1997) *Hear! Hear! Promoting Children's and Young People's Democratic Participation in Local Government*. London: Local Government Information Unit.

World Commission on Environment and Development (1987) *Our Common Future*. New York: World Commission on Environment and Development/Oxford University Press.

6   **ALAN DYSON**

Inclusive education

KEY MESSAGES

- Inclusive education depends on ensuring that every part of the education system is aligned with inclusive values – that is, values to do with ensuring that *all* children are educated in ways that are equitable and ensure their full participation in learning.
- Different bodies of research, reaching somewhat different conclusions, have considered the question of what makes an inclusive school. However, it is likely that such a school needs to be able *both* to employ proven strategies at the group level for students whose difficulties are related to their social and economic disadvantage *and* to problem-solve ways of meeting the needs of individuals who cannot have their needs met through such strategies.
- An inclusive pedagogy is almost certainly one that is built on principles that see the learner as an active constructor of knowledge. However, such a pedagogy can also draw on techniques through which the teacher intervenes vigorously with students who might learn little if left purely to their own devices.
- Schools can only become inclusive within the context of an inclusive education system. Such a system has to have structures (in the form of a legislative framework, curriculum and assessment and funding mechanisms) that are themselves

inclusive and has to deliver support to schools in developing their own inclusive approaches.

- The education system itself has to play a part in developing a more 'inclusive' society. This means that it has to make some specific contribution and that the work of every level of the system, including schools, has to be shaped around this contribution.

INTRODUCTION

Our current state of knowledge about maintaining students with significant special educational needs in mainstream schools arises from more than 30 years of experience of what happens when such students are placed alongside their peers rather than in the special schools that have historically been regarded as the only possible setting in which they can be educated. This evidence was admirably summarized for the Barnardo's 'what works' series by Sebba and Sachdev (1997).

Debates about the pros and cons of 'inclusion' in this sense continue to rage; see, for instance, Hornby (1999) in the UK and Kauffman and Hallahan (1995) in the USA. Moreover, there is a series of problems that need to be addressed wherever more inclusive provision is attempted: how and where to educate students whose behaviour challenges their teachers and schools; how to deliver therapies and other non-educational services most efficiently when students are 'scattered' throughout mainstream schools; whether to opt for 'neighbourhood school' or 'resource base' models of inclusion; and how to respond to parental preferences for non-inclusive provision. These difficulties should not be minimized. However, as Sebba and Sachdev's (1997) overview demonstrates, although we do not have answers to all of the problems of inclusion, we do have very considerable knowledge of much of 'what works'. Moreover, reviews of the evidence over many years appear to indicate that, given reasonable 'good practice', students with special educational needs *tend* to do no worse in inclusive settings and might do somewhat better than they did in their special schools (Galloway and Goodwin 1987; Hegarty 1993; Lipsky and Gartner 1997; Crowther *et al.* 1998).

In one sense, therefore, there is no urgent need for yet another review of the evidence. However, this only holds good if we see the field of inclusive education as unchanging and as no more than a continuation under another label of the integration movement of the 1970s and 1980s. In fact, inclusion is a notoriously slippery concept (Booth 1995) and, although this can sometimes be frustrating for commentators and practitioners alike, it also tends to make it extremely dynamic, constantly developing in the light of new thinking, new policies and new contexts. In this chapter, therefore, I set out to address a series of questions that reflect the current context:

- How has thinking about inclusion changed in recent years and what could we now use as a good definition of 'inclusive education'?
- What are the implications of this definition for the nature of 'inclusive schools'? In particular, what characteristics of these schools enable them to respond to the needs of widely differing groups of marginalized students?
- What sort of pedagogy facilitates the participation of all students in shared learning experiences while at the same time maximizing their attainments?
- What are the characteristics of education systems that enable them to develop and maintain inclusive schools?
- What contribution does an inclusive education system make to an 'inclusive society'?

DEVELOPMENTS IN THINKING ABOUT INCLUSIVE EDUCATION

It is probably true to say that the origins of the inclusive education movement (in so far as it constitutes a coherent 'movement') lie in the progressive extension of the integration agenda during the 1980s and, in particular, in the case made in the USA for a complete 'merger' of special and mainstream education (Gartner and Lipsky 1987, 1989). Since then, thinking has developed in three ways:

First, there has been a marked politicization of the issue of disability (Oliver 1990), which has led to separate special education coming to be seen in some quarters as part of the systematic oppression (Abberley 1987) of disabled people. As a result, inclusive education for disabled children is not so much a matter of effectiveness, efficiency or professional judgement, but rather a matter of civil and human rights (see, for instance, CSIE, undated).

Second, the concept of inclusion has, by some commentators at least, been broadened so that it extends beyond a concern simply with the *presence* of students with a disability or special needs label in mainstream schools. Instead, the focus in more recent thinking has been on *participation* rather than presence and on *all* students rather than those with particular labels [see, for instance, UNESCO's (1994) seminal Salamanca Statement and the more recent 'Index for Inclusion' issued to all schools with DfEE support (Booth *et al.* 2000)].

Third, the 'New' Labour government from 1997 onwards have promoted an alignment of the concept of inclusive education with the wider concept of 'social' inclusion. David Blunkett, Secretary of State for Education from 1997 to 2001, argued (Blunkett 1999a,b, 2000) that high educational attainment is the pathway to full 'inclusion' in society – particularly through successful participation in the labour market – and that schools are needed, therefore, which are 'inclusive' in the sense of maximizing the attainments of groups who have traditionally done badly in the education system. These groups include, but are by no means restricted to, children with disabilities or special educational needs.

MAKING SENSE OF INCLUSION

There is no doubt that these competing 'discourses of inclusion' (Dyson 1999) bring with them considerable potential for confusion and misunderstanding. In particular, what seems to have happened is the bringing together under the label of 'inclusive education' of some very specific issues in the field of disability with some equally specific issues in the field of social and educational disadvantage, alongside some more general concerns to do with traditional 'liberal values' (Clark *et al.* 1997) of equity and participation. In turn, this means that the evidence-base that grew out of the integration movement in the 1970s and 1980s is no longer adequate to address this wide range of issues. Instead, finding out 'what works' in inclusive education now involves bringing together evidence from quite different fields that have not previously been related to each other in any systematic way.

The approach that I propose to adopt here is to agree with Tony Booth in arguing that inclusive education should be seen as part of the continuing attempt in England (and, to differing extents, in the UK as a whole) to develop comprehensive community education (Booth 1995, 1996). Such an attempt is predicated upon the broad 'liberal values' to which we alluded above, rather than on a particular set of organizational structures or pedagogical techniques. Inclusive education, therefore, is about seeking to develop schools and education systems in which all children can participate and which are able to educate all children in a way that is recognizably equitable. Inevitably, these broad values have to be worked out in terms of their detailed meanings for different groups of children in different contexts; those meanings may well vary significantly. Inevitably, too, different forms of inequity will come to prominence at different times. Not long ago, for instance, concerns about equity in access and placement were prominent; now it is concerns about equity in respect of attainment that dominate the agenda. The task that faces those who are committed to inclusive education, therefore – whether as practitioners, researchers, policy makers or advocates – is to bear with the fluid and dynamic nature of the field and to find ways of holding together the diverse principles, issues and practices out of which it is constituted.

INCLUSIVE SCHOOLS

By far the greatest volume of evidence we have is that which relates to the characteristics of 'inclusive schools'. It is important to exercise some caution here, for two reasons in particular. First, although it is common to think of schools as being unequivocally either inclusive or non-inclusive, the evidence suggests a far more complex pattern. Schools change over time; teachers within the same school have different values and practices; schools act across a broad range of areas and their actions are by no means always consistent with one another. At best, therefore, particular schools are more inclusive in some aspects of their practices at some times and less inclusive in other aspects at other times (Booth 1995; Skidmore 1999; Dyson and Millward 2000).

Second, although the evidence is great, much of it arises from studies of schools that are inclusive primarily in the sense that they educate students with special educational needs who might otherwise be placed in special schools. There is no certainty that schools that do well in this respect also do well in educating other groups of students or vice versa (Reynolds 1995; Lunt and Norwich 1999). Moreover, there must be some doubts about the robustness of the evidence that is available. By and large, it is derived from case studies of schools judged to be inclusive by pro-inclusion researchers, without any comparisons with other schools or any 'hard' measures of inclusivity (Dyson and Millward 2000). When schools are researched from a more sceptical position, the findings can be markedly different (see, for instance, Baker and Zigmond 1995).

Nonetheless, there is a broad consensus as to what the characteristics of an 'inclusive school' are. Lipsky and Gartner (1999: 17–18), for instance, argue that the evidence points to the following key features:

- *School-wide approaches*: 'The philosophy and practice of inclusive education is accepted by all stakeholders'.
- *All children can learn*: 'Inclusive schools have a belief that all children can learn and that all benefit when that learning is done together'.
- *A sense of community*.
- *Services based on need rather than category*: 'Each student is recognized as an individual, with strengths and needs, not as a label or as a member of a category'.
- *Natural proportions*: students with special needs attending their neighbourhood school and being distributed across regular classrooms.
- *Supports are provided in general education*.
- *Teacher collaboration*.
- *Curriculum adaptation*: 'Drawing from the school's general curriculum, inclusion provides adaptations to enable all students to benefit from the common curriculum'.
- *Enhanced instructional strategies*.
- *Standards and outcomes*: 'The learning outcome for students with disabilities is drawn from that expected of students in general'.

Essentially, this list comprises three basic characteristics: a set of inclusive values that are shared across the school; a set of specific policies and practices which realize these values; and a high level of teacher collaboration. This last characteristic is emphasized in particular (albeit in different ways) by writers such as Tom Skrtic (1991) and Mel Ainscow (1999), who believe that schools can only become inclusive if they see student diversity positively, as a challenge to reform existing practices and find new ways of responding to students' individual characteristics. Hence, Ainscow produces a list of school characteristics that is different from, although complementary to, that produced by Lipsky and Gartner. Schools that can successfully meet the challenge of inclusion, he argues, will be characterized by:

- **effective leadership**, not only by the headteacher but spread through-out the school;
- **involvement** of staff, students and community in school policies and decisions;
- a commitment to **collaborative planning**;
- attention to the potential benefits of **enquiry and reflection**; and
- a policy for **staff development** that focuses on classroom practice.

(Ainscow 1999: 124, emphases in original)

The rationale for this view of inclusive schools is that inclusion is not about the implementation of a set of particular structures or techniques. On the contrary, it is about teachers working together to solve the problems of practice that are generated by the need to respond to student diversity. It is the quality of these problem-solving processes – devolved leadership, collaboration, enquiry and reflection – rather than the presence of one or other form of organization or practice that makes schools inclusive.

However, although Ainscow in particular subscribes to the sort of extended notion of inclusive education we have adopted here, a somewhat different perspective on school characteristics has been adopted by American researchers studying schools serving poor urban areas. Typically, such schools have to deal with the interrelated impacts of poverty, racial oppression and cultural and linguistic diversity and so they, too, are inclusive in our sense. Writing recently on the evidence arising from America's 'Title 1' – effectively, a federal compensatory education programme – Robert Slavin (2001) argues that schools in such circumstances should embrace a whole-school reform programme. They should choose from a range of carefully evaluated models of proven effectiveness that could have an impact on:

all aspects of school functioning: instruction, curriculum, school organiza-tion, provision of supplementary services, family support, professional development, and so on ... [I]n choosing a program with evidence of effectiveness in schools such as theirs, school staffs can have confidence that if they implement the program as designed, they are likely to see the same kinds of gains produced in the evaluations. When well implemented, comprehensive programs unite school staffs around common goals, giving them a consistent, well-integrated approach to most aspects of school functioning.

(Slavin 2001: 241)

This is a very different model of the 'inclusive school' from that offered by Ainscow (1999), Skrtic (1991) and others working primarily from a special needs or disability perspective. It is much more concerned with raising attain-ment ('effectiveness' and 'gains') and with establishing a coherent approach through the implementation of a clearly specified 'program' rather than through collaborative problem-solving. To some extent, this simply reflects differences that have arisen within the overall school improvement field between models which are tightly specified and stress fidelity of implementation on the one hand, and those which are less tightly specified and stress the development of shared values and aims on the other (Reynolds *et al.* 2000). However, it may also reflect the different sorts of approach that are needed as schools seek to respond to different groups of students.

Put crudely, many students who are low-attainers or under-achievers and who live in adverse social circumstances bring with them resources that enable them to engage in only limited ways with school learning as traditionally understood. This is not, of course, to say that they do not bring other kinds of resources, but it does mean that they will learn school-related knowledge and skills more effectively where they are given maximum support to do so. Such support, as Slavin (2001) suggests, takes the form of consistent and coherent teaching approaches, the creation of a stable and purposeful learning environment in the school, the enlistment of family and community support for learning and intervention in students' out-of-school problems where necessary.

On the other hand, students with the sort of disabilities and other deep-seated difficulties that tend to form the basis of special educational needs may, in many cases, benefit from a different kind of approach. Although they can learn a great deal in the right circumstances, it may be unrealistic to expect that vigorous teaching approaches will be capable of overcoming their difficulties to any significant extent. The issue instead will be how to offer them the same learning opportunities as their non-disabled peers, how to give them 'access' in some meaningful way to the common curriculum and how to enable them to participate in social and learning activities with their peers. This will be much more a matter of taking careful account of their individual characteristics, providing individually appropriate 'supports' and making individually appropriate 'adaptations' to the environment, to the curriculum and to teaching methods. Hence, as Ainscow and others suggest, the importance of the *willingness* of the school to do this – its 'inclusive values' – and of the opportunities that are provided for staff to work together to 'problem-solve' their way towards the best approach in each individual case.

A truly 'inclusive' school has to be able to do both of these things – to apply well-founded and coherent strategies to the relatively large numbers of children who are at risk of exclusion because of their limited social resources and to respond creatively to individuals who do not fit neatly into these large-scale strategies and demand a more individualized response. Relatively little work has been done on identifying schools that undertake this dual and potentially contradictory task effectively. Some researchers claim to have attempted a synthesis of the available evidence from both of these fields (Lipsky and Gartner 1997; Wang *et al.* 1997; Mittler 2000; National Institute for Urban School Improvement, undated) although it can sometimes be difficult even here to determine whether evidence from both fields is weighted equally and where evidence ends and advocacy begins. Nonetheless, the general consensus appears to be that there is no inherent contradiction between inclusive approaches for children with disabilities and 'special educational needs' on the one hand and for children experiencing other forms of disadvantage and marginalization on the other. On the contrary, approaches that differentiate at a categorical level between children experiencing different forms of exclusion tend to reinforce that exclusion by limiting schools' capacity to respond to differences at an individual level and within the context of common entitlements. As Wang *et al.* put it, reviewing research on educational 'resilience':

> Educational environments that are responsive to human diversity treat differences among students as strengths that can be built upon or as needs that must be accommodated. Unresponsive and ineffective systems of delivery ignore individual differences or, even worse, treat student differences in a stigmatizing manner that reduces learning opportunities. Research on educational resilience stresses the importance of responding to children's differences, not as deficiencies, but as starting points for uniting the resources, talents, and efforts of families, teachers, schools, and communities in order to overcome adversity and promote learning success.
>
> (Wang *et al.* 1997: 11)

AN INCLUSIVE PEDAGOGY

This principle, of treating individual differences as positives rather than negatives, is one that commands consensus across a good deal of literature on inclusive education. As a general principle, it brings together a commitment to valuing diversity, a recognition of the rights of the child and a notion of educational entitlement and enrichment. It also leads us towards identifying the basis for an inclusive pedagogy. The 'talent development model', for instance, developed at the Center for the Education of Students Placed at Risk (CRESPAR) in the USA, is, as its name suggests, predicated on the assumption that even the most disadvantaged students have 'talent' which can be developed. It therefore emphasizes the claim that 'all students can learn in demanding high-expectation academic settings. This goal is reachable', CRESPAR argues, 'if schools are committed to implementing multiple, evidence-based activities to "overdetermine success", and if all relevant stakeholders are genuinely involved, supportive and held accountable' (Boykin 2000: 3).

At first, this sounds like a highly directive and highly interventionist approach. However, the talent development model also places emphasis on the resources that all children bring with them into school and, therefore, on approaches to teaching and learning that are best placed to capitalize on those resources:

> To be sure, all children must learn basic skills, yet there must also be a focus on the development of higher order and critical thinking skills, on

creative problem-solving skills, on critical analysis and self-reflection . . .
There must be more active academic task engagement. Students must
spend more time in classrooms actively engaged in writing, reading, and
acquiring numeracy skills, rather than in passively listening to teachers or
other students . . . The greater the amount of active task engagement, the
greater the learning outcomes . . . Rather than treating children as passive
receptacles for knowledge, where learning is conceived as a pouring in
and pouring out process, children must come to be active co-constructors
of their knowledge and skill base.

(Boykin 2000: 11–12)

It is at this point where inclusive thinking about disability and special needs
coincides with inclusive thinking about social and educational disadvantage.
Didactic views of teaching and learning – what Freire (1972) calls the 'banking'
concept of education – are predicated on the teacher 'depositing' knowledge in
students. Given that students are typically taught in large groups, this requires
that everyone in the group does more or less the same thing at the same time
and the same pace. Inevitably, therefore, groups have to be constructed around
notions of 'like-ability', which means that students who learn differently from
(perhaps more slowly than) their peers have to be placed in separate groups
or, indeed, in separate schools. This banking notion of education, therefore,
cannot be inclusive in any real sense.

The talent development model, however, explicitly commits itself to a view
of learning that starts with what students already know and encourages them
to play an active role in constructing their own knowledge (Poplin and Stone
1992). This 'constructivist' view places particular emphasis on the social nature
of learning (i.e. learning through interaction with one's peers) and on the role
of the teacher as supporter of the students' efforts to make sense of their world
rather than as deliverer of knowledge. Such a view not only makes the participation of students with learning difficulties in ordinary classrooms possible, it
also makes it necessary if they are to learn from and with their peers – and if
their peers are to learn from and with them (for an exploration of these links,
see Ware 1995; Udvari-Solner 1996). Moreover, constructivist views also enable
and require the participation of students who may not have learning difficulties
per se but who are marginalized in other ways. Although, according to the
'banking' concept of education, such students are often seen as bringing little
knowledge and few skills with them into the classroom, this does not, construc-
tivists would argue, disbar them from participation. As the talent development
model makes clear, they too start from where they are and actively build
knowledge through interaction with peers and teachers.

In recent years, there has been significant interest in techniques that suggest
that the alternative to rigid didactic teaching styles need not be confined to the
equally inflexible approach of leaving children to 'discover' things for themselves, unaided by the teacher. Without recourse to didacticism, for instance,
students can be engaged and guided vigorously by their teachers through 'whole
class interactive teaching' (Reynolds and Farrell 1996) or can be taught 'thinking

skills' in a way that increases the resources they can bring to bear on the construction of knowledge (Feurstein *et al.* 1980; Blagg *et al.* 1991; Adey and Shayer 1994). Much remains to be discovered about how, precisely, these and similar strategies can best be used and there is a real danger of 'faddism' as new techniques are adopted and abandoned in quick succession. However, it is likely that a broadly constructivist approach, operationalized through a series of structured and supportive pedagogical techniques, offers the prospect not only of 'including' marginalized students, but of providing them with high levels of support and guidance, which make it more likely that they will learn as effectively as their more advantaged peers. It is probably worth adding, moreover, that some of the 'supports and adaptations' – classroom assistants, differentiated materials, use of instructional technology, and so on – which are traditionally presented as the basis for inclusion (see Lipsky and Gartner 1997: 12), only make sense in the context of a more fundamental approach of this kind.

AN INCLUSIVE SYSTEM

It is sometimes assumed that inclusive education can be achieved simply through the sorts of actions outlined above – that is, through the creation of 'inclusive schools' using an 'inclusive pedagogy'. However, it has become clear that schools' attempts at becoming inclusive can be undermined by the shortcomings – or, indeed, the anti-inclusive values – of the wider education system (Booth *et al.* 1997, 1998; Rouse and Florian 1997). It makes more sense, therefore, to suggest that inclusive schools can *only* develop and be maintained in the context of a wider education system that is itself supportive of inclusion.

One of the fullest analyses of how national and local education systems can support inclusion is emerging from an ongoing project sponsored by UNESCO. The 'Open File on Inclusive Education' (UNESCO 2001) is a collaborative effort, coordinated at the University of Newcastle, to provide guidance to national and local administrators and decision makers seeking to promote inclusive education. It is based on contributions from experts around the world who have identified the major features of systems in which inclusive schooling becomes possible:

- The effective management of the transition to inclusive education; for instance, through the building of public and professional consensus and the development of an appropriate legislative framework.
- Professional development strategies developing the necessary skills, knowledge and values in the teaching force.
- Assessment systems that recognize the learning of all students.
- The availability of support for both learners and teachers from beyond the school.
- The involvement of families and communities in the education process.

- The development of a curriculum in which all learners can participate meaningfully.
- The establishment of resourcing and funding systems that deliver resources efficiently to mainstream schools and do not include perverse incentives for placing students in non-mainstream settings.
- Systems for managing student transitions between phases of education and on into the adult world.
- Strategies and mechanisms for working with schools to develop inclusive approaches.

These facilitators of inclusive education can perhaps best be seen as dividing into two main groups: the structures of the education system and the supports available to schools.

The structures of the education system

This group is concerned with the legislative framework, with funding systems and with curriculum and assessment. Although these structures and their management in support of inclusive education are extremely complex, at bottom they present a simple alternative: the education system can be organized on one of two assumptions – that the full range of students is educated in mainstream schools or that mainstream schools are established to meet the needs of the *majority* of students with a minority left to fit in as best they can or, failing that, to be educated separately (Ainscow and Sebba 1996).

The nature of the school curriculum is a good example of this. The National Curriculum in England, for instance, was introduced through a consultation document in which there was almost no acknowledgement that many students had 'special educational needs' or other sorts of difficulty (DES 1987). It was not surprising, therefore, that schools initially struggled to teach such students in the context of a curriculum that was, effectively, not designed for them (Swann 1992; Bines 1993). Successive governments have loosened the curriculum framework, particularly in secondary schools (Dearing 1994; DfEE 2001), and have offered guidance as to how it can be delivered in an 'inclusive' manner (for instance, the inclusion statement in DfEE/QCA 1999). However, the consequence has been a curriculum that is increasingly differentiated for different groups and the return to a partially segregated 'vocational' curriculum for low-attaining students (DfEE 2001: 4.40; Hackett 2001). It is arguable that in neither case has the English system succeeded in developing a curriculum framework that facilitates inclusive approaches in schools.

Similarly, there is growing evidence that the way schools are funded impacts on their capacity and willingness to become inclusive (see Parrish 1997; Meijer 1999; Parrish *et al.* 1999). The *inclusive* assumption is that all students will be in mainstream schools and therefore that funding will be delivered efficiently to those schools, in proportion to the demand in their populations, so that they can make appropriate provision. The *exclusive* assumption is that some students will not be in mainstream schools, or will be there only exceptionally, so that appropriate funding is available only outside the mainstream or through complex and bureaucratic processes. The current policy in England displays characteristics of both assumptions. On the one hand, it remains committed to a high level of individual 'pupil-bound' budgets (Pijl and Dyson 1998) – via, for instance, statements of special educational need – which are cumbersome to access. On the other hand, it seeks to deliver as much funding as possible directly to schools in the form of both a relatively constant annual sum for the education of all students (weightings take into account differences in school populations) and additional funding tied to specific initiatives and priorities, such as Excellence in Cities (DfEE 1999b).

Curriculum and funding systems, of course, are governed by a wider legislative framework, which can be more or less inclusive in effect. It is not enough for official policy statements to contain declarations of commitment to inclusive principles if the legislative framework supports exclusive structures (on how this contradiction undermines very powerful commitments to inclusion in South Africa, see Sayed and Carrim 1998; for a more wide-ranging critique of special education policies, see Fulcher 1989). Suffice it to say that in England an avowed commitment to inclusive education sits alongside legislation that protects the existence of special schools, permits the exclusion of students from schools for disciplinary reasons and encourages a system of 'parental choice' that seems grossly inequitable in its operation (Ball 1993; Gold *et al.* 1993; Gewirtz *et al.* 1995; Reay and Ball 1997, 1998).

Support for schools

The second set of systemic factors concerns the extent to which the system offers tangible support for schools in developing and implementing inclusive approaches. Such supports include the range of professional advice and intervention available to schools and the extent to which they are enabled to engage with families and communities. The point here is that schools inevitably have a limited range of resources in-house, not just in terms of funding and material resources, but also of the expertise of their teachers. It follows that, if they are to educate a wider range of students, they need to be able to call on additional resources to meet these new demands. Traditionally, the UK education systems have relied on a range of 'intermediary bodies' (Cordingley and Kogan 1993), forming part of the system of local government, to deliver these resources. However, local government reorganization and the progressive narrowing of this local role means that there has been a good deal of rethinking as to how this function will be performed in the future (see Audit Commission 1990, 1999; Housden 1993; Millward and Skidmore 1995; DfEE 1999a; Sofer 2000). What seems to be emerging from these debates is that local authorities and other 'intermediary bodies' have a key role to play strategically – charting an overall direction, ensuring that resources are available, monitoring provision, and so on – but that they should avoid becoming front-line deliverers of services, which might best be delivered by schools themselves (Dyson *et al.* 2000). In particular, they have to achieve a delicate balance between ensuring that schools are enabled to become inclusive and taking over responsibilities from schools in such a way that they remove all incentive for them to be inclusive.

The contribution to inclusive approaches by agencies outside education has long been recognized – and long recognized as problematic (Dyson *et al.* 1997, 1998). The source of these problems is that the needs of students and their families do not neatly coincide with the traditional boundaries between service delivery agencies. Put simply, whether a student learns effectively in school depends to a significant extent on non-educational factors: whether he or she is healthy, safe and supported outside of school, for instance. The educational progress of *all* students, therefore, depends on broad social policies (in law and order, health and the environment) that create optimum conditions for development. For some students, these universal policies need to be supplemented by preventive work or by direct problem-solving interventions.

In all of these cases, the key seems to be that service providers should be able to work together towards common goals and that this involves overcoming the barriers created by professional cultures, by separate legislative and funding frameworks and by the professional 'turf wars' that are endemic to this field. In an inclusive system, there is an additional imperative that services are able to work in and with mainstream schools and to support the presence and participation of students in those schools. The limited success of traditional strategies for achieving these apparently simple aims has spawned a series of alternatives. One is the reorganization of the agencies themselves so that institutional barriers between them are removed (Dyson and Millward 2001; Levis 2001). Another is through locating services in or close to schools so that they can work together to offer holistic support to children (Dreyfoos 1994; Scottish Office 1998; van Veen *et al.* 1998). A third is to enable schools themselves to work collaboratively so that they can supplement each other's resources and constitute larger units with which external agencies can work more efficiently (Lunt *et al.* 1994; Evans *et al.* 1999). All of these appear to offer ways forward and it is not too difficult to envisage the emergence, in the not too distant future, of groups of schools operating as the base for multi-service provision to meet the needs of all children and families in their areas.

The engagement of schools with families and, to a lesser extent, communities, is equally well-researched and equally problematic (for a review of activities, see Ball 1998; for reviews of UK and international research evidence, respectively, see Dyson and Robson 1999; Moss *et al.* 1999). The broad outlines of the evidence are clear. Many schools seek to involve the families of their students and, when they are successful in doing so, there is a positive impact on attitudes and attainments. However, engagement with families and communities tends to be dominated by the interests of the school and takes place very much on its terms. This is a problem where family and community interests diverge significantly from those of professionals. Moreover, students who are already vulnerable to exclusion are more likely to come from families and communities which schools find it difficult to engage. They are, therefore, doubly disadvantaged by this lack of engagement. Again, it may be that a closer alignment of groups of schools with particular communities and a formalization of the responsibilities of such groups for *all* children and families in their communities might go some way to addressing these difficulties.

WIDER SOCIAL ISSUES

This last set of issues is only occasionally touched on in the inclusive education literature – that is, the relationships between inclusive schooling, the wider life-chances of individual students and the broad social and economic structures that shape those life-chances. At its simplest, do inclusive schools, even if set within inclusive education systems, lead to participation in an 'inclusive society', as indicated, for instance, by access to adult services, employment, a full social life, and so on? The evidence we have is not encouraging. Certainly, schooling in general leads many young people into what has been called a 'wasted youth' (Pearce and Hillman 1998) and there is evidence that inclusive schools do not necessarily provide effective support for young people with disabilities as they enter the adult world (Dyson and Millward 1999). It may be that a more structured system of support, such as the new Connexions Service (DfEE 2000), which itself has some basis in research (Social Exclusion Unit 1999), may prove to be more effective.

The issue, however, is wider than this. Inclusive schools are only likely to contribute to an 'inclusive' society if they form part of a coherent set of policies for developing such a society and if, therefore, all of their work is directed towards this end. This has some specific implications. For instance, if access to employment is an important marker of participation in an 'inclusive' society, then schools have to produce young people with the necessary skills and attitudes, while other social and economic policies have to ensure that employment opportunities are made available.

This issue has been brought home vividly through research, sponsored by the Joseph Rowntree Foundation, that colleagues and myself are undertaking into the role of schools in area regeneration. Although the usual focus of research is on how well schools manage students from disadvantaged areas within their own four walls, or, perhaps, how assiduous they are in developing links with the local community, we are focusing on how schools support economic regeneration strategies that operate at whole-authority or, indeed, at regional level. Some of those strategies demand that schools maintain a 'hard-line' focus on raising attainments, even if this means spending less time on working with the community or on dealing with problems in students' out-of-school lives (Dyson *et al.* 2001). There are, of course, other, very different approaches. Some inclusion advocates would see the contribution of inclusive schools much more in terms of the development of inclusive values within society (UNESCO 1994; Skrtic 1995; Thomas 1997). The point – at what is still an early stage in this debate – is that the purpose of inclusive education cannot simply be to produce inclusive schools; it also has to contribute in some tangible way to the development of an 'inclusive society', however that problematic term might be defined.

WHAT WE DO NOT KNOW

Reviewing the evidence presented here, there is a sense in which we know everything and nothing about inclusive education. We know everything because inclusive education is, in effect, synonymous with 'good' education or, indeed, simply with 'education'. It draws on everything we know about educating children, but is simply insistent that 'children' should mean *all* children. On the other hand, this emphasis on *all*, in so far as it means all children being offered similar experiences in similar settings with a view to producing similar outcomes, is a very recent one. There is, therefore, a good deal of critique of non-inclusive systems on which we can draw and a good deal of advocacy for a new system, but very little rigorous analysis of how such a new system might actually 'work' in practice (Clark *et al.* 1995, 1998).

It is arguable, therefore, that the most urgent needs are two-fold. First, there is a need for a synthesis of what we already know. In so far as 'inclusive education' is simply a revitalization of long-standing concerns about issues of equity, participation, diversity and disadvantage in education, a thorough-going attempt is required to assemble the evidence we have, to scan it for synergies and contradictions and to try to build from it a more holistic knowledge base. This chapter is, in however small and imperfect a way, an attempt to do just that.

Second, in so far as inclusive education is indeed something new, there is a need to find out *what works* by studying in some detail inclusive education *at work*. We now have increasing numbers of schools, colleges and other education settings, in increasing numbers of education systems, where 'inclusion', however weakly articulated, is an avowed aim. We ought, therefore, to be in a position to move beyond advocacy, beyond the glowing description of exemplars of outstanding inclusive practice and beyond the separate study of discrete groups of marginalized students towards repeated studies of what inclusive education looks like on the ground, what sustains it and what outcomes it has.

SOME IMPLICATIONS AND CONCLUSIONS

I have tried, throughout this chapter, to keep one eye on the multiple implications for policy and practice of what we already know about inclusive education. If, however, there is a single, dominant message, it is about the importance of what we might call 'alignment' in the development of inclusive education.

By this I mean that all aspects of the education system, from the detail of teachers' classroom practice, through school organization and local authority support to national policy, have to be 'aligned' with the principles of inclusion. In this sense, the argument alluded to at the start of the chapter – that inclusive education is about permeating inclusive values through the system rather than about implementing particular techniques – appears to be justified.

There are two reasons for emphasizing this principle of alignment. The first is that inclusive education means nothing unless and until it is experienced by students at risk of exclusion. There is, therefore, no point in having grandiose statements of support for inclusion at the centre of education systems unless those statements are turned into practical policy, those policies are implemented within schools and teachers practice in inclusive ways within their classrooms. Equally, inclusive education is about enabling teachers and schools to work inclusively in the face of challenges from student diversity, which have historically led them to marginalize particular groups of learners. This will only happen if each level of the education system offers the support to the levels 'below' it which make it practicable for them to meet these challenges effectively.

REFERENCES

Abberley, P. (1987) The concept of oppression and the development of a social theory of disability, *Disability, Handicap and Society*, 2(1): 5–19.

Adey, P. and Shayer, M. (1994) *Really Raising Standards: Cognitive Intervention and Academic Achievement*. London: Routledge.

Ainscow, M. (1999) *Understanding the Development of Inclusive Schools*. London: Falmer Press.

Ainscow, M. and Sebba, J. (eds) (1996) Developments in inclusive education, *Cambridge Journal of Education*, 26(1) (special issue).

Audit Commission (1990) *Losing an Empire, Finding a Role*. London: HMSO.

Audit Commission (1999) *Held in Trust: The LEA of the Future*. London: Audit Commssion.

Baker, J.M. and Zigmond, N. (1995) The meaning and practice of inclusion for students with learning disabilities: themes and implications from the five cases, *Journal of Special Education*, 29(2): 163–80.

Ball, M. (1998) *School Inclusion: The School, the Family and the Community*. York: Joseph Rowntree Foundation.

Ball, S.J. (1993) The market as a class strategy in the UK and US, *British Journal of Sociology of Education*, 14(1): 3–19.

Bines, H. (1993) Curriculum change: the case of special education, *British Journal of Sociology of Education*, 14(1): 75–90.

Blagg, N., Ballinger, M. and Gardner, R. (1991) *Somerset Thinking Skills Course*. Oxford: Blackwell in association with Somerset County Council.

Blunkett, D. (1999a) Excellence for the many, not just the few: raising standards and extending opportunities in our schools, the CBI President's Reception Address by the Rt. Hon. David Blunkett MP, 19 July 1999. London: DfEE.

Blunkett, D. (1999b) Social exclusion and the politics of opportunity: a mid-term progress check, a speech by the Rt. Hon. David Blunkett MP. London: DfEE.

Blunkett, D. (2000) Raising aspirations for the 21st century, a speech to the North of England Education Conference, Wigan, 6 January 2000. London: DfEE.

Booth, T. (1995) Mapping inclusion and exclusion: concepts for all?, in C. Clark, A. Dyson and A. Millward (eds) *Towards Inclusive Schools?* London: David Fulton.

Booth, T. (1996) A perspective on inclusion from England, *Cambridge Journal of Education*, 26(1): 87–99.

Booth, T., Ainscow, M. and Dyson, A. (1997) Understanding inclusion and exclusion in the English competitive education system, *International Journal of Inclusive Education*, 1(4): 337–54.

Booth, T., Ainscow, M. and Dyson, A. (1998) England: inclusion and exclusion in a competitive system, in T. Booth and M. Ainscow (eds) *From Them to Us: An International Study of Inclusion in Education*. London: Routledge.

Booth, T., Ainscow, M., Black-Hawkins, K., Vaughan, M. and Shaw, L. (2000) *Index for Inclusion: Developing Learning and Participation in Schools*. Bristol: Centre for Studies on Inclusive Education.

Boykin, A.W. (2000) The talent development model of schooling: placing students at promise for academic success, *Journal of Education for Students Placed at Risk*, 5(1&2): 3–25.

CSIE (Centre for Studies on Inclusive Education) (undated) *What is Inclusion?* http://inclusion.uwe.ac.uk/csie/csiefaqs.htm (CSIE) (accessed 2 July 2001).

Clark, C., Dyson, A. and Millward, A. (1995) Towards inclusive schools: mapping the field, in C. Clark, A. Dyson and A. Millward (eds) *Towards Inclusive Schools?* London: David Fulton.

Clark, C., Dyson, A., Millward, A. and Skidmore, D. (1997) *New Directions in Special Needs: Innovations in Mainstream Schools*. London: Cassell.

Clark, C., Dyson, A. and Millward, A. (1998) Theorising special education: time to move on?, in C. Clark, A. Dyson and A. Millward (eds) *Theorising Special Education*. London: Routledge.

Cordingley, P. and Kogan, M. (1993) *In Support of Education: The Functioning of Local Government*. London: Jessica Kingsley.

Crowther, D., Dyson, A. and Millward, A. (1998) *Costs and Outcomes for Pupils with Moderate Learning Difficulties in Special and Mainstream Schools*, RR89. London: DfEE.

Dearing, R. (1994) *The National Curriculum and its Assessment: Final Report, December 1993*. London: School Curriculum and Assessment Authority.

Department for Education and Employment (1999a) *Code of Practice: LEA–School Relations*. London: The Stationery Office.

Department for Education and Employment (1999b) *Excellence in Cities*. London: DfEE.

Department for Education and Employment (2000) *Connexions: The Best Start in Life for Every Young Person*. London: DfEE.

Department for Education and Employment (2001) *Schools Building on Success: Raising Standards, Promoting Diversity, Achieving Results*. London: The Stationery Office.

Department for Education and Employment/Qualifications and Curriculum Authority (1999) *The National Curriculum: Handbook for Primary/Secondary Teachers in England*. London: DfEE/QCA.

Department of Education and Science/The Welsh Office (1987) *The National Curriculum 5–16: A Consultation Document*. London: DES.

Dreyfoos, J. (1994) *Full-Service Schools*. San Francisco, CA: Jossey-Bass.

Dyson, A. (1999) Inclusion and inclusions: theories and discourses in inclusive education, in H. Daniels and P. Garner (eds) *World Yearbook of Education 1999: Inclusive Education*. London: Kogan Page.

Dyson, A. and Millward, A. (1999) Falling down the interfaces: from inclusive schools to an exclusive society, in K. Ballard (ed.) *Inclusive Education: International Voices on Disability and Justice*. London: Falmer Press.

Dyson, A. and Millward, A. (2000) *Schools and Special Needs: Issues of Innovation and Inclusion*. London: Paul Chapman.

Dyson, A. and Millward, A. (2001) *Preliminary Evaluation of Hertfordshire's Children Schools and Families Service*. London: DfES.

Dyson, A. and Robson, E. (1999) *School, Family, Community: Mapping School Inclusion in the UK*. Leicester: Youth Work Press for the Joseph Rowntree Foundation.

Dyson, A., Lin, M. and Millward, A. (1997) *Effective Communication between Schools, LEAs, Health and Social Services in the Field of Special Educational Needs*. Newcastle: Special Needs Research Centre, University of Newcastle DfEE and Department of Health.

Dyson, A., Lin, M. and Millward, A. (1998) Inter-agency cooperation for children with special educational needs: an analytical framework, in D. van Veen, C. Day and G. Walraven (eds) *Multi-service Schools: Integrated Services for Children and Youth at Risk*. Leuven: Garant.

Dyson, A., Clark, J., Hall, E., Hall, I. and Roberts, B. (2000) *Increasing the Attainments of Under-achieving Groups*. http://www.local-regions.detr.gov.uk/beacon/year2/research/04/index.htm (DETR) (accessed 14 December 2000).

Dyson, A., Millward, A. and Robson, E. (2001) Participation and democracy: what's inclusion got to do with it?, *International Colloquium on Inclusive Education*, 26–29 June 2001, University of Stirling.

Evans, J., Lunt, I., Wedell, K. and Dyson, A. (1999) *Collaborating for Effectiveness: Empowering Schools to be Inclusive*. Buckingham: Open University Press.

Feurstein, R., Rand, Y., Hoffman, M.B. and Miller, R. (1980) *Instrumental Enrichment: An Intervention Programme for Cognitive Modifiability*. Baltimore, MD: University Park Press.

Freire, P. (1972) *Pedagogy of the Oppressed*. Harmondsworth: Penguin.

Fulcher, G. (1989) *Disabling Policies? A Comparative Approach to Education Policy and Disability*. Lewes: Falmer Press.

Galloway, D. and Goodwin, C. (1987) *The Education of Disturbing Children: Pupils with Learning and Adjustment Difficulties*. London: Longman.

Gartner, A. and Lipsky, D.K. (1987) Beyond special education: toward a quality system for all students, *Harvard Educational Review*, 57(4): 367–95.

Gartner, A. and Lipsky, D.K. (1989) *The Yoke of Special Education: How to Break It*. Rochester, NY: National Center of Education and the Economy.

Gewirtz, S., Ball, S.J. and Bowe, R. (1995) *Markets, Choice and Equity in Education*. Buckingham: Open University Press.

Gold, A., Bowe, R. and Ball, S. (1993) Special educational needs in a new context: micropolitics, money and 'education for all', in R. Slee (ed.) *Is There a Desk With My Name On It? The Politics of Integration*. London: Falmer Press.

Hackett, G. (2001) Pupils to quit at 14 to work, *The Sunday Times* (London), 24 June, pp. 1–2.

Hegarty, S. (1993) Reviewing the literature on integration, *European Journal of Special Needs Education*, 8(3): 194–200.

Hornby, G. (1999) Inclusion or delusion: can one size fit all?, *Support for Learning*, 14(4): 152–7.

Housden, P. (1993) *Bucking the Market: LEAs and Special Needs*. Stafford: NASEN.

Kauffman, J.K. and Hallahan, D.P. (eds) (1995) *The Illusion of Full Inclusion*. Austin, TX: PRO-ED.

Levis, N. (2001) Hertfordshire ground-breakers, *Times Educational Supplement* (London), 22 June, pp. 1–3.

Lipsky, D.K. and Gartner, A. (1997) *Inclusion and School Reform: Transforming America's Classrooms*. Baltimore, MD: Paul H. Brookes.

Lipsky, D.K. and Gartner, A. (1999) Inclusive education: a requirement of a democratic society, in H. Daniels and P. Garner (eds) *World Yearbook of Education 1999: Inclusive Education*. London: Kogan Page.

Lunt, I. and Norwich, B. (1999) *Can Effective Schools Be Inclusive Schools?* London: Institute of Education.

Lunt, I., Evans, J., Norwich, B. and Wedell, K. (1994) *Working Together: Inter-School Collaboration for Special Needs*. London: David Fulton.

Meijer, C.J.W. (ed.) (1999) *Financing of Special Needs Education: A Seventeen-country Study of the Relationship between Financing of Special Needs Education and Inclusion*. Middlefart, Denmark: European Agency for Development in Special Needs Education.

Millward, A. and Skidmore, D. (1995) *Local Authorities' Management of Special Needs*. York: YPS.

Mittler, P. (2000) *Working Towards Inclusive Education: Social Contexts*. London: David Fulton.

Moss, P., Petrie, P. and Poland, G. (1999) *Rethinking School: Some International Perspectives*. Leicester: Youth Work Press for the Joseph Rowntree Foundation.

National Institute for Urban School Improvement (undated) *Improving Education: The Promise of Inclusive Education*. http://www.edc.org/urban/publicat.htm#improvinged (NIUSI) (accessed 2 July 2001).

Oliver, M. (1990) *The Politics of Disablement*. London: Macmillan.

Parrish, T.B. (1997) Fiscal issues relating to special education, in D.K. Lipsky and A. Gartner (eds) *Inclusion and School Reform: Transforming America's Classrooms*. Baltimore, MD: Paul Brookes.

Parrish, T.B., Chambers, J.G. and Guarino, C.M. (eds) (1999) *Funding Special Education: Nineteenth Annual Yearbook of the American Education Finance Association*. Thousand Oaks, CA: Corwin Press.

Pearce, N. and Hillman, J. (1998) *Wasted Youth: Raising Achievement and Tackling Social Exclusion*. London: IPPR.

Pijl, S.J. and Dyson, A. (1998) Pupil-bound budgets in special education: a three-country study, *Comparative Education*, 34(3): 261–79.

Poplin, M.S. and Stone, S. (1992) Paradigm shifts in instructional strategies: from reductionism to holistic/constructivism, in W. Stainback and S. Stainback (eds) *Controversial Issues Confronting Special Education: Divergent Perspectives*. Boston, MA: Allyn & Bacon.

Reay, D. and Ball, S.J. (1997) 'Spoilt for choice': the working classes and education markets, *Oxford Review of Education*, 23: 89–101.

Reay, D. and Ball, S.J. (1998) Making their minds up: family dynamics of school choice, *British Educational Research Journal*, 24(4): 431–48.

Reynolds, D. (1995) Using school effectiveness knowledge for children with special needs – the problems and possibilities, in C. Clark, A. Dyson and A. Millward (eds) *Towards Inclusive Schools?* London: David Fulton.

Reynolds, D. and Farrell, S. (1996) *Worlds Apart? A Review of International Surveys of Educational Achievement Involving England.* London: Ofsted.

Reynolds, D., Teddlie, C. with Hopkins, D. and Stringfield, S. (2000) Linking school effectiveness and school improvement, in C. Teddlie and D. Reynolds (eds) *The International Handbook of School Effectiveness Research.* London: Falmer Press.

Rouse, M. and Florian, L. (1997) Inclusive education in the market-place, *International Journal of Inclusive Education,* 1(4): 323–36.

Sayed, Y. and Carrim, N. (1998) Inclusiveness and participation in discourses of educational governance in South Africa, *International Journal of Inclusive Education,* 2(1): 29–43.

Scottish Office (1998) *New Community Schools: The Prospectus.* Edinburgh: The Stationery Office.

Sebba, J. and Sachdev, D. (1997) *What Works in Inclusive Education.* Ilford: Barnardo's.

Skidmore, D. (1999) Divergent discourses of learning difficulty, *British Educational Research Journal,* 25(5): 651–63.

Skrtic, T.M. (1991) *Behind Special Education: A Critical Analysis of Professional Culture and School Organization.* Denver, CO: Love.

Skrtic, T.M. (ed.) (1995) *Disability and Democracy: Reconstructing (Special) Education for Postmodernity.* New York: Teachers College Press.

Slavin, R.E. (2001) How Title I can become the engine of reform in America's schools, in G.D. Borman, S.C. Stringfield and R.E. Slavin (eds) *Title I: Compensatory Education at the Crossroads.* Mahwah, NJ: Lawrence Erlbaum Associates.

Social Exclusion Unit (1999) *Bridging the Gap: New Opportunities for 16–18 Year Olds Not in Education, Employment or Training.* London: The Stationery Office.

Sofer, A. (2000) LEAs: the problem or the solution?, in T. Cox (ed.) *Combating Educational Disadvantage: Meeting the Needs of Vulnerable Children.* London: Falmer Press.

Swann, W. (1992) Hardening the hierarchies: the national curriculum as a system of classification, in T. Booth, W. Swann, M. Masterton and P. Potts (eds) *Curricula for Diversity in Education.* London: Routledge.

Thomas, G. (1997) Inclusive schools for an inclusive society, *British Journal of Special Education,* 24(3): 103–7.

Udvari-Solner, A. (1996) Theoretical influences on the establishment of inclusive practices, *Cambridge Journal of Education,* 26(1): 101–19.

UNESCO (1994) *Final Report. World Conference on Special Needs Education: Access and Quality.* Paris: UNESCO.

UNESCO (2001) *The Open File on Inclusive Education.* Paris: UNESCO.

van Veen, D., Day, C. and Walraven, G. (eds) (1998) *Multi-Service Schools.* Leuven: Garant.

Wang, M.C., Haertel, G.D. and Walberg, H.J. (1997) Fostering educational resilience in inner-city schools, *Children and Youth,* 7: 119–40.

Ware, L. (1995) The aftermath of the articulate debate: the invention of inclusive education, in C. Clark, A. Dyson and A. Millward (eds) *Towards Inclusive Schools?* London: David Fulton.

7

BRYONY BERESFORD

Preventing the social exclusion of disabled children

KEY MESSAGES

- The evidence on 'what works' in the social care of disabled children is still minimal; there is even less research on effective approaches to tackling the social exclusion of disabled children.
- Social exclusion permeates the lives of disabled children with long-term consequences that are hard to reverse.
- The experiences of social exclusion increase as children grow older.
- Recent studies suggest that disabled children do not view themselves as intrinsically different to other children, but their treatment by others and their experiences of a disabling environment promote a sense of difference.
- Several factors contribute to the social exclusion of disabled children and young people that are both frequently overlooked by service providers and are under-researched. These include transport, social and leisure needs, housing issues and involvement in decision making.
- Accessible transport systems are fundamental to social inclusion.
- Survey data show that disabled children and young people are significantly less likely to participate in sport and leisure activities, particularly out of school.

- Disabled children spend far more time in the home than non-disabled children, yet, for many, the physical and social environment within the home is highly restrictive.
- Although initiatives such as Quality Protects are actively promoting the greater involvement of disabled children in assessment and decision-making processes, considerable work is still to be done.
- The evidence emerging from practice, particularly from inclusive play and leisure projects, suggests that social inclusion, to a greater or lesser extent, can be achieved *in those settings*. The wider and long-term impacts of these projects have yet to be evaluated.
- Three factors are important for inclusive play: the training of *all* staff, resources and a suitable environment.
- Evaluation of pilot schemes aiming to promote inclusion highlights the importance of careful planning and consultation with children, including those with speech impairments.
- Disabled children most value services that support or promote 'ordinary', everyday activities and experiences.
- An agenda seeking to promote social inclusion has implications for both policy and practice. In particular, it challenges us to address the debate regarding the pros and cons of specialist versus mainstream social care provision. As yet, this debate lacks the research evidence from which to make authoritative assertions.
- Tackling social exclusion requires short- and longer-term measures for change within individual attitudes and behaviours, the physical and social environment and the policies and practice governing the way services are provided.

INTRODUCTION

This chapter synthesizes what is known about what works in preventing the social exclusion of disabled children, drawing on research concerned with such children who are living at home. The focus is deliberately on how social care can support and promote social inclusion in the communities where the majority of disabled children live. That is not to say that what is covered here does not apply to children in special and residential schooling. After all, most of these children also live in the family home, even if only during school holidays. Furthermore, in working towards the inclusion of disabled children, those who are currently most likely to be segregated into residential schools (those with complex needs or challenging behaviour) will hopefully, in the future, find they can stay at home.

In the past, the inter-relationships between social care provision and social exclusion were not considered. Because families with a disabled child were excluded from the ordinary sources of having a 'break' (childcare, play and leisure services/facilities), specialist provision – typically respite care in residential, segregated settings – was seen as the solution (Morris 1998a). This was not viewed as a service to the child but as a means of respite for the parent. It became clear, however, that this was not what children (or their parents) wanted (Oswin 1984). In recent years, there have been significant improvements in provision, with a move to family-based (and hence more inclusive) short-term care services and far more positive reports from children and their parents about residential short-term care (Crisp *et al.* 2000). However, short-term care will always remain a 'special' service; the challenge for social care is to look at how it can minimize its 'specialness' and look to providing services that promote or support inclusion.

The evidence on what works in the social care of disabled children is still minimal (Beresford *et al.* 1996) and has focused on 'special' services. Work on identifying effective ways of preventing social exclusion is even less developed. At the moment, it is limited to looking at specific areas of service provision and interventions at an individual rather than at a community level. This current imbalance of the evidence should not be taken to imply that the issues discussed here are the only issues. There is a lot more work to be done; this is merely the baseline from which we can move forward.

EXCLUSION

The experience of social exclusion

Social exclusion is an experience that permeates the lives of disabled children. Besides the compelling argument that exclusion is a human rights issue, and that a number of basic rights are being denied to disabled children, the consequences of social exclusion are long-term and hard to reverse. This has significant implications for the quality of life of disabled young people and the future generation of disabled adults, and on the demands made on statutory and other support services.

Two recently completed studies provide detailed insight into the lives of disabled children and young people (Watson and Priestley 1999; Connors and Stalker 2000). These studies are particularly valuable as they sought to explore and record in a holistic way the daily lives of disabled children and young people, as opposed to focusing on a particular issue or form of service provision. Although the researchers are keen to point out the positive accounts that emerge, there are also consistent findings across the projects of what characterizes the day-to-day lives of disabled children. What is significant is that these findings predominantly fall within the dimension of exclusion/ inclusion.

A key finding, from these and other projects, is that disabled children do not perceive themselves as intrinsically different to non-disabled children. Rather, it is the way they are treated by others (children and adults), or their experiences of a disabling physical environment, that promotes a sense of difference or of being disabled.

Several specific issues or experiences arise from the accounts of disabled children and young people involved in these studies. Many reported difficulties in accessing social facilities. This problem was more keenly experienced by older children and young people who could not access public transport or age-appropriate leisure spaces, such as fast-food outlets. In terms of local provision to improve access, improvements had been made for adults but not for children. Connors and Stalker (2000) report that one of the boys participating in their study found that his local Shopmobility scheme didn't have children's wheelchairs. The lack of opportunities to do the sorts of things non-disabled children do in their spare time was the reason behind reports of boredom and loneliness. Indeed, we know from a national comparative survey of young people's sport and leisure activities that disabled children and young people spend their spare time differently to non-disabled young people. More time is spent watching television and videos than among the general population of young people and half the amount of time is spent playing sport (Finch *et al.* 2001).

Another prominent theme, and one commonly found in other research involving disabled children, is reports of bullying and hostility (verbal and non-verbal) from peers and members of the public. The impact on the children and young people's well-being from experiences such as these are not difficult to predict: a sense of exclusion and isolation and not being valued by society are the feelings commonly reported in research (e.g. Noyes 1999).

Watson and Priestley (1999) were particularly struck by the limited opportunities to spend time with other children (disabled or non-disabled) without an 'active' (or controlling) adult presence (the presence of special needs assistants in mainstream education was given as an example). In addition, the lack of inclusive out-of-school activities or facilities means that disabled children spend more time at home with their parents than non-disabled children typically do (Mulderij 1996). Watson and Priestley (1999: 16) concluded:

> Although disabled children wanted to locate themselves in the world of children, there were various barriers to their full participation. As well as the adult surveillance discussed above, these included physical barriers such as access to playgrounds and facilities and attitudinal barriers on the part of other children.

They argue that this exclusion from the world of childhood means disabled children spend much of their time in a disablist, childist adult world.

An alternative way of exploring disabled children's needs and priorities is to identify the types of services that are viewed positively. This was the approach adopted by Mitchell and Sloper (2001) and supports the conclusions drawn by other researchers. When Mitchell and Sloper asked disabled children and young people about the services they valued and what they felt made a good-quality service, it was services which protect and promote friendships and those which offer opportunities to develop independence skills in a fun, informal setting that were most frequently nominated. Other priorities identified by this project also strongly relate to inclusion. The young people talked about the need to be able to go out into the community and join in regular age-appropriate leisure activities and be included in decision making.

The consequences of exclusion

Exclusion from everyday mainstream activities has an impact on excluded children's abilities to become included once they have the opportunity to do so. Following their study of the out-of-school lives of disabled children, Petrie *et al.* (2000) argued that attendance at special school/special units in mainstream school meant that disabled children had no experience of 'the cultural norms of children who interact through mainstream education' (p. 78). They cite research from Denmark (Kampman 1997) that developed the notion of children having to serve a 'play apprenticeship' to become experts in play culture: the way play is structured, the unspoken rules, appropriate group entry behaviour. This lack of exposure to other children and surveillance by adults means that disabled young people can end up finding they relate far more easily to adults than their peers (Robinson 1997)

What appears to happen is that exclusion increases as the child grows older. In the pre-school years, disabled children may not use 'special' provision, attending 'mainstream' parent and toddler groups, play groups and using parks and other leisure facilities alongside non-disabled children. Although some children then move on to mainstream primary school, the start of school is the time for many when the process of exclusion begins; upon transfer to secondary school, an even greater proportion of disabled children are 'segregated'. At the same time, their access to other activities within their local community becomes increasingly difficult or impossible. Thompson *et al.* (2000) describe this as 'fracturing neighbourhood friendships'. While the recent analysis of the second-year Quality Protects Management Action Plans noted improvements in terms of inclusion (at least at a strategic level) of young disabled children in mainstream provision through Sure Start and Early Years programmes (Council for Disabled Children 2000), this does not seem to progress through to 'later years' services.

There is clear evidence, both qualitative and quantitative, of the long-term consequences of this exclusion. Hirst and Baldwin's (1994) work on reaching adulthood compared the outcomes of disabled young people with their non-disabled peers. They found significant differences between young disabled and young non-disabled people in their lifestyles, living circumstances and expectations for the future. They identified differences between the two groups in the extent to which the necessary steps to independence had been achieved; namely, employment (and conversely dependence on social security), control of one's own finances, skills necessary for independent living and moving out of the family home. The researchers also noted that, compared with their non-disabled peers, the disabled young people had lower self-esteem and were more likely to report a lack of control over their lives.

These discrepancies in the circumstances and self-perceptions of disabled and non-disabled young people are the product of living a life, virtually from birth, characterized by social exclusion. Mulderij (1996), in her study of young disabled children, concluded that the 'lifeworlds' of young physically disabled children are smaller and more restricted than those of non-disabled children. This exclusion is experienced at all levels or areas of the child's life, from schooling to opportunities to participate in everyday childhood and teenage activities (Cook *et al.* 1996; Mulderij 1996; Petrie *et al.* 2000). Petrie *et al.* (2000), in summarizing their findings on the out-of-school lives of disabled children, used three phrases: 'confinement', 'lack of companions' and 'rejection'.

The costs of exclusion are high and long-term, affecting individuals, families, communities and society at large. Using the case of special educational provision, Middleton (1999) argues that excluding disabled children from the everyday experiences of childhood and adolescence means that their eventual 're-entry' into mainstream society becomes extremely difficult, if not impossible, demanding considerable resources and with a potential long-term cost in individual self-esteem. The alternative is continued exclusion.

Addressing exclusion: the issues

In addition to the way the current systems of educational and specialist social care might be contributing to the social exclusion of disabled children, other issues have been identified as playing an important role in inclusion, including transport, housing, social/leisure opportunities, information and decision making. (There are, of course, other factors, such as public attitudes, which have not received research attention.)

Transport issues

Accessible transport systems are fundamental to social inclusion and equality of opportunity (Hine and Mitchell 2001). For many older disabled children and young people, being able to use public transport (preferably independently) becomes a high priority (DoH/JRF/The Children's Society 2001). Transport and travel has received little research attention, although disabled adults' experience of travel has been summarized as one of 'constraint and compromise' (Porter 2000). There is clearly a need for a focus on transport and travel in future research, policy and practice on issues of social exclusion and disabled children. Access to *locations* is fundamentally linked to access to *transport*: Porter cites Meadows' (1992) notion of a 'transport chain'. It is pointless having an accessible leisure centre if it is not serviced by accessible transport; similarly, the value of accessible transport is lessened if inadequate equipment or unsuitable housing mean individuals cannot leave their home unaccompanied. Although transport and travel issues may not fall into the remit of social services departments, the Children Act 1989 does place responsibility on them to oversee the needs of disabled children. An holistic approach to the assessment of the needs of disabled children and young people has to include the issue of transport, given its pivotal role in so many aspects of young people's lives.

Social and leisure needs

There is compelling evidence that disabled children and young people face significant discrimination and are excluded from enjoying the range of play and leisure opportunities afforded to their non-disabled peers. Yet it is widely acknowledged that participation in sport has the potential to promote the social inclusion of disabled young people and have positive benefits for their physical and mental well-being.

A recent survey, the first of its kind, has detailed the involvement in, and access to, sport and leisure activities by disabled children and young people (Finch *et al.* 2001). The survey involved more than 2200 disabled children and young people aged 6–16 years; the results were compared to those from a survey of non-disabled children and young people. The findings show significant and consistent under-participation in sport and leisure activities by disabled children and young people compared with their non-disabled counterparts. Differences in participation in non-school sports clubs are particularly striking. Just over one in ten disabled young people was a member of a non-school sports club, compared with just under half of non-disabled young people. Barriers to participation reported by participants in the research included: a lack of money, unsuitability of or no local facilities, a lack of accessible transport and hostile staff or members of the public using the facilities. Most disabled young people who took part in the survey said they minded being excluded from sport and leisure opportunities.

Housing

Most research of the social exclusion of disabled children has been concerned with issues outside the home environment. There has been a greater recognition of the importance of housing for disabled adults; this has been driven in part by the consistent message from disabled adults and older people that housing is the cornerstone of effective community care (Bochel *et al.* 1999). In addition, there is a body of research that clearly illustrates that the physical features of the homes of disabled adults can act as barriers to independent living (Stark 2001).

For disabled children, however, the issue of housing has been neglected. There is little awareness within social services departments of the effects of housing on the lives of disabled children and their families (Beresford and Oldman 2000), and the need to assess family's housing are not routinely mentioned in Social Services Inspectorate (SSI) reports on disabled children's services (SSI 1994).

Yet, apart from the time spent at school, home is where children spend much of their time. Indeed, for the reasons already discussed, disabled children are likely to spend more of their spare time within the home environment than non-disabled children (Mulderij 1996). Research in the USA has shown that children's homes can be their most restrictive environments (Brotherson *et al.* 1995). A piece of recent in-depth research (Oldman and Beresford 1998) explored the impact of the home environment on the lives of disabled children and found that physical barriers within the home had the effect of excluding children from everyday childhood activities. The places where the children played and what they played was dependent on their ability to move independently about the home and to have access to all parts of the home. Some children had very restricted play lives. Barriers in the home also meant that the children could be excluded from developing self-care or life skills (such as making snacks and drinks) and contributing to family life by helping out in the kitchen. Finally, a lack of equipment or adaptations meant some children were denied the right to privacy when using the toilet or bathing. What also emerged from this research were the ways that the attitudes or behaviour of parents influenced the child's use of, or access to, parts of the home (there were lots of concerns about safety in the kitchen, for example). Parents could also assume control over the use of equipment (installed to assist the child), as well as making unilateral decisions about the adaptations made to the home.

Parents were also involved in this project and it was very clear from their accounts that resolving housing issues could substantially improve families' quality of life. Some parents were adamant that if they lived in housing that suited all the family's needs, there would be less need for specialist (non-inclusive) services such as short-term care.

Information and decision making

Access to information is central to promoting and supporting inclusion. Information is fundamental for disabled children to manage their day-to-day lives, to make informed decisions, to provide informed consent, to make choices and to plan for the future (Alderson and Montgomery 1996; Beresford and Sloper 1999). The sorts of information needed by a disabled child include information about a medical condition, managing the psychosocial aspects of having a long-term condition or impairment, rights and entitlements and sources of support and opportunities both in the present and the future.

A key area where disabled children have been excluded is in the process of assessment and decision making both preceding and integral to service provision. Having their wishes respected and being able to make choices are features of service provision that disabled children and young people value highly (Morris 1999; Noyes 1999; Crisp *et al.* 2000; Mitchell and Sloper 2001). Although initiatives such as Quality Protects are actively promoting greater involvement in assessment and decision-making processes, there is considerable work to be done to ensure disabled children and young people are fully consulted and involved (SSI 1994; Lenehan 2000).

> Failure to respect the right of disabled children to be heard represents a fundamental denial of their status as people. It disempowers them, it renders them vulnerable to abuse and exploitation by adults, it means their experience and knowledge fails to inform decisions that affect them, and it denies them the opportunities for personal development and growth associated with the process of participating.
>
> (UN Committee on the Rights of the Child 1997: 2)

This ongoing denial of the right to be heard affects the skills and confidence children and young people acquire in their abilities (and expectations) to make their views heard and to make choices and decisions. This helps to widen the gap between disabled children and their non-disabled peers.

INCLUSION

Promoting inclusion: the evidence from practice

Increasingly, social exclusion is informing the sorts of services being provided to disabled children and their families. At the present time, this is most clearly observed in projects being set up by voluntary sector organizations where there is, perhaps, wider scope for innovation. A glance through the appointments pages in local and national pages is testament to the growth in 'social inclusion' posts within disabled, children's and 'mainstream' organizations. (An example I came across when I was writing this chapter was a full-time post to enable inclusion of local young disabled people in a community-based boat club.)

This growth in practice is not reflected in, and hence not informed by, any (systematic) research into how to implement and manage an inclusive service. Thus while legislation (e.g. the Disability Discrimination Act) and government initiatives (e.g. Quality Protects) may support, if not demand, inclusive practice in social care, the means by which this is to be achieved is not clear and, at the moment, cannot draw on a body of evidence. In addition, there is little evidence on the outcomes to services users of services aimed at promoting social inclusion. Do they work? There are two questions that need to be addressed: how to develop and run an inclusive service (the process) and whether the service achieves what it sets out to do (the outcome). The following section reports on what we *do* know and draws primarily on the area where there has been most research, namely inclusive play and leisure services (that is, providing an inclusive *service*), and more general work on promoting the inclusion of disabled children and young people in *communities*. The 'levels' at which these two types of provision are operating are different and, therefore, are useful in providing evidence for the different ways that promoting or supporting inclusion can, or should be, approached.

Inclusive play and leisure services: the lessons learnt

Inclusion is something that has to be supported. For instance, attendance at the same play scheme, while representing some measure of integration between disabled and non-disabled children, does not mean that they end up playing together. Certain things need to be in place within an organization so that inclusion, as opposed to integration, can take place (Newton 1997; Petrie *et al.* 2000; Thompson *et al.* 2000). Three factors appear important:

- *Training.* Staff training has repeatedly been shown to be a key factor in providing inclusive services. These training needs include: knowledge of medical conditions; practical issues (managing toileting, feeding, medication, etc.); awareness/skills in providing or facilitating appropriate activities; and dealing with challenging behaviour. Within any scheme there is a need to have strategies in place to ensure that *all* staff (volunteers and paid workers) are trained. A similar message comes from research on supporting children in mainstream school settings; the need for teaching staff to have adequate knowledge of the condition and its management has been shown to be a key factor in ensuring a child's positive school experience (Cavet 1998; Lightfoot *et al.* 1999).
- *Resources.* There are differing views on how much adults need to be involved in children's play. The fact that some disabled children need assistance to join in activities makes resolving this issue more complex. Research on inclusive play services consistently points to the need for adequate staffing levels to support or facilitate inclusive play. In some circumstances, for example, an adult may need to be present to enable a child to move about. At a different level, an adult may, by direct intervention, facilitate play between disabled and non-disabled children. Petrie *et al.* (2000) tentatively concluded that this sort of intervention acted as a useful 'icebreaker' between children and meant they were more likely, subsequently, to interact on their own initiative.
- *A suitable environment.* As well as basic issues of access, the provision of play environments that are 'barrier-free' and blur the differences in abilities of the children is important. A soft play room is a good example. Petrie *et al.* (2000), in observing disabled and non-disabled children in such an environment, noted that it was difficult to distinguish between so-called disabled and non-disabled children. This is a powerful example of the way the physical environment can enable or include as well as disable or exclude.

Finally, another positive outcome of providing inclusive services is that families begin to expect all local community services to be inclusive; these sorts of expectations and demands from families can only help to drive provision in that direction (Thompson *et al.* 2000).

Promoting inclusion in the community: lessons from the Children in Need Programme

In 1996, The Children's Society began a programme of work on inclusion of children and young people in their local communities (Perry 1998). The purpose of the programme was to look at the role of community-based support systems in promoting inclusion for disabled children and young people. To do this, several projects were evaluated both to assess their effectiveness in promoting inclusion and to look at lessons learnt in setting up such projects. Three projects were identified as being 'well-established models of good practice' in promoting the inclusion of disabled children and young people:

- *Student Scheme: PACT Yorkshire.* This scheme involves a rolling programme of links between student volunteers from universities and local families. The assistance provided by the volunteer is geared to suit the individual needs of the family. Typically, it includes helping a young person access local leisure facilities and home-based support during the busy after-school period.
- *Take 10 and the Spice Group: PACT Yorkshire.* These are two groups (one established more than eight years ago, one more recently) of disabled teenagers and young adults who regularly meet to discuss disability issues and to find ways of expressing their views to a wider audience. For example, the Take 10 group produced a video about their lives and views, which was then presented to the local council's Children's Services Working Group as part of a wider consultation process.
- *SPACE (Suffolk Partnership Achieving Choice and Experience).* Established in 1990, SPACE enables young people with learning difficulties to meet and socialize with non-disabled young people through supporting access to local community and leisure facilities.

Evaluation of these and other, more embryonic, schemes highlighted several key issues for promoting the inclusion of disabled children and young people. First, there is a need for careful planning and the presence of adequate resources to support inclusion strategies. Perry argues that work to enable inclusion has to be *intentional*. Second, disabled children and young people need to be involved in the planning and development of 'services' to support inclusion. This *consultation* needs to include children with a wide range of impairments, including those who do not use speech to communicate. Third, the *ordinariness* of the activities that are, most potently, what inclusion means to disabled children and young people: having friendships, going out with friends, enjoying family outings. Fourth, as well as supporting inclusion at an individual level, the *presence* of disabled children and young people in community environments also influences and changes community perceptions. This argument is supported by the experiences of the manager of an inclusive play and leisure service (Out and About, Ipswich), which has been in existence for more than 15 years. Her observation was that, in her locality, the presence of physically disabled children in community settings is no longer unusual and negative reactions from members of the public are extremely rare.

Promoting inclusion: increasing the evidence base

'Evidence-based' social care is now a familiar phrase and we need to think what it means to develop an evidence base for promoting the inclusion of disabled children and young people. There are several levels of evidence that need to be collected. At one level, some fundamental work is needed on identifying what disabled children and young people want from social care services – that is, user-defined outcomes. There are also more specific issues, such as identifying effective ways of supporting inclusion at individual, group and community levels. Research should also seek to collect process and/or outcome data about a service to answer the question: What 'intervention' works for whom and in what circumstances? Finally, practitioners (with or without the support of researchers) should be gathering evidence in the course of developing, implementing, running and evaluating a service. Across all this research, it is important that all stakeholders (children, parents, practitioners, members of the community) are involved, so that a complete picture of the evidence is obtained.

IMPLICATIONS FOR POLICY

When it first appeared on the statute books, the Children Act 1989 was seen to promote inclusion. Indeed, Morris (1998b) has identified how some rights to inclusion stipulated by the UN Convention on the Rights of the Child are covered within the Children Act 1989 (see Table 7.1).

The problem has been that local authorities have continued to locate the 'problem' of exclusion in the disabled child rather than considering the external factors (social, physical, service and organizational) that contribute to exclusion. In other words, the traditional medical model informed local interpretation of the policy framework despite its potential to tackle exclusion:

> it is the medical model's focus on impairment as the 'problem', as what people are 'suffering' from, which takes attention away from the problems of disabling attitudes and unequal access which, according to disabled people themselves, are much more important in determining life chances and the quality of life.
>
> (Morris 1998b: 14)

Table 7.1 The Children Act 1989 and disabled children's rights to inclusion

Disabled children have the human right to be included in their local community and do the kinds of things non-disabled children do. They have a right to support to help them do this	UN Convention on the Rights of the Child, Article 23 (1), (3) Children Act 1989, Schedule 2, Paragraph 6
Disabled children have the human right to take part in play and leisure activities and to freely express themselves in cultural and artistic ways. They have the right to equal access to cultural, artistic, recreational and leisure activities	UN Convention on the Rights of the Child, Article 31 Children Act 1989, Schedule 2, Paragraph 8
Disabled children have the human right to live with their parents unless it is not in their best interests. They have the right to services to make it possible for their families to look after them	UN Convention on the Rights of the Child, Article 9 Children Act 1989, Section 17(1)
Disabled children have the human right to express their views and for these to be taken into account. They also have the right to freedom of expression	UN Convention on the Rights of the Child, Articles 12 and 13 Children Act 1989 Guidance and Regulations: Vol. 6, Paragraphs 6.6 and 6.7

Source: Morris (1998b: 9, 10).

Since the Children Act 1989, two key pieces of legislation have been implemented that have the potential to further promote social inclusion: the Disability and Discrimination Act 1999 and the Carers and Disabled Children Act 2000.

At this point in time, do we need new or more policy concerning the social exclusion of disabled children? New policies do not guarantee change in the quality of individuals' lives or, indeed, in service provision and delivery. Whenever research looks at the way policy is implemented across different authorities, considerable differences are found. Some local authorities are making significant progress in improving services to disabled children and, within that, addressing social exclusion (Council for Disabled Children 2000). This suggests the issue is more about the willingness or desire to change and move forward to address social exclusion. There is certainly a job still to be done in educating relevant groups and individuals at local and national levels about disabled children and the imperative that the elimination of social exclusion needs to be prioritized and resourced.

The importance of multi-agency working is highlighted later in this chapter. However, at a national level, the cross-departmental or joint guidance for implementing policy is perceived by managers and practitioners as a powerful tool for promoting multi-agency working at a local level (Beresford and Oldman 2000). There is an argument, however, for legislation and policy guidance about equipment and transport issues needing to be more informed by the disabled children/social exclusion agenda. However, this requires a research base, which at the moment is very limited.

IMPLICATIONS FOR PRACTICE

Morris's (1998b) analysis of the way forward for the role of social care services in promoting and supporting social inclusion for disabled children and young people points to basic areas of change: holistic, needs-led assessment (steered by notions of inclusion and the opportunity to live as normal a life as possible) and changes in the types of service and, therefore, where resources are directed:

> Unfortunately, the most common way that Social Services Departments attempt to meet their obligations towards disabled children is by providing care outside their home, away from their families, in ways which also take children away from their local community. This can be prevented by adopting a needs-led approach to assessment and service provision which also addresses disabling barriers.
>
> (Morris 1998b: 55)

This raises the issue of whether services should continue to be specialized or whether resources should be channelled into improving the accessibility of disabled children and young people to mainstream provision.

Specialist versus mainstream provision

In terms of the debate over specialist versus mainstream social care provision, the available research evidence is inadequate for authoritative statements to be made. What we do know is that focusing resources exclusively on specialist or segregated provision appears to result in different standards being applied for eligibility and access. For instance, disabled children are excluded from mainstream play and leisure services because of inadequate provision and resources, and attendance at specialist play services is rationed. This contrasts with play provision for non-disabled children, which is widely available and 'rationed' to a much lesser extent. The paradox is that disabled children are, under the Children Act 1989, 'children in need' and local authorities have an *obligation* to provide resources for them; local authorities are, in contrast, only given *permission* to provide for non-disabled children who are not 'in need' (Petrie *et al.* 2000). It is also argued that maintaining an emphasis on specialist provision – typically, short-term care services – drains resources that might be more effectively used to develop or adapt community-based services or tackle the disabling barriers in the child's home or local environment.

We also know that disabled children and young people value contact with each other (Barlow and Harrison 1996; Morris 1998a; Beresford and Sloper 1999). Specialist provision, such as short-term residential care and special play schemes, offer opportunities for this sort of contact. Perhaps the issue is more about what is being provided under the specialist provision umbrella – the philosophy, aims and quality of the services on offer and, in particular, the extent to which they seek to achieve social inclusion. For example, a senior practitioner recently told me of her visits to two residential short-term care centres. At the first, no-one was in: the young people were out in the community doing various activities. At the second, the young people were in the centre with very little to do and no opportunities for external activities.

Thus, with respect to the specialist versus mainstream debate at the present time, there is a sense that there is a danger of throwing the baby out with the bathwater. Maybe it is a case of wanting to pull the plug too early. Certainly the research evidence is incomplete, as are the choices and opportunities within mainstream provision.

Multi-agency working

Throughout this chapter, the way that the different needs of children and young people interrelate has been stressed. Social exclusion is not just an issue for social services departments, but one for all local and national government departments. In addition, the examples of transport and housing have been used to illustrate that change or intervention within specific areas will only have limited effects if other aspects or needs of a young person's life remain unchanged. Although responsibility for providing housing and transport services is not generally within the remit of Social Services, the Children Act 1989 stipulates that there is a clear role and responsibility to ensure the needs of disabled children are met. There is, perhaps, a danger of viewing this as a legislative burden, although it can also be seen as a lever for championing and promoting a socially inclusive approach to service provision. In addition, within that process of change must be a commitment to taking a multi-agency approach to resolving the issues that a social inclusion agenda necessarily raises.

Lifting and handling

Finally, it is necessary to draw attention to the increasing impact of the Manual Handling Operations Regulations 1992. Initially, this did not seem to have much impact on community-based services. However, the subsequent development of case law and the Royal College of Nursing's (RCN) guidance on manual handling (1996) has, inappropriately it is argued, begun to have a significant effect on community-based services for disabled children and their families, in particular the provision of family-based short-term care and mainstream play and leisure services. A survey by the Shared Care Network in

2000 (Lenehan 2000) found community-based short-term care services were being suspended or restricted because of moving and handling issues. This is alarming, because the RCN guidelines concentrate almost exclusively on handling ill people in hospital settings rather than individuals with ongoing care needs who live in community settings. A discussion paper issued by the Council for Disabled Children (Lenehan 2000) argues that current practice 'either forces children back into large residential settings or leaves them in unacceptably vulnerable situations'. With respect to the latter, Lenehan provided the example of a child who had been sexually abused by a family member remaining in the home because the local authority did not have any foster carers trained in lifting and handling techniques and with accessible accommodation.

There is clearly a pressing need for practice guidelines and training to be developed for lifting and handling children and adults in community settings based on principles of inclusion, independence and respect. There are also questions about the availability and suitability of design of current equipment (which tends to be static or fixed) for use by disabled children and young people in a range of community settings.

CONCLUSIONS

Tackling social exclusion requires both short- and long-term measures; the domains in which change needs to take place include individual attitudes and behaviours, features of the physical and social environments of local communities and local policy and practice in the way services are provided. Such changes need to be driven and supported by national policy, with legislation and, where necessary, cross-departmental guidance for its implementation (Beresford and Oldman 2000).

In addition, any change must take place within the context of true consultation with all sections of the population of disabled children. We need to know what disabled children want or need to live their lives as they want to live them – the essence, surely, of what social inclusion is all about. The development of new ways of meeting the needs of disabled children and young people has to be subject to rigorous research so that we can answer the questions: what works, for whom and in what circumstances? In addition, and mirroring what is being called for in social care practice, this research should fall within mainstream childhood research. Indeed, some basic comparative work on disabled and non-disabled children's experiences and perceptions would be helpful (Watson and Priestley 1999).

Finally, some of the issues and ideas reported in this chapter are beginning to be addressed – in small ways and at a local level. It shows it can be done. For many of these innovative projects, the challenge will be to roll out pilot 'schemes' into mainstream services. What is important is that systems are put in place so that different agencies and organizations can learn from each other, so that time is not wasted in 'reinventing' the wheel.

REFERENCES

Alderson, P. and Montgomery, J. (1996) *Health Care Choices: Making Decisions with Children*. London: Institute for Public Policy Research.

Barlow, J. and Harrison, K. (1996) Focusing on empowerment: facilitating self-help in young people with arthritis through a disability organisation, *Disability and Society*, 11(4): 539–51.

Beresford, B. and Oldman, C. (2000) *Making Homes Fit for Children: Working Together to Promote Change in the Lives of Disabled Children*. Bristol: Policy Press.

Beresford, B. and Sloper, P. (1999) *The Information Needs of Chronically Ill and Physically Disabled Children and Young People*. York: Social Policy Research Unit, University of York.

Beresford, B., Sloper, P., Baldwin, S. and Newman, T. (1996) *What Works in Services for Families with a Disabled Child?* Barkingside: Barnardo's.

Bochel, C., Bochel, H. and Page, D. (1999) Housing: the foundation of community care?, *Health and Social Care in the Community*, 7(6): 492–501.

Brotherson, M.J., Cook, C.C., Cuconan-Lahr, R. and Wehmeyer, M. (1995) Policy supporting self-determination in the environments of children with disabilities, *Education and Training in Mental Retardation and Developmental Disabilities*, 1: 3–14.

Cavet, J. (1998) *People Don't Understand: Children, Young People and Their Families Living with a Hidden Disability*. London: National Children's Bureau.

Connors, C. and Stalker, K. (2000) 'It's part of me and I quite like me' – children's experience of disability, paper presented to the conference on *Working Together? Supporting Disabled Children and Their Families*, organized by the Joseph Rowntree Foundation and Pavillion, Edinburgh, 16 November.

Cook, C.C., Brotherson, M.J., Weigel-Garry, C. and Muze, I. (1996) Home environments to support children with disabilities, in M. Wehmeyer and D. Sands (eds) *Self-determination Across the Life Span: Theory and Practice*. Baltimore, MD: Brookes.

Council for Disabled Children (2000) *Quality Protects: Second Analysis of Management Action Plans with Reference to Disabled Children and Families*. London: Department of Health.

Crisp, A., Marchant, R. and Jones, M. (2000) *Quite Like Home: What You Told Us about Fairlawn, The Croft and Southdowns. Young People's Views about Residential Respite Care Services in Kent*. Brighton: Triangle and Kent County Council.

Department of Health, Joseph Rowntree Foundation and the Children's Society (2001) *Ask Us!: A CD-Rom Summary of a National Consultation Programme with Disabled Children and Young People*. London: The Children's Society.

Finch, N., Lawton, D., Williams, J. and Sloper, P. (2001) *Disability Survey 2000: Young People with a Disability and Sport*. London: Sport England.

Hine, J. and Mitchell, F. (2001) Better for everyone? Travel experiences and transport exclusion, *Urban Studies*, 38(2): 319–32.

Hirst, M. and Baldwin, S. (1994) *Unequal Opportunities: Growing Up Disabled*. London: HMSO.

Kampman, J. (1997) Relations between adults and children, unpublished seminar paper presented at the *ENSAC 8th International Conference*, Trondheim, Norway, August.

Lenehan, C. (2000) *Lifting and Handling: A Paper for Discussion*. London: Council for Disabled Children.

Lightfoot, J., Mukherjee, S. and Sloper, P. (1999) Supporting pupils in mainstream school with an illness or disability, *Child: Care, Health and Development*, 25(4): 267–83.

Meadows, T. (1992) Transport chains, paper presented at *COMOTRED*, Lyons, June.

Middleton, L. (1999) The social exclusion of disabled children: the role of the voluntary sector in the contract culture, *Disability and Society*, 14(1): 129–39.

Mitchell, W. and Sloper, P. (2001) Quality in services for disabled children and their families: what can theory, policy and research on children's and parents' views tell us?, *Children and Society*, 15: 237–52.

Morris, J. (1998a) *Still Missing? Vol. 1. The Experiences of Disabled Children and Young People Living Away from Their Families*. London: Who Cares? Trust.

Morris, J. (1998b) *Accessing Human Rights: Disabled Children and the Children Act*. Barkingside: Barnardo's.

Morris, J. (1999) *Hurtling into a Void: Transition to Adulthood for Young People with Complex Health and Support Needs*. York: Joseph Rowntree Foundation/ Pavilion.

Mulderij, K.J. (1996) Research into the lifeworld of physically disabled children, *Child: Care, Health and Development*, 22(5): 311–22.

Newton, D. (1997) *Play Choice: Inclusion in the Early Years*, a report on the work of a partnership between Save the Children and Birmingham Social Services. Birmingham: Birmingham City Council and Save the Children.

Noyes, J. (1999) *Voices and Choices. Young People Who Use Assisted Ventilation: Their Health and Social Care and Education*. London: The Stationery Office.

Oldman, C. and Beresford, B. (1998) *Homes Unfit for Children: Housing, Disabled Children and Their Families*. Bristol: Policy Press.

Oswin, M. (1984) *They Keep Going Away: A Critical Study of Short-term Residential Care Services for Children with Learning Difficulties*. London: King's Fund.

Perry, F. (1998) *Children Belong Together: Working Towards the Inclusion of Children and Young People with Disabilities in Their Communities*, a report of the work of the Children's Society's Children in Need Programme. London: The Children's Society.

Petrie, P., Egharevba, I., Oliver, C. and Poland, G. (2000) *Out-Of-School Lives, Out-Of-School Services*. London: The Stationery Office.

Porter, A. (2000) Playing the 'disabled role' in local travel, *Area*, 32(1): 41–8.

Robinson, J. (1997) Listening to disabled youth, *Childright*, 140, October, pp. 5–6.

Royal College of Nursing (1996) *Introducing a Safer Patient Handling Policy*. London: Royal College of Nursing.

Social Services Inspectorate (1994) *Services to Disabled Children and Their Families*. London: HMSO.

Stark, S. (2001) Creating disability in the home: the role of environmental barriers in the United States, *Disability and Society*, 16(1): 37–49.

Thompson, B., Taylor, H. and McConkey, R. (2000) Promoting inclusive play and leisure opportunities for children with disabilities, *Child Care in Practice*, 62: 108–23.

United Nations Committee on the Rights of the Child (1997) general discussion paper on children with disabilities, 6 October (unpublished).

Watson, N. and Priestley, M. (1999) *Life As A Disabled Child: A Qualitative Study of Young People's Experiences and Perspectives*, final project report to ESRC. Leeds: Disability Research Unit, University of Leeds.

8

DAVID UTTING
JULIE VENNARD
SARA SCOTT

Young offenders in
the community

KEY MESSAGES

- Research suggests that community-based programmes generally yield a greater average reduction in recidivism than those in custodial settings.
- Effective interventions with young offenders are:

  - designed to improve personal and social skills;
  - focused on changing behaviour;
  - multi-modal programmes combining several different approaches.

- The more effective programmes:

  - target high- and medium-risk offenders;
  - are well-structured and 'high dosage';
  - challenge ways of thinking as well as behaving;
  - are tailored to an assessment of the needs and risk factors of individuals;
  - address the full range of offending-related problems, including family and environmental factors as well as personal deficits;
  - adhere to agreed objectives and procedures.

- Forms of intervention which show an average increase in recidivism include vocational counselling and deterrent or 'scared straight' programmes, such as shock incarceration.

- Protective factors that reduce the likelihood of reoffending include: strong social and emotional bonds; families and schools sharing beliefs and standards that oppose crime; and opportunities and skills for young people to contribute positively to their community and to receive recognition and praise.
- Optimism about the rehabilitative potential of interventions with young offenders is based largely on research studies that have used systematic review and statistical meta-analysis techniques to explore 'what works'.
- There are, however, considerable gaps and limitations in relation to existing knowledge – particularly in relation to work in Britain – and a need for effective evaluation of current initiatives.

INTRODUCTION

Over the last few years, new opportunities have arisen for better coordinated and less punitive responses to young offenders in Britain. Policy changes, in particular the Crime and Disorder Act 1998, and a new emphasis on the importance of 'joined-up' government have combined to provide a clearer focus on the prevention of offending and reoffending across a range of services. However, successful outcomes can only be assured through careful attention to the effectiveness of interventions aimed at preventing young people from becoming involved in criminal activities and at redirecting young offenders away from further involvement in crime. This chapter provides a summary of the current evidence base in relation to the effectiveness of community-based programmes that target young offenders and those 'at risk' of becoming involved in criminal activities. It suggests that the state of knowledge concerning risk factors, protective factors and effective interventions provides grounds for optimism about the potential for preventing offending and reoffending. However, it also highlights the considerable limitations of existing knowledge, particularly in relation to work in Britain, and the very real need for effective evaluation of current initiatives.

YOUTH CRIME: PATTERNS AND RESPONSES

One in four offenders cautioned by police or found guilty by the courts in England and Wales are aged 10–17 years and the vast majority of their crimes are against property. Eight out of ten young offenders are male (Home Office 1998). The 'peak' age at which young women in a Home Office survey were most likely to commit offences was 16; it was 21 for young men, suggesting, contrary to the received wisdom that young offenders generally 'grow out of crime' in their late teens, that many young men do not in fact desist from such activities until their mid-20s (Graham and Bowling 1995).

Most young offenders who admit their offences are cautioned by the police and it is widely recognized that dealing with first offenders outside the formal court system works well, as most first offenders who are cautioned do not reoffend within two years (Audit Commission 1996). The small percentage of young people who commit crime repeatedly are responsible for a wholly disproportionate number of offences. In the most recent Home Office Youth Lifestyles Survey, 10 per cent of offenders claimed responsibility for committing nearly half of all the offences admitted by respondents (Flood-Page *et al.* 2000).

Since coming to power in 1997, the Labour government has made youth crime a priority. The 1998 Crime and Disorder Act established a statutory principal aim for the youth justice system in England and Wales of preventing offending by children and young people. This aim is consistent with evidence that those who begin offending at an early age are disproportionately likely to become serious and persistent offenders (Yoshikawa 1994; Loeber and Farrington 1998; Rutter *et al.* 1998). Community intervention is seen as playing a major role in the government's programme of reform and the legislation gives youth courts new powers to make orders on reparation and parenting, as well as requiring young offenders to comply with community-based action plans designed to tackle their criminal behaviour. In addition, inter-agency youth offending teams have been established in England and Wales to address the causes of a young persons' offendings and to deliver suitable community-based interventions.

The Youth Justice and Criminal Evidence Act 1999 builds on the ideas concerning restorative justice in the Crime and Disorder Act 1998 by establishing new Youth Offender Panels. These panels are expected to negotiate contracts with offenders convicted for the first time (and their families), the conditions of which may include reparation to victims. An individually tailored package of activities might also include drug or family counselling, unpaid community work and regular school attendance. In addition, the Crime (Sentences) Act 1997 allows the court to impose curfew orders with electronic monitoring on 10- to 15-year-old offenders.

The new panels and the range of interventions available to them bring practice in England and Wales somewhat closer to that of the Scottish Children's Hearing System, which treats offending by children and young people aged 8–15 as primarily a welfare issue. Under this system, conditions 'in the interests of the child' that can be attached to a supervision requirement include restrictions on where the young offender lives, regular school attendance and a possible curfew.

EFFECTIVE INTERVENTIONS

The present climate of cautious optimism about the rehabilitative potential of community sentences follows a period during which many politicians and academics subscribed to the view that, when it came to rehabilitation, 'nothing works' (Martinson 1974; Lipton *et al.* 1975; Brody 1976; Blagg and Smith 1989). This view has been challenged by research studies during the past ten years that have used systematic review and statistical meta-analysis techniques to explore 'what works' in the intervention and rehabilitation of young offenders (Lipsey 1992, 1995; Sherman *et al.* 1997; Lipsey and Wilson 1998).

Meta-analyses of the results from evaluation studies of community-based programmes for young offenders have identified types of intervention that have proved more effective in reducing reoffending than others. In Mark Lipsey's synthesis of the results of 440 evaluations (Lipsey 1992, 1995), 'treatment' groups of young offenders were compared with non-treated 'control' groups. Three types of programme showed an average reduction in recidivism rates of 20 per cent or more: programmes designed to improve personal and social skills; programmes focused on changing behaviour; and multiple service programmes combining several different approaches. Ineffective types of intervention associated with an increase in offending were vocational counselling, outward-bound type programmes and deterrent or 'scared straight' programmes, such as shock incarceration.

In a more recent study, in which Lipsey and Wilson (1998) narrowed their focus to programmes designed for young offenders convicted of serious and violent crimes, a similar pattern emerged. The types of community-based programme found to 'work' for serious and violent young offenders are generally the same as those that show effectiveness with young offenders in general, although the average decrease in recidivism dropped to 12 per cent.

Meta-analysis has also shown that interventions are generally more effective when the implementation is carefully monitored to ensure programme 'fidelity' and where the intervention provided for young offenders is 'high dosage', in that the programme is intensive and sustained over several months. James McGuire (1995) has used the findings from such research to identify some broad principles for improving the effectiveness of programmes:

- *Risk classification*: more effective programmes match the level and intensity of intervention to an assessment of the seriousness of offending and the risk that individual offenders will commit further offences.
- *Criminogenic needs*: when assessing an individual offender's needs, programmes should distinguish between those that support or contribute to offending and those that are more distantly related or unrelated.
- *Responsivity*: programmes work best when they are carefully structured and the learning styles of the offenders and the staff working with them are well-matched. The learning styles of offenders tend to require active, participatory methods of working.

- *Community base*: research suggests that, on balance, community-based programmes yield more effective outcomes than those in custodial settings. The implied advantage of a community setting is that learning takes place in the 'real world' close to the offender's home environment, family and friends. Even so, programmes that incorporate the other principles of effective intervention can reduce offending in any treatment setting (see also Andrews 1995).
- *Intervention modality*: the results of meta-analyses suggest that the most consistently effective programmes are multi-modal, tackling the multiple needs of offenders with multiple services. Programmes are also more effective where their content and methods are skills-oriented, concentrating on problem solving and other personal and social interaction. Approaches with a cognitive or behavioural (or 'cognitive-behavioural') focus also tend to be more effective.
- *Programme integrity*: effective programmes have a clear rationale linking their stated aims to the methods being used. They are adequately resourced to achieve those aims and staff are appropriately trained and supported. Monitoring and evaluation are an integral part of the programme.
- *Dosage*: programmes must be of sufficient intensity and duration to achieve their aims, especially with those who are chronic or serious offenders, or who are at high risk of becoming so.

That rehabilitation programmes are more likely to succeed in reducing reoffending when they are tailored to an assessment of needs and risk factors in the lives of individual young offenders suggests that risk-profiling techniques offer a potentially valuable tool for designing and evaluating programmes as well as matching young offenders to appropriate interventions. In accordance with such an assessment, the Home Office has recently adopted a single risk-assessment instrument ('Asset') for use throughout England and Wales.

Knowledge of the factors in children's lives associated with an increased risk of offending and reoffending is beginning to drive new community-based initiatives, such as 'Communities that Care' (Communities that Care UK 1997). The major risk factors have been identified using evidence from longitudinal research on both sides of the Atlantic (Howell *et al.* 1995; Farrington 1996; Rutter *et al.* 1998). They include:

- *Family factors*: low income; poor parental supervision; harsh or erratic discipline; having parents whose attitude condones antisocial behaviour and law breaking.
- *School factors*: low educational achievement, starting in primary school; aggressive or disruptive behaviour; truancy; a disorganized school.
- *Community factors*: availability of illegal drugs; growing-up in a disadvantaged area with a high population turnover.
- *Individual/peer factors*: hyperactivity and impulsivity; early involvement in crime (under 14); friends involved in crime and/or whose attitude condones law breaking.

Graham and Bowling (1995) have shown that the likelihood of desisting from crime is strongly related to some of these risk factors. According to their self-report study of offending by young people, young men were less likely to desist if they had high rates of previous offending, if siblings, partners or peers had been in trouble with the police, or if they took drugs or drank heavily. Research has also identified protective factors in children and young people's lives which help explain why some young people start to offend, whereas others, in what appear to be equally adverse circumstances, do not. Michael Rutter and others have defined a range of factors that appear to buffer children who are exposed to multiple risks (Garmezy 1985; Rutter *et al.* 1998). Several individual characteristics fall into this grouping, including (female) gender, an outgoing disposition and high intelligence. But so, also, do relationships with family, friends and the wider community. Protective factors include: strong social and emotional bonds; families and schools sharing beliefs and standards that oppose crime; and opportunities and skills for young people to contribute positively to their community and to receive recognition and praise (Howell *et al.* 1995).

PROMISING PRACTICE WITH YOUNG OFFENDERS

Existing evidence of 'what works' and 'what's promising' relies heavily on research carried out in the USA and Canada. Relatively few community-based programmes for young offenders have been convincingly evaluated in Britain. However, a template for the classification of evaluative evidence developed by Lawrence Sherman and colleagues (1997) for the US Congress has been adopted by Home Office researchers in Britain (Goldblatt and Lewis 1998) and provides a way of ranking evaluations according to their design. This template describes as 'promising' programmes found to be effective in at least one non-randomized study of comparable groups (where one participated in a programme and the other did not), but where the certainty is too low to support conclusions that can be generally applied. This chapter includes examples of interventions with young offenders that would at least be classified as 'promising' on the Sherman scale. Also included are programmes which draw heavily on previously evaluated initiatives in Canada and the USA and those which, despite a lack of rigorous evaluation, reflect the evidence and established principles of 'what works'.

Parenting programmes

Inconsistent and harsh discipline, together with inadequate supervision, has been clearly linked with an increased risk of young people becoming young offenders (Farrington 1996; Rutter *et al.* 1998). Poverty and family conflict appear to diminish parental abilities to support and set boundaries for children

(Utting *et al.* 1993). In addition, a trajectory has been observed that links disrupted parenting and severe childhood behaviour problems with early offending (Patterson *et al.* 1998). Parenting skills programmes for parents whose children exhibit such problems in pre-adolescence have achieved positive outcomes (Tremblay *et al.* 1995; Webster-Stratton 1996; Hawkins *et al.* 1999).

In relation to adolescents, 'functional family therapy' and 'multi-systemic therapy' – two interventions evaluated in the USA – have led to behavioural improvements and reduced reoffending among young people mandated to take part, with their parents, by the courts. One evaluation of functional family therapy showed that, in families who had experienced the intervention two-and-a-half years previously, younger siblings were half as likely as those referred to other forms of family therapy (or where there had been no intervention) to have appeared in court (Alexander and Parsons 1973, 1980; Klein *et al.* 1977). An interactive CD-Rom based on functional family therapy called *Parenting Wisely* has been developed and evaluations by the programme's creator are positive (Gordon, in press). This programme is currently being piloted by four UK youth offending teams in the context of the Parenting Order introduced as part of the Crime and Disorder Act 1998 and will be evaluated over a two year period.

Multi-systemic therapy combines family and behavioural therapy strategies with intensive family support services delivered by multidisciplinary teams on call 24 hours a day. One four year study found the re-arrest rate for violent and other offences was substantially lower among participants in this form of therapy than among those randomly allocated to individual therapy (Borduin *et al.* 1995). The apparent success of the programme is attributed to a combination of the content, the focus on behaviour in the context of problematic family relations and delivery at home or in the local community. Given its replicated effectiveness in the USA, multi-systemic therapy deserves to be implemented and evaluated in the UK.

Fostering

Fostering schemes for young offenders build on evidence that parents and 'significant' adults who use positive reinforcement and consistent sanctions can reduce antisocial behaviour by children and young people. Evaluations of a 'Treatment Foster Care' scheme in the USA found that young offenders placed with specially trained and supported foster parents were less likely to be imprisoned subsequently than those given alternative community placements. Recidivist young offenders were less likely to be arrested following fostering than youths placed in 'group care' accommodation (Chamberlain 1998).

There is a growing number of remand fostering schemes in England and Wales which have succeeded in recruiting and retaining foster parents. There are indications that a high proportion of serious and repeat offenders placed on remand with foster parents succeed in staying out of trouble during their placement. An assessment of a community remand project run jointly by NCH

Action for Children and Wessex (Hampshire) youth offending team undertaken by the Dartington Social Research Unit identified the strengths of the scheme as its ability to divert troubled youngsters from custody and to give them a glimpse of a more rewarding, less antisocial lifestyle. Weaknesses included a high rate of first placements breaking down and the adjustment problems that young people faced on returning to their own homes. Even so, it was concluded that the programme had uncovered a 'rich seam' of foster families and established a new and positive model for the development of specialist community services for young offenders (Dartington Social Research Unit 1993).

Cognitive-behavioural interventions

Cognitive-behaviourism is the name given to a range of interventions that recognize that cognitive deficits and inappropriate ways of behaving are rooted in the social conditions affecting individual development (McGuire 1996). The main components of cognitive-behavioural programmes are typically behaviour modification, moral reasoning enhancement and training in social skills, self-instruction ('inner speech'), social problem solving and anger control. Combined 'multi-modal' programmes are increasingly favoured.

Meta-analyses and other reviews of evaluation studies have identified cognitive-behavioural approaches as among the most consistently effective community-based programmes in reducing recidivism among young offenders, including those involved in serious and violent crime. For example, in an analysis of programmes for young offenders, Lipsey (1992) concluded that those which were skills-oriented and used concrete behavioural techniques had the most impact within and outside the juvenile justice system; typically, a 10–16 per cent reduction in recidivism against matched control groups. Similarly, Lösel (1995) estimated from an overview of meta-analytic studies that programmes which yielded the best results with young offenders (on average a reconviction rate 10 per cent lower than for a matched control group) were cognitive-behavioural, skills oriented and 'multi-modal'.

Despite the widespread use of cognitive-behavioural programmes with young offenders in the UK, there have been few rigorous evaluations of their content and effectiveness. Where programmes have been subject to independent evaluation, the number of participants has tended to be too small for reliable statistical analysis of differences in reconviction rates compared with comparison groups.

Notwithstanding the limitation of sample size, however, evaluations of two intensive programmes in Scotland, which take a multi-modal, skills-oriented and cognitive-behavioural approach, show promising results (see Jamieson 1998; Lobley et al. 2001). Both the Inverclyde and Freagarrach projects targeted persistent offenders at high risk of receiving a custodial sentence or a secure accommodation order. The Freagarrach project, managed by Barnardo's, has adopted a strong multi-agency approach. In the year after they started to attend Freagarrach, the overall rate of offending by the young people decreased by between 20 and 50 per cent. The programme involved constant contact with committed staff, individualized work programmes and an accepting and caring culture.

Education, training and employment

Research has consistently linked educational under-achievement and a lack of commitment to school to an increased risk of offending and of reoffending (Graham and Bowling 1995). In the light of this, several programmes in the UK seek to reintegrate juvenile offenders and 'at risk' youth into mainstream schooling or involve them in further education, training or employment. Little evidence is available concerning their effectiveness.

An evaluation of the Apex CueTen programme in Scotland suggests that programmes based on multi-agency partnerships can engage persistent young offenders and sustain their involvement. However, the evaluation highlighted the importance of staff being adequately prepared for the range of family and social problems that young people bring with them (Lobley and Smith 1999). The extent to which such programmes have a long-term influence over employment and reoffending may depend on how well young people are supported once their involvement with the programme has ended.

Mentoring

Mentoring programmes are increasingly popular as a way of offering friendship and non-judgemental support through frequent contact with an adult or older peer who serves as a role model. In Britain, there are several mentoring programmes working with young people referred for poor school attendance and antisocial behaviour, including young offenders. These include the Dalston Youth Project run by Crime Concern and projects supported by the Divert Trust, such as the Nottingham-based 'Lifting the Exclusion Zone' that works with African-Caribbean youth from three inner-city schools. In the absence of more rigorous evaluation, there is some evidence from 'before and after' monitoring of arrest rates of reoffending being reduced (Webb 1997).

Another mentoring scheme, 'Youth at Risk', has worked in partnership with local authorities and probation services in several areas to deliver a 12 month programme for 14- to 19-year-olds whose problems in terms of emotional adjustment and behaviour are especially severe. Participants typically include a high proportion of young people who have been 'looked after' by the local authority and recidivist offenders. A somewhat controversial feature of the programme is its use of an intensive, one-week residential programme where participants are encouraged to confront difficult personal issues, including antisocial behaviour. This leads to a nine month 'follow-through' period when participants meet regularly with their volunteer mentors ('committed partners') and work towards personal goals, including school attendance, qualifications and employment. They also attend weekly group sessions concerned with personal development and topics such as anger management, problem solving, drug misuse and sexual health. Monitoring suggests reductions in the numbers of participants involved in drugs and crime and in the frequency of offending during the course. However, there has been no independent evaluation of 'Youth at Risk' on which issues such as its longer-term effectiveness and the use of 'confrontation therapy' can be assessed (Utting 1996; Day 1998).

Evaluation in the USA shows that mentoring programmes do address some of the major risk factors associated with offending and can help to reduce reoffending. However, research messages are clouded by the fact that studies have focused on 'at risk' youth or on mixed groups of 'at risk' youth and young offenders. There is also cautionary evidence that mixing groups of convicted offenders with 'at risk' youth as part of a mentoring scheme can have negative consequences for the latter in terms of offending (O'Donnell 1992). Evidence from one study suggests that mentoring programmes are more likely to change antisocial behaviour if they include contingencies – rewards that depend on good behaviour and weekly targets being met (Fo and O'Donnell 1974).

A physical focus

Leisure pursuits, sports and other demanding physical activities are popular and prominent components in a range of programmes for young offenders in Britain, but have been subject to very little independent evaluation (Coalter 1988; Taylor *et al.* 1999). The hope is that such activities will foster socially valued skills, increase self-esteem, self-discipline, responsibility and respect for rules, provide acceptable outlets for energy and frustration and thereby reduce offending behaviour.

Lipsey and Wilson's (1998) meta-analysis identified 'wilderness' and outdoor challenge programmes among the least effective types of intervention programmes for serious and violent young offenders, whether in community or institutional settings. A review by Jon Barrett (1996) cites American programmes showing some reduction in the frequency and severity of offending, but found little research concerned with longer-term outcomes. One exception was a project in the 1960s, where the impact appeared greater for late-onset offenders with fewer convictions than for recidivists (Kelly and Baer 1971; Baer 1975). Reoffending declined in the short term for a participation group compared with a matched control group, but less so over five years. Other reviews of programmes in the USA and New Zealand found that some outdoor adventure programmes had reduced reoffending, but could have done better if short-term effects were reinforced by follow-up programmes in the community (Winterdyk and Griffiths 1984; Fyfe 1990, cited in Barrett 1996; McKay 1993).

A study of demanding physical activity programmes carried out for the Home Office (Taylor *et al.* 1999) emphasizes the need for schemes to have a clear rationale and for participants to spend enough time on the programme for personal and social development objectives to be reached. Its proposals for a best practice 'toolbox' include high-speed referrals to minimize the risk of drop-out and arrangements for continuing the learning process once participants have completed the programme. Indications that demanding physical activities may work best as ingredients of multi-modal interventions are, meanwhile, supported by what is known about Fairbridge, a national programme that includes a 'wilderness' expedition.

Fairbridge is a national voluntary organization working in partnership with youth justice, probation and other statutory agencies from 11 urban centres. Its aims are to foster core personal and social skills, including self-awareness, negotiation and goal setting, among young people 'at risk'. Participants aged 14–25 are brought together in groups that deliberately mix young people from different backgrounds, including offenders and non-offenders. One in five participants are probation clients. The programme is voluntary and includes a two day induction followed by a one-week basic course. They transfer to a residential centre where teams take part in climbing, canoeing, abseiling, orienteering and other outdoor pursuits. Follow-through takes place in the community when young people are helped by a staff mentor to prepare and implement a personal development plan, including goals such as desisting from offending, gaining educational or training qualifications or finding a job. Workshops and group activities are arranged, as well as opportunities to participate in further outdoor and constructive leisure pursuits.

While no rigorous evaluation of Fairbridge has yet been conducted using comparison groups, research by Kent Probation Service into reoffending among clients referred to Fairbridge suggests that 48 per cent committed further offences compared with a predicted rate of 85 per cent (Whitfield 1995).

Motor projects

Widely used by the probation service, youth justice and the voluntary sector, motor projects typically provide training in car mechanics and may include the restoration of old vehicles that can be used for 'banger' racing. A survey of probation-run programmes (Martin and Webster 1994) found that most were challenging the offending behaviour of participants in group sessions which utilized McGuire and Priestley's (1985) sourcebook of cognitive-behavioural techniques.

The impact of motor projects on reoffending is unclear, since few have been independently evaluated. Difficulties in assessing their effectiveness arise from such factors as the wide variation in the age of participants, poor record keeping and the short duration of the project. A reconviction study based on motor projects surveyed by the Home Office (Martin and Webster 1994) reported that almost 80 per cent of offenders who took part were reconvicted within two years, the vast majority of them for further motoring offences. A second reconviction study based on the long-established Ilderton Motor Project in London, which used matched groups of participating and non-participating offenders, produced more promising results (Wilkinson and Morgan 1995;

Wilkinson 1997). However, neither of these studies provide any information about the factors which contributed to, or detracted from, success, such as the age range and offending background of participants and the components of the programme. It may be, for example, that motor projects have the greatest impact when combined with group work on offending behaviour, victim awareness, driving and the law.

Restorative justice

Restorative justice has evolved as a means of 'diverting' repeat offenders from the formal criminal justice system. Its primary aims are to attend to the needs of victims, enable offenders to assume responsibility for their actions and involve families and the wider community in preventing reoffending. Marshall (1998) describes restorative justice as 'a problem-solving approach which involves the parties themselves and the community generally in an active relationship with statutory agencies' (p. 5).

In practice, restorative justice schemes may involve one or more meetings between victims and offenders to reach agreement as to the form that reparation might take. It could involve an apology, an explanation as to how the behaviour came about, or a plan to make good the losses or harm caused by the crime. The offender may also agree to make a financial payment to the victim or undertake some form of work for the victim or for the community. Not all 'restorative justice' schemes so named prioritize face-to-face contact between perpetrators and their victims. Those that do not tend rather to rely on general 'victim awareness' sessions and initiatives in which offenders write letters of apology. Meetings do, on the other hand, enable victims to express the full emotional impact of the offence to those responsible, while bringing home to offenders the harmful consequences of their behaviour. At the same time, offenders can be offered support to tackle the problems associated with their offending. It is, however, crucial that meetings between victims and offenders are facilitated by skilled, trained mediators whose impartiality is protected.

Family group conferences give greater priority to tackling offending behaviour and its causes than is usually the case with victim–offender mediation. A key purpose of family group conferences is to agree a plan of rehabilitation for the offender and to engage the support of family and other influential acquaintances in helping the offender to stay out of trouble. Family group conferences are allied to the concept of 'reintegrative shaming' by which offenders are encouraged to experience shame for their behaviour in the context of efforts to reintegrate them into the community (Braithwaite 1989). This is contrasted with the stigmatizing and alienating shame resulting from prosecution in court.

Under the Crime and Disorder Act 1998, courts in England and Wales must consider imposing reparation orders on young offenders in all cases where they do not impose a compensation order. The new Action Plan Order, a three month intensive programme of community intervention, may include reparation. Reparation should also be considered as an element of the police 'final warning' that replaces cautioning for young offenders following a first or second offence. Moreover, from April 2000, all first-time offenders who plead guilty in the youth courts in a number of pilot areas will be referred to Youth Offending Panels. Under the Youth Justice and Criminal Evidence Act 1999, these panels will agree the contract terms with young offenders and their families, that include a strong element of apology and reparation. The panels are likely to be implemented throughout England and Wales by 2003.

Victim–offender mediation can take place at different stages of the criminal process. Some schemes, such as that undertaken by the Northamptonshire Diversion Unit, take the form of a pre-court 'Caution Plus'. Others are court-based, as with schemes in Leeds, Coventry and Wolverhampton, where mediation is taken into account in sentencing. Evaluation of both approaches suggests they are generally welcomed by victims and cost considerably less than a successful prosecution (Marshall and Merry 1990; Hughes *et al.* 1996). Unfortunately, there is a shortage of evidence concerning the effects of any restorative justice programmes on reoffending. Available research casts doubt on the ability of mediation or conferencing to influence recidivism unless they result in action to tackle relevant risk factors in the lives of individual offenders. The most recent evaluation of seven UK programmes (five of these young offender programmes) commissioned under the Crime Reduction Programme found clear evidence of success in reducing reoffending in only one programme, that undertaken by the West Yorkshire Victim Offender Unit, which works with serious adult offenders. There was no evidence that any of the youth offending schemes had any impact on rates of recidivism (Miers *et al.* 2001). It should, however, be noted that the schemes examined were very uneven in their provision and:

> Many schemes operated with few paid staff, relying upon volunteers and a few, key charismatic individuals. The work they were doing was, in most cases, non-statutory; so there was no requirement for offenders (and, of course, victims) to become involved. Finally, one of the adult schemes was almost entirely inactive due to cuts in resources, while most of the juvenile schemes were severely disrupted by preparations for the introduction of Youth Offending Teams (YOTs) in Spring, 2000.
>
> (Miers *et al.* 2001: vii)

The Thames Valley scheme operated by the police is subject to a major three year evaluation funded by the Joseph Rowntree Foundation, results of which will not be available until April 2002.

DISCUSSION

The Crime and Disorder Act 1998 in England and Wales has established a new framework for a multi-agency youth justice system where the statutory principal aim is prevention. As the accompanying Home Office framework document explains:

> Action to prevent children and young people offending should not start or finish with the youth justice system. The first objective of any youth crime reduction strategy should be to stop children and young people ever becoming involved in crime.
>
> (Home Office 1998)

In pursuit of this, it lays down six key objectives:

1 The swift administration of justice so that every young person accused of breaking the law has the matter resolved without delay.
2 Confronting young offenders with the consequences of their offending, for themselves and their family, their victims and the community and helping them to develop a sense of personal responsibility.
3 Intervention which tackles the particular factors (personal, family, social, educational or health) that put the young person at risk of offending and which strengthens 'protective factors'.
4 Punishment proportionate to the seriousness and persistence of the offending.
5 Encouraging reparation to victims by young offenders.
6 Reinforcing the responsibilities of parents.

These objectives acknowledge the accumulating evidence that criminality is preventable and that rehabilitation can be made to work. The 'what works' movement has succeeded in promoting the need for evidence-based policy, although its very success in disseminating the principles of effective practice has, at the same time, highlighted the limitations of existing knowledge.

In addressing the question 'What works in community-based programmes for young offenders?', this chapter has frequently referred to reviews using the statistical techniques of meta-analysis to assess the strength of various approaches that have been evaluated. These show that, across the board, rehabilitative programmes with young offenders have achieved recidivism rates that are a modest improvement over 'treatment as usual'. The most effective community-based programmes have done considerably better, achieving average reductions in recidivism at least 20 per cent lower than the rates for control groups (Lipsey 1992, 1995).

Meta-analytic studies necessarily produce broad-brush findings with regard to the ingredients of successful interventions; more needs to be known about the content, duration and intensity of programmes that have most impact and the most effective combinations of programmes to be placed on the menu within 'multi-modal' packages. Although some practitioners are experienced and undoubtedly skilled in working with young women offenders and young ethnic minority offenders, there is little research literature concerning promising approaches with these groups. There is also more to be learned about which kinds of programme are most appropriate with offenders in different age groups and posing different levels of risk of offending. For example, further research is needed to unravel the finding that 'individual counselling' has only modest and inconsistent effects in community programmes for all types of young offenders (Lipsey 1992), yet is shown to be among the most effective interventions for those guilty of serious and violent offences (Lipsey and Wilson 1998).

Although research has not identified any one approach as suitable for all young offenders, there are clear indications that programmes that follow what are now widely termed the 'what works' principles can reduce reoffending. Generally speaking, the more effective programmes:

- target high- and medium-risk offenders;
- are well-structured;
- use an approach that challenges ways of thinking as well as behaving;
- address the full range of offending-related problems, including family and environmental factors as well as personal deficits;
- adhere to agreed objectives and procedures.

One major review of crime prevention studies allocated their findings to four categories, depending on the rigour of the evaluation and whether the results had been confirmed by further studies (Sherman *et al.* 1997). As a rule of thumb, the resulting 'What works', 'What doesn't work', 'What's promising' and 'What's unknown' are salutary, not least in highlighting the negative evidence concerning punitive programmes, such as 'boot camps' using military basic training and 'shock' incarceration programmes. Simple checklists are less helpful where the key to effective (or ineffective) practice lies in the detail. In the case of community mentoring, for example, there has been a succession of American evaluations yielding unimpressive results (Howell *et al.* 1995). One study did suggest that mentoring can reduce reoffending when a consistent system of contingent rewards and sanctions is applied (Fo and O'Donnell 1974). But the results from a replication reveal some negative effects for unconvicted young people 'at risk' when grouped together in a programme with young offenders (O'Donnell 1992). Too bald a view of this evidence could either lead to the rejection of mentoring, on the basis of too many inconclusive evaluations, or its endorsement on the basis of the one positive study involving young offenders.

The problem is more basic in the UK, where very few programmes have been adequately evaluated in the first place. Small numbers of participants and limited duration (often due to short-term funding) have been common features of projects, contributing to the lack of an evaluation 'culture' in Britain. Few evaluations of UK programmes included a comparison group to increase confidence that positive (or negative) outcomes were attributable to intervention. Future studies should be large enough to achieve high standards in terms of sampling and research design if they are to yield findings that can be generalized.

Outcome evaluations need to gather information on reconviction rates, preferably over a period of two years or more. But they also need to look for any changes in attitudes towards offending behaviour and problems associated with offending, as varied as improved literacy or reduced drug dependence. Process evaluation is also essential to ensure that programmes are being implemented as intended, to identify any difficulties in achieving objectives and to understand which ingredients and delivery methods are most successful. Few of the evaluations reviewed in this chapter go beyond 'what works' to why and how it works. Future evaluations need to identify the 'active ingredients' which, in certain contexts, influence and enable particular young offenders and their families to make different choices.

Central government has an important part to play – a fact that is currently acknowledged by the £250 million Crime Reduction Programme. Projects funded, with an in-built commitment to evaluation, include:

- early interventions to reduce the risks of young people from becoming involved in crime;
- action on social conditions that foster crime;
- intervention with offenders under community supervision or in custody to ensure that reoffending is reduced.

In addition, the Youth Justice Board is funding the youth offending teams in England and Wales to develop parenting support, mentoring, education, training and employment and cognitive-behavioural and restorative justice programmes. Development money has also been provided for bail supervision and support schemes in which mentoring and remand fostering are expected to play a prominent part (Youth Justice Board 1999). This broadly reflects the evidence concerning the most promising approaches. Recognition of the influence of families on adolescent antisocial behaviour is especially appropriate given the evidence that young offenders are more likely to improve their cognitive skills and to learn socially acceptable ways of behaving when parents and siblings are involved in the programme.

That current knowledge concerning 'what works' and 'what's promising' relies heavily on programmes delivered and evaluated in North America inevitably raises issues relating to the different structural and cultural contexts. Factors as varied as the availability of firearms, a higher minimum age for purchasing alcohol, a lower minimum age for driving motor vehicles, the existence of a gang culture and heavier use of custody may mean that promising community-based programmes in the USA are not altogether transferable. Their effectiveness in Britain cannot be assumed without further evaluation.

Moves to devise more reliable screening of the risks presented by individual young offenders raise the possibility that meaningful evaluation could become a routine and relatively straightforward procedure. Instruments such as 'Asset', developed for the Youth Justice Board by the Probation Studies Unit at Oxford University's Centre for Criminological Research, can be used as a 'before' measurement of a range of criminogenic risk factors. Progress in preventing reoffending and reducing its associated risks can be measured by repeating the assessment 'after' young offenders have completed the programme. Widespread use of a screening tool would, in turn, generate a national database whose 'normative' prediction scores could provide a reliable and accessible benchmark for the effectiveness of local programmes.

The advantages that better screening promises to confer on evaluation are really a by-product of its greatest potential benefit, which is an improved ability to match individuals with interventions most likely to prevent (re)offending. Careful targeting of high- and medium-risk offenders requires effective systems for assessing the level of risk posed by individuals. The risk of reconviction can already be predicted with a fair degree of accuracy on the basis of type of offence, age, sex and previous offending history. But such indicators fail to take account of the personal and social problems associated with juvenile offending. Research suggests that these risk factors and 'criminogenic needs' must be recognized if programmes are to have any lasting, rehabilitative impact. Young people at high risk of reoffending tend to experience a wide variety of problems and disadvantages, including family dislocation, failure at school, drug and alcohol dependence. Such problems, if left unaddressed, are liable to undermine any long-term benefit from cognitive-behavioural and other interventions. Improved assessment instruments should not only result in more effective targeting, but also improved tailoring in terms of the different 'packages' that can be assembled within multi-modal programmes for individual offenders. They will help to plug the gaps in current knowledge about the optimum duration and intensity of the various components. They will also help the courts and those who supervise young offenders to move away from any simple equation between the immediate offence and the appropriate intervention. A young man guilty of 'joy riding' could, for example, present a level of risk and criminogenic need that a motor project would be wholly incapable of meeting.

The prize that better screening could eventually deliver is the ability to identify and provide effective early intervention for the relatively small group of young offenders at risk of becoming chronic, serious or violent adult criminals. As Rolf Loeber and David Farrington (1998) point out in their review of knowledge concerning the latter two categories, serious and violent juvenile offenders tend to develop a range of behaviour problems from childhood and to commit numerous delinquent acts in addition to more serious offences. The offences that first bring them to the attention of the youth justice system may, therefore, give little hint of the risk that they pose, unless additional screening is available.

The best available evidence may not, for the most part, be home grown. But it does justify genuine excitement about the potential not only for preventing reoffending, but also for making it less likely that children and young people will turn to crime in the first place. In the USA, research knowledge concerning risk factors, protective factors and effective intervention is already being brought together in support of the Comprehensive Strategy for Serious, Violent and Chronic Juvenile Offenders (Office of Juvenile Justice and Delinquency Prevention 1995). The Communities that Care programme is the US government's preferred model for achieving neighbourhood action to reduce risks and enhance protection for children in the relevant domains of family, school and the wider community. This holistic approach to prevention is already being piloted in more than 25 locations in the UK (Communities that Care UK 1997).

Opportunities are being created in Britain for a less punitive, but similarly seamless approach. The crime prevention potential of support services, such as the Sure Start programme for pre-school children in disadvantaged neighbourhoods, is explicitly acknowledged. Similarly, youth justice policy has been given an unequivocal focus on prevention. Community-based programmes are poised to assume new prominence in the treatment of young offenders as use of secure accommodation is restricted to the most serious or persistent. In the long term, success may ensure fewer victims of crime, lower costs of crime and fewer troubled young people whose law-breaking drives them deeper into social exclusion. But success is far from assured unless careful attention continues to be paid to evidence concerning what really works with young offenders.

REFERENCES

Alexander, J.F. and Parsons, B.V. (1973) Short-term behavioral intervention with delinquent families: impact on family process and recidivism, *Journal of Abnormal Psychology*, 18: 219–25.

Alexander, J.F. and Parsons, B.V. (1980) *Functional Family Therapy*. Monterey, CA: Brooks/Cole.

Andrews, D.A. (1995) The psychology of criminal conduct and effective treatment, in J. McGuire (ed.) *What Works? Reducing Reoffending*. Chichester: Wiley.

Audit Commission (1996) *Misspent Youth: Young People and Crime*. London: Audit Commission.

Baer, D.J. (1975) Instruction ratings of delinquents after outward bound survival training and their subsequent recidivism, *Psychological Report*, 36: 547–53.

Barrett, J. (1996) *A Review of Research Literature Relating to Outdoor Adventure and Personal and Social Development with Young Offenders and Young People at Risk*. Ravenglass: Foundation for Outdoor Adventure.

Blagg, H. and Smith, D. (1989) *Crime, Penal Policy and Social Work*. London: Longman.

Borduin, C.M., Mann, B.J., Cone, L.T. *et al.* (1995) Multisystemic treatment of serious juvenile offenders: long-term prevention of criminality and violence, *Journal of Consulting and Clinical Psychology*, 63(4): 560–78.

Braithwaite, J. (1989) *Crime, Shame and Reintegration*. Cambridge: Cambridge University Press.

Brody, S. (1976) *The Effectiveness of Sentencing*, Research Study No. 35. London: Home Office.

Chamberlain, P. (1998) *Treatment Foster Care*, Juvenile Justice Bulletin, December. Washington, DC: Office of Juvenile Justice and Delinquency Prevention.

Coalter, F. (1988) *Sport and Anti-Social Behaviour*, Research Report No. 2. Edinburgh: Scottish Sports Council.

Communities that Care UK (1997) *Communities That Care: A New Kind of Prevention Programme*. London: Communities that Care UK.

Dartington Social Research Unit (1993) *Taking Forward Specialist Services for Young Offenders: The Hampshire Young Offender Community Support Scheme*. Totnes: Dartington Social Research Unit.

Day, M. (1998) *An Evaluation of the Youth At Risk Programme on behalf of Smith's Charity and the Linbury Trust*. London: Centre for Youth Work Studies, School of Education, Brunel University.

Farrington, D.P. (1996) *Understanding and Preventing Youth Crime*. York: Joseph Rowntree Foundation.

Flood-Page, C., Campbell, S., Harrington, V. and Miller, J. (2000) *Youth Crime: Findings from the 1998/1999 Youth Lifestyles Survey*, Research Study No. 209. London: Home Office.

Fo, W.S.O. and O'Donnell, C.R. (1974) The buddy system: relationship and contingency conditioning in a community intervention program for youth with nonprofessionals and behavior change agents, *Journal of Consulting and Clinical Psychology*, 42: 163–9.

Garmezy, N. (1985) Stress-resistent children: the search for protective factors, in J.E. Stevenson (ed.) Recent Research in Developmental Psychopathology, supplement to the *Journal of Child Psychology and Psychiatry*, 4: 213–33.

Goldblatt P. and Lewis, C. (eds) (1998) Annexe A, in *Reducing Offending: An Assessment of Research Evidence on Ways of Dealing with Offending Behaviour*, Research Study No. 187. London: Home Office.

Gordon, D.A. (in press) Intervening with troubled families: functional family therapy and parenting wisely, in J. McGuire (ed.) *Treatment and Rehabilitation of Offenders*. Chichester: Wiley.

Graham, J. and Bowling, B. (1995) *Young People and Crime*, Research Study No. 145. London: Home Office.

Hawkins, J.D., Catalano, R.F., Kosterman, R., Abbott, R. and Hill, K.G. (1999) Preventing adolescent health risk behaviors by strengthening protection during childhood, *Archives of Pediatrics and Adolescent Medicine*, 153: 226–34.

Home Office (1998) *Youth Justice: The Statutory Principal Aim of Preventing Offending by Children and Young People*. http://www.homeoffice.gov.uk/cdact/youjust.html (accessed 28 July 2001).

Howell, J.C., Krisberg, B., Hawkins, J.D. and Wilson, J.J. (1995) *A Sourcebook: Serious, Violent & Chronic Juvenile Offenders*. London: Sage.

Hughes, G., Pilkington, A. and Leisten, R. (1996) *An Independent Evaluation of the Northamptonshire Diversion Unit*. Milton Keynes: The Open University.

Jamieson, J. (1998) *Evaluation of the NCH Inverclyde Intensive Probation Unit*. Stirling: Social Work Research Centre, University of Stirling.

Kelly, F.J. and Baer, D.J. (1971) Physical challenge as a treatment for delinquency, *Crime and Delinquency*, 17: 437–45.

Klein, N.C., Alexander, J.F. and Parsons, B.V. (1977) Impact of family systems intervention on recidivism and sibling delinquency: a model of primary prevention and program evaluation, *Journal of Consulting and Clinical Psychology*, 45: 469–74.

Lipsey, M.W. (1992) Juvenile delinquency treatment: a meta-analytic inquiry into the variability of effects, in T.D. Cook, H. Cooper, D.S. Cordray *et al.* (eds) *Meta-analysis for Explanation: A Casebook*. New York: Russell Sage Foundation.

Lipsey, M.W. (1995) What do we learn from 400 research studies on the effectivenes of treatment with juvenile delinquents?, in J. McGuire (ed.) *What Works: Reducing Re-offending*. Chichester: Wiley.

Lipsey, M.W. and Wilson, D.B. (1998) Effective intervention for serious juvenile offenders: a synthesis of research, in R. Loeber and D.P. Farrington (eds) *Serious and Violent Juvenile Offenders: Risk Factors and Successful Interventions*. London: Sage.

Lipton, D., Martinson, R. and Wilks, J. (1975) *The Effectiveness of Correctional Treatment: A Survey of Treatment Evaluation Studies.* New York: Praeger.

Lobley, D. and Smith, D. (1999) *Working with Persistent Juvenile Offenders: An Evaluation of the Apex CueTen Project.* Edinburgh: The Scottish Office Central Research Unit.

Lobley, D., Smith, D. and Stern, C. (2001) *Freagarrach: An Evaluation of a Project for Persistent Juvenile Offenders*, Crime and Criminal Justice Research Findings No. 53. Edinburgh: Scottish Executive Central Research Unit.

Loeber, R. and Farrington, D.P. (eds) (1998) *Serious and Violent Juvenile Offenders: Risk Factors and Successful Interventions.* London: Sage.

Lösel, F. (1995) Increasing consensus in the evaluation of offender rehabilitation? Lessons from recent research syntheses, *Psychology, Crime and Law*, 2: 19–39.

Marshall, T. (1998) *Restorative Justice: An Overview*, unpublished Paper for the Home Office. London: Home Office.

Marshall, T. and Merry, S. (1990) *Crime and Accountability: Victim–Offender Mediation in Practice.* London: HMSO.

Martin, J.P. and Webster, D. (1994) *Probation Motor Projects in England and Wales.* Manchester: Home Office.

Martinson, R. (1974) 'What works? Questions and answers about prison reform, *The Public Interest*, 10: 22–54.

McGuire, J. (ed.) (1995) *What Works: Reducing Re-offending.* Chichester: Wiley.

McGuire, J. (1996) *Cognitive-Behavioural Approaches: An Introductory Course on Theory and Research*, Course Manual. Liverpool: Department of Clinical Psychology, University of Liverpool.

McGuire, J. and Priestley, P. (1985) *Offending Behaviour: Skills and Stratagems for Going Straight.* London: Batsford.

McKay, S. (1993) Research findings related to the potential of recreation in delinquency intervention, *Trends*, 30(4): 27–30.

Miers, D., Maguire, M., Goldie, S. *et al.* (2001) *An Exploratory Evaluation of Restorative Justice Schemes, Final Report.* London: Home Office.

O'Donnell, C.R. (1992) The interplay of theory and practice in delinquency prevention: from behavior modification to activity settings, in J. McCord and R.E. Tremblay (eds) *Preventing Antisocial Behavior: Interventions from Birth Through Adolescence.* New York: Guilford Press.

Office of Juvenile Justice and Delinquency Prevention (1995) *Guide for Implementing the Comprehensive Strategy for Serious, Violent, and Chronic Juvenile Offenders.* Washington, DC: OJJDP.

Patterson, G.R., Forgatch, M.S., Yoerger, K.L. and Stoolmiller, M. (1998) Variables that initiate and maintain an early-onset trajectory for juvenile offending, *Development and Psychopathology*, 10: 531–47.

Rutter, M., Giller, H. and Hagell, A. (1998) *Antisocial Behavior by Young People.* Cambridge: Cambridge University Press.

Sherman, L., Gottfredson, D., MacKenzie, D. *et al.* (1997) *Preventing Crime: What Works, What Doesn't, What's Promising: a Report to the United States Congress.* Washington, DC: US Department of Justice, Office of Justice Programs (www.ncjrs.org. or www.preventingcrime.org).

Taylor, P., Crow, I., Irvine, D. and Nicholls, G. (1999) *Demanding Physical Activity Programmes for Young Offenders Under Probation Supervision.* London: Home Office.

Tremblay, R.E., Pagani-Kurtz, L., Mâsse, L.C., Vitaro, F. and Pihl, R.O. (1995) A bimodal preventive intervention for disruptive kindergarten boys: its impact through mid-adolescence, *Journal of Consulting and Clinical Psychology*, 63(4): 560–8.

Utting, D. (1996) *Reducing Criminality Among Young People: A Sample of Relevant Programmes in the United Kingdom*, Research Study No. 161. London: Home Office.

Utting, D., Bright, J. and Henricson, C. (1993) *Crime and the Family: Improving Child-rearing and Preventing Delinquency*, Occasional Paper No. 16. London: Family Policy Studies Centre.

Webb, J. (1997) *Dalston Youth Project Programmes 1, 2 and 3 for Young People Aged 15–18 Years: Summary of the Evaluations*, report prepared for Crime Concern and the Dalston Youth Project. Nottingham: Janice Webb Research.

Webster-Stratton, C. (1996) Early intervention for families of preschool children with conduct problems, in M.J. Guralnik (ed.) *The Effectiveness of Early Intervention: Second Generation Research*. Baltimore, MD: Paul H. Brookes.

Whitfield, D. (1995) Partners in crime, article in the Fairbridge magazine *Challenger*.

Wilkinson, J. (1997) The impact of Ilderton Motor Project on motor vehicle crime and offending, *British Journal of Criminology*, 37(4): 568–81.

Wilkinson, J. and Morgan, D. (1995) *The Impact of Ilderton Motor Project on Motor Vehicle Crime and Offending*. London: Inner London Probation Service.

Winterdyk, J. and Griffiths, C. (1984) Wilderness experience programmes: reforming delinquents or beating around the bush?, *Juvenile and Family Court Journal*, 35(3): 35–44.

Yoshikawa, H. (1994) Prevention as cumulative protection: effects of early family support and education on chronic delinquency and its risks, *Psychological Bulletin*, 115(1): 28–54.

Youth Justice Board (1999) *Invitations to Tender*. http://www.youth-justice-board.gov.uk/grants.html (accessed 28 July 2001).

DIANA McNEISH
TONY NEWMAN

Involving children and young people in decision making

KEY MESSAGES

- The involvement of children and young people has become an increasingly important trend, promoted by a series of policy initiatives.
- There is a growing body of research and practice literature providing important lessons for effective processes of participation.
- There are several models of participation that differentiate between approaches on the basis of the amount of power that is shared or transferred.
- Approaches to involvement need to be informed by the context in which it is taking place; that is, for the individual child and for children and young people collectively.
- There are some common themes emerging from research and practice which suggest that the following issues are important:

  - addressing the attitudinal barriers to participation;
  - creating participatory structures and processes;
  - achieving inclusive participation;
  - encouraging motivation.

- Although there has been a burgeoning of research and practice literature in recent years, there are still some important gaps, including a lack of information on whether participation is having an impact on outcomes.

INTRODUCTION

The involvement of children and young people as active participants in decision making has become an increasingly important trend. There is a move from a wholly paternalistic approach to welfare towards one which recognizes that organizations providing services have a responsibility to involve the people that use them. Early approaches to participation focused largely on adults based on the assumption that, by involving parents or concerned adults, the best interests of children would automatically be served. This is much the same attitude taken towards women and voting at the start of the twentieth century. Today, it is widely acknowledged that the involvement of children and young people as participants in their own right is equally important. The debate has moved on from *whether* to involve children and young people to *how* such involvement can be achieved and *what* approaches are most appropriate in which situations. A series of policy developments have placed firm expectations on planners and service providers to involve children and young people in the decisions that affect their lives.

This chapter reviews the evidence from research and practice addressing 'what works' in involving children and young people. Although there has been a burgeoning research (as well as policy and practice) interest in this area, few studies have systematically evaluated the processes of participation. There has been even less research on the outcomes of participation. Current evidence can tell us a little about what seems to work best in the process of engaging children and young people in decision making; it can tell us virtually nothing about whether the outcomes for children are better as a result of their engagement. But participation is such a fundamental human right that we can assume for the purposes here that engagement in the processes, as a first step, is worthwhile. After all, we do not need to evaluate the outcomes for individuals or society to conclude that universal suffrage is a good thing. Nevertheless, there are several topics it would be good to have researched in more depth, including the impact of participation on the effectiveness of services.

For the moment, the research evidence we have is largely exploratory and descriptive, providing accounts of different approaches to participation and their perceived advantages and disadvantages from the point of view of the main stakeholders. The value of this growing body of evidence should not be diminished. From knowing virtually nothing a few years ago, we now have sufficient information from research and practice to make some confident assertions about the factors to be addressed in planning and implementing participatory approaches to service development and delivery. This chapter aims to summarize these lessons.

WHAT IS PARTICIPATION AND WHY IS IT IMPORTANT?

The reasons for involving children and young people range from the moral to the political and pragmatic. The growth of participation can be traced through several parallel developments:

1 *The growth of the power of the 'consumer'.* From the 'Patients Charter' to 'Best Value', the voice of the service user has become central to modernizing public services.
2 *Pressure from young people's user groups.* Early attempts to involve user groups frequently failed to hear the voices of the most marginalized and disadvantaged groups. This was particularly true for children and young people until groups such as NAYPIC (National Association of Young People in Care) began to challenge assumptions about young people's capabilities. Supported by a growing number of children's rights advocates, young people's pressure groups gradually had an impact on policy.
3 *The United Nations Convention on the Rights of the Child.* Article 12 sets out the rights of children and young people to express their views about anything which affects them and there are a number of other articles in the Convention (for example, concerning the rights to freedom of conscience and religion) asserting the rights of children to hold views independently of adults. The Convention has probably had its greatest impact as a rallying point for children's rights advocates who have used it to keep young people's participation firmly on the policy agenda.
4 *The Children Act 1989 and subsequent inquiry reports.* Implemented in 1991, the Children Act for England and Wales made it a legal requirement for the views of young people to be taken into account in any decision affecting them. The importance of listening to young people has been reinforced by successive inquiries into the abuse of children, particularly those in the looked after system. A recurring theme of these has been the failure of adults to listen to young people. This concern has led to an interest in more effective ways of empowering young people as a protective strategy, central to the Quality Protects initiative, which aims to transform both the management and delivery of social services for children and requires mechanisms for children's and young people's views to be heeded.
5 *The growth of 'citizenship' as a policy issue.* Government commitment to a 'stakeholder democracy' and the resurgence of interest in the concept of citizenship has contributed to a search for new ways of involving young people as members of their communities and as citizens, such as the development of youth councils and youth parliaments.

In addition to the above providing a policy push for participation, there are several other incentives to promote the involvement of children and young people. Writers such as Cooper (1993), Davie and Galloway (1996), Gersch (1996), Treseder (1996) and Hennessy (1999) have highlighted the benefits of participation for organizations and for young people themselves. It is argued that participation: enables resources to be targeted more effectively – it can avoid wasting time and money on services young people don't want to use; improves quality; gives young people greater ownership and commitment to services; and enhances skills of adults involved in planning and providing them. For children and young people, involvement helps them to support and positively influence each other, provides opportunities for them to gain experience, skills and confidence and encourages young people to take responsibility and control of their own lives. It is also argued that participation benefits society more generally. As Lansdown (1995) has pointed out, participation is essential for a healthy society:

> Participation is a fundamental right of citizenship. The creation of a society which combines a commitment to respect for the rights of individuals with an equal commitment to the exercise of social responsibility must promote the capacity of individuals from the earliest possible age, to participate in decisions that affect their lives.
>
> (Lansdown 1995: 4)

The drawbacks of participation are mainly practical. It is generally acknowledged that involving young people in decision-making processes takes time, involves developing new skills for adults and young people, requires an investment of resources, can entail a major shift of attitude on the part of organizations and, like any process of negotiation, it can make decision making slower.

Some commentators have also drawn attention to some potential risks of participation for young people. Examples include: imposing responsibilities for which young people have not been prepared; exposing them to over-intensive peer pressure; involving them in tasks for which they do not have the confidence or skills; involving them in public presentations or media activities where they have not fully understood the possible implications; and involving them in project activities to the exclusion of other interests in their lives. These risks are not inherent in participation itself, but can result from ill-conceived or poorly planned processes. It is not difficult to envisage these disadvantages occurring when service providers are exhorted to involve children and young people without the necessary time and resources to do it properly.

WHAT IS PARTICIPATION?

All of the above begs the question of 'what is participation?' As Boyden and Ennew (1997) point out, there are two interpretations of the term 'participation'. It can mean simply 'taking part in', or being present; or it can mean a form of empowerment, having a real say in decisions. Although it is primarily the second definition of participation with which we are concerned, the first is by no means easy to achieve, particularly when working with excluded groups. Some disabled children and young people, for example, lack the opportunity even to participate in everyday activities, as amply illustrated by Bryony Beresford in this book.

Several writers have developed typologies of participation (Arnstein 1969; Brager and Specht 1973). These models have recently been adapted to the participation of children and young people by Hart (1992, 1997), Thoburn *et al.* (1995) and Shier (2000), neatly summarized in the Quality Protects Research Briefing by Sinclair and Franklin (2000). These models generally make hierarchical distinctions between approaches according to the amount of *power* sharing. However, successful participation is not simply a matter of organizations being willing to share their power with young people and allow them to have a voice. It also involves young people themselves making a *choice* to get involved. Participation is a two-way process.

Most of the principles of participation apply both to adults and young people, but there are some extra considerations in the involvement of young people:

- *The impact of adult attitudes* and the assumptions made about young people's capabilities and what they should and should not get involved in.
- *Relative power.* Socially and legally young people do not have the same amount of autonomy as adults.
- *Changing interests and capacities.* Young people change more rapidly than adults; what is appropriate for a young person aged 12 may not be the same as for a 15-year-old.
- *Time is experienced differently.* A year may be regarded as a realistic timescale for action within an organization; it is likely to feel like a lifetime to many young people.

Hart (1992, 1997) highlights four common examples of non-participation:

- *Manipulation*: where adults involve children or their work to illustrate an adult point of view.
- *Deception*: where adults, with good intentions, deny their own involvement in a project because they want others to think that it was done entirely by young people.
- *Decoration*: where children are used to promote a cause but have little notion of what the cause is about and no involvement in organizing the event.
- *Tokenism*: this often occurs when adults are keen to give young people a voice without thinking through the implications. Examples include the involvement of children at an event without adapting the proceedings to enable meaningful participation, and the selection of young people to sit on panels or committees with little opportunity for them to consult with the peers whom they are supposed to represent. Here, young people are performing a symbolic function. Their presence serves to reassure adults present that their views are being taken into account without any meaningful attempt to actually do so.

Drawing from the models developed by Hart and others, it is possible to identify five levels of genuine participation:

Levels of genuine participation

Information. Adults retain full control over the planning and implementation of a project; young people are involved purely as recipients of services. The value of providing good information should not be diminished, as it enables young people to make informed choices about whether or not a service is appropriate for them.

Providing information is the minimum level of participation and is a prerequisite of good practice. The main issue is to ensure that it is the right information reaching the right young people.

Consultation. Adults retain control over the planning and implementation of a project but do so while taking into account the views of young people. Consultations can occur before something is set up to inform its development, during the life of a project to ensure it is meeting young people's needs or when a project has ended as part of a closing evaluation.

Consultations have become a popular means of involving young people and there are different ways of carrying them out. The main issue is to ensure that the approach taken is fit for the purpose by asking the right questions of the right young people. A consultation done badly (or over-consulting young people) can be as bad as not consulting at all.

Representation. Adults set up a project but involve some young people in planning and/or running it. This may or may not be accompanied by a consultation with a wider group of young people.

Representation often involves the inclusion of some young people on a steering group or management committee. The main issues to consider are how young people are selected (for example, whether they are chosen by adults or by their peers) and whether they are truly expected to represent the views of a wider group of young people or simply put forward their own viewpoints. In reality, it is often not feasible to expect young people to represent the views of others.

Partnership. Where projects are developed in partnership, adults and young people work together to plan and run the project. Partnership denotes a degree of real power sharing, so young people should be involved in all the key decisions of the project, including the financial ones.

There are a growing number of examples of partnership initiatives, many of which started as adult-led but gradually moved towards an increased sharing of power and responsibility between adults and young people. The main issues are which young people are involved and how power and responsibility are shared.

Self-management. Projects that are self-managed by young people may be initiated by adults or young people, but ultimately they are planned and managed by young people themselves. They may choose to engage the help of adults or to employ adults to run aspects of the project for them.

There are few examples of fully self-managed projects and those that exist are often fairly small. This is hardly surprising given the practical and financial obstacles involved for young people who wish to run a project independently of adults. However, there are increasing numbers of projects where the balance of control has shifted away from adults towards young people or where aspects are fully self-managed.

One danger of models of participation, particularly those presented as ladders or hierarchies, is that they can imply that all projects should aspire to the highest level. Several writers (e.g. Treseder 1996) have argued this interpretation is a mistake. Participation needs to be appropriate to its context and take account of the issues involved, the objectives sought and the young people who make up the target group. Different kinds of participation might be appropriate for different parts of a project or at different stages in its development.

THE DIFFERENT CONTEXTS OF DECISION MAKING

It is important to distinguish between involving young people in decisions about their lives as individuals and their participation in issues affecting young people collectively. The different contexts of participation can be summarized as follows:

- *Participation in individual decision making*: the involvement of individual young people in reaching decisions about aspects of their own lives. This is particularly relevant when considering the involvement of children in giving consent for medical treatment, in decisions about where children should live and with whom (after a divorce, for example) and in reviewing the care plans of children looked after.
- *Participation in service development and provision*: the involvement of young people individually or collectively as consumers of services. Young people can plan, shape, deliver or evaluate services at different levels.
- *Participation in research*: the involvement of young people in research as consultants, commissioners or researchers. Young people can formulate the questions to form the basis of a consultation exercise, design questionnaires or conduct interviews. We do not discuss these areas here, though there is now a collection of material providing ethical and practical guidance to those intending to involve young people in research (Alderson 1995; Morrow and Richards 1996; Boyden and Ennew 1997; McAuley 1998; Kirby 1999; Christensen and James 2000).
- *Participation in communities*: the involvement of young people as members of a neighbourhood community or community of interest. This dimension is explored in more depth by Gary Craig in this book.

- *Participation in influencing policy or public awareness*: the involvement of young people in shaping and delivering messages to the public or policy makers via their participation in campaigning groups, involvement with the media, and so on.

These contexts are not mutually exclusive. However, when exploring the resources and skills required on the part of organizations, workers and young people themselves, it is worth considering the context and purpose of participation. The challenges are different for young people making decisions about their individual lives to those encountered by young people participating at the community or civic levels and different strategies are required to overcome them.

PARTICIPATION IN INDIVIDUAL DECISION MAKING

There are many sets of circumstances in which young people participate in decisions affecting their lives as individuals, including decisions taken at home within the family. The participation rights of children within the family are frequently overlooked, although as Lansdown (1997) points out: 'Ultimately, if we are to challenge the low status of children in our society, their vulnerability to abuse, exploitation and neglect and create a social environment of respect for children, it is with the family that we must start' (p. 138). The ambivalence with which children's rights within the family are regarded is illustrated by the reaction of many adults to the campaign to remove the rights of parents to smack their children.

Morrow's (1998) research on children's perspectives on family life suggests that children themselves are aware that decision making in families can be complex. Some children involved in the research felt that they had a say in family decision making, others did not. Morrow points out that even young children could understand and talk about the notion of 'rights' and being listened to, and that although some children reflected that they would like a say in the process of decisions, they did not necessarily want ultimate control or to make decisions on their own. This is supported by a survey of young people's social attitudes, which found that the majority of young people accept the age-related restrictions on their autonomy (Newman 1996). There is a growing body of research exploring the discourses of family life and the ways in which the autonomy of children and young people is negotiated (Mayall 1994; Brannen and O'Brien 1996). Other research is shedding light on how children are involved in decisions following parental separation and divorce (Neale and Smart 1998). Such research may be overlooked by social care professionals, yet it has some important lessons for those trying to work with families at times of crisis. The research which is beginning to emerge on family group conferencing is starting to draw these lessons together (Connolly and McKenzie 1999).

For people working in the field of social care, the decisions faced by and for children are often extremely difficult, frequently involving a lot of adults, sometimes including circumstances where the views and interests of children and young people are different to those of parents and professional carers. Examples include a child being asked to consent to medical treatment, a young person looked after by the local authority involved in reviewing their placement, and a decision being made in court about where a young person should live and with whom.

We know that attempts to involve young people in such decisions sometimes go wrong. This can be because the adults concerned are not sufficiently committed to the participation of children, or they don't know how to involve children properly, or because the decision-making processes and structures make it very difficult for children to be fully involved. This is illustrated by research by Thomas and O'Kane (1998) of children and decision making in the looked after system. They found that, although children are now more likely to participate in decision-making meetings, there is still considerable variation, with some children being totally excluded, others simply told of the outcome and some invited but without preparation and support. Older children were more likely to be involved in decision-making meetings than younger ones. Advocacy was rarely available to children. Yet the children involved in this study wanted to be given more opportunities to have their say and to be listened to. Thomas and O'Kane's research echoes the findings of others, including Gardner (1987), who considered children's involvement in reviews, and Schofield and Thoburn (1996), whose study focused on involvement in child protection decisions.

An overview of research literature, especially that concerning children looked after (Wheal and Sinclair 1995; Willow 1996; Grimshaw and Sinclair 1997; Hill 1997; Horgan 1998; Thomas and O'Kane 1998), enables us to highlight important factors in involving young people in individual decision making (see box opposite).

PARTICIPATION IN SERVICE DEVELOPMENT, PROVISION AND EVALUATION

Children and young people collectively are now more frequently involved in identifying needs and in planning services. This may be done through consultation processes with young people from the target group of the service or through the more active involvement of young people working alongside planners. Many agencies providing services to young people now involve young people in an advisory or management capacity. A common example is the involvement of young people on management or advisory committees. These may be exclusively of young people or mixed groups of adults and young people. Other ways in which young people can be involved in managing projects are in selecting staff, writing project policies and giving presentations on the work of the project.

Key factors in individual decision making with young people

- The importance of *information* for children and young people to make an informed decision.
- *Time and explanation* for children to properly understand the issues.
- Ongoing *consultation*: decision making is a process not to be confined to the one-off meeting.
- The availability of *support* for the young person to talk through options in a non-judgemental environment.
- *Appropriate settings* for decision making that are accessible, comfortable, private and appropriate to the young person's culture. Many children find the usual style of meetings uncomfortable.
- If a young person is to be involved making decisions with adults present, opportunities should be made available for him or her to *prepare* beforehand and talk things through afterwards.
- *Even-handedness* in the handling of differences of view, for example between the young person and a parent or other adult.
- Attention to the *child's own priorities*, which may be different to the adults concerned and may be regarded as less significant than those of adults.
- Access to an *advocate* or supporter to help a child represent their point of view.
- Attention to *any special needs* a child may have, including communication needs.
- The importance of *feedback* and discussion on the outcomes of decisions. This is particularly important, since many children, although they feel listened to, often feel that their views have little impact on the outcomes of decisions.

There are now a growing number of established practice examples where young people are involved in the development and evaluation of services. These include care leavers carrying out reviews of local authority provision (Hazlehurst 2000), young people involved in the education and training of staff (Boylan *et al.* 2000) and young people directly providing support to other young people (Rhodes 2000). Although, on the whole, the voluntary sector was the first to enter the field, with early accounts of participatory practice emerging mainly from organizations such as Save the Children and The Children's Society, statutory organizations are rapidly catching up with some creative examples from such diverse areas as Kirklees (Pickford 1996), Milton Keynes (Morgan 1999) and the London Borough of Camden (McGee 2001). Many of these initiatives have benefited from a voluntary/statutory partnership and it has been noted that voluntary agencies can have an important role as a catalyst for participation and in sustaining developments over time (McNeish *et al.* 2000).

Reviews of different approaches to involving children and young people in service delivery (Cohen and Emanuel 1998; McNeish 1999; McNeish *et al.* 2000; Alpeki 2001) enable us to identify some common themes and lessons emerging from practice:

- *The need to develop the skills and confidence of staff.* If participation is to become a mainstream rather than a marginal activity, then it cannot be left to a few participation 'experts' who have the confidence and skills to work with young people in this way.
- *The need to develop skills for children and young people.* Young people also need preparation and training to be effective in their role.
- *Providing motivation and reward.* We deal with this theme later in the chapter.
- *Building in the links with decision makers.* To be effective in bringing about change, there has to be commitment at a senior level and there needs to be regular active links with the people who ultimately have the power.
- *Addressing organizational culture, structures and processes.* These are often very adult-focused but some are more conducive to the involvement of children.

Where young people are involved as direct providers of services, reviews of different approaches (Cohen and Emanuel 1998; McNeish *et al.* 2000) highlight the following lessons:

- The importance of clarity of expectations and boundaries.
- The need to equip young people with the information and training they need to carry out their role.
- The importance for young people of having access to sufficient support.
- Asking the 'what if' questions: do young people know who to go to if they are concerned about something or something is going wrong?
- Building in motivating factors to attract and retain young people's involvement.
- Ensuring that young people have the required time and commitment to see the job through.
- Planning ahead to train other young people so that the service does not rely too heavily on the same group.
- Addressing confidentiality issues, especially where young people may have access to sensitive information about peers.

YOUNG PEOPLE AS MEMBERS OF COMMUNITIES AND AS CITIZENS

Young people may be members of a geographical community (or neighbourhood) or a community of interest, although 'community involvement' often refers to the first of these. In the past, community participation tended to focus on the role of adults. The interests of young people may have been addressed but these were often identified and mediated via parents. Recently, there has been more emphasis on the direct involvement of young people in communities and in urban regeneration, and there are now several recorded examples at a local level (see, for example, McGee 2001) in addition to a growing number of reports and articles providing guidance as well as practice examples (Wellard *et al.* 1997; Kitchin 2000; Speak 2000). The different considerations needed to involve young people in communities were highlighted by Fitzpatrick *et al.* (1998), who concluded that:

- The level of support needed to sustain young people's involvement is greater than that needed for adults. This requires substantial resources and dedicated staff time.
- The participation of young people should be scheduled early in the life of a project to allow young people enough time to develop the skills and confidence to become effective participants.

There have also been several reviews of approaches to promote participation in local governance (Willow 1997) and some attention to the pros and cons of various structures, such as youth forums and councils (Fitzpatrick *et al.* 1998; Matthews *et al.* 1998).

A synthesis of the research and practice literature on the collective involvement of young people suggests the following issues are important.

THE ELEMENTS OF EFFECTIVE PARTICIPATORY PROCESSES

Addressing attitudinal barriers

Attitudes to young people's participation hinge on beliefs about:

- the competence of young people to participate as autonomous individuals;
- how young people develop competence with age and maturity;
- rights versus protection, in particular about young people's vulnerability and adult responsibilities to safeguard and protect them.

One reason for the failure to involve children is a prevalent adult belief that children are not competent to make difficult decisions. Alderson's work (1993) on children's consent to surgery challenges this. She concludes that very young children can be capable of making wise choices.

Adults' beliefs about the capabilities of young people can be inconsistent and contradictory, particularly on sensitive topics. Organizations wishing to engage the participation of young people need to understand their values and assumptions. Health and social care organizations historically have been steeped in values emphasizing the vulnerability of young people. These often live on in current organizational culture and pose hidden barriers to participation.

One of the challenges facing social workers and others is that they are working with some of the most vulnerable children and young people and they somehow have to balance the participation rights for young people with their own responsibilities to provide care and protection. The need for such a balance is recognized within both the UN Convention and the Children Act 1989. Achieving the balance is difficult and will be recognized by any parent or worker who has tried to encourage a young person to make their own decisions, while protecting them from the potentially harmful outcomes of risky behaviour.

As well as the attitudes of adults, the attitudes of children and young people can help or hinder involvement. Young people may have fixed views about adults as out of touch, not really interested, not to be trusted, and so forth. If adults and young people are to work together, some time may need to be set aside to explore these attitudes and generate a positive relationship.

Creating more participatory structures and processes

Most organizations are adult-focused and function with hierarchical structures and processes not naturally lending themselves to the active participation of young people. Even where organizations have made an overt commitment to greater participation, the required shift in processes, systems and values often fails to occur. The common consequence is workers who are highly committed to participation operating in the face of very persistent, and sometimes hidden, organizational barriers.

Research that has looked at recent practice suggests that getting the processes right involves the following elements:

Creating participatory processes

1 *Clarifying objectives.* Organizations and individuals need to be clear about why they are seeking participation, what they want it to achieve and what level of participation is appropriate. These aims need to be agreed with participants and revisited at regular intervals so that progress can be evaluated. There needs to be honesty about which decisions are open to change and which are not. If an issue is not negotiable, it is important to say so from the start.
2 *Setting a realistic time-scale.* Participation is not a quick fix; it involves planning and preparation. In all likelihood, a participatory approach will take longer than you think, especially at first.
3 *Meetings or what?* Adult decision making tends to occur in meetings. This may not be the best means of engaging with young people. If meetings are to be used, issues to be considered include their timing and location, the way in which they are conducted and the provision of opportunities for participants to get to know each other and feel

comfortable and confident. Ensuring that young people have an opportunity to influence the agenda is important, as is providing them with the support and information to get to grips with the issues to be discussed and consult with other young people. It is particularly important to have sufficient numbers of young people present at meetings; having a couple of young people amidst a sea of adults is not likely to constitute meaningful participation.

4 *Investing resources*. Participation needs to be underpinned by the resources to provide training, support and skill development for both staff and young people. Some of the practical barriers to participation have financial implications: the costs of transport, child care, providing resources and equipment for groups, ensuring that young people are compensated for their time and effort.

5 *Providing support to staff*. Participation requires commitment from all parts of the organization, not just staff in direct contact with young people. Front-line staff need to know that they have the organizational backing to work in more participatory ways.

6 *Providing support to young people*. Young people require support, information and skill development to help them become active participants. Issues to consider include ensuring that information is shared with young people, avoiding jargon and finding ways to communicate information that does not rely entirely on written formats.

7 *Building in involvement as soon as possible*. Participation can often be a bit of an afterthought or it can be tempting to get something started by adults with a view to bringing young people on board later. This can make it very difficult for young people to shape decisions, as it is usually harder to make changes once something has started. Early involvement can appear risky to adults, who may not want to raise expectations or subject young people to the uncertainties of plans in their infancy.

Achieving inclusive participation

Young people are not a homogeneous group. Just as generalizations about 'young people' need to be avoided, similar care needs to be applied before generalizing about groups of young people who share particular characteristics, such as age, gender, ethnicity, sexual orientation or disability. Nevertheless, some consideration needs to be given to how some young people's experience of participation is affected by these factors and experiences of past exclusion. Some studies provide insights into the issues to be addressed in involving excluded groups (Morris 1998), but there is still a considerable research gap. There is also much more research and practice experience relating to older children and young people than younger children, although some accounts are beginning to emerge (Day Care Trust 1998). If organizations are serious about reducing the social exclusion of young people, then ensuring that *all* young people are enabled to participate is an essential prerequisite. As Bryony Bereford illustrates in her chapter in this book, the failure to heed the participation rights of disabled children, for example, is having enormous and permanent negative consequences.

Motivating young people to be involved

One of the challenges facing organizations seeking to involve young people is to motivate their involvement. Young people have competing pressures on their time and being involved in service development for a local authority or voluntary organization may not be top of their list of priorities.

Practice experience and research seeking the views of young people suggests that there are several important factors in motivating young people's involvement. Research by ourselves and our colleagues (McNeish *et al.* 2000) has elicited a number of ideas from young people about what motivated their involvement:

Encouraging motivation

1 *The issue needs to be relevant and important*: fairly obviously, young people are more likely to get involved in an issue they see as important. Unfortunately, adults and young people do not always share the same priorities.
2 *The activities need to be interesting and fun*: a fairly common comment from young people who have been active participants is that meetings set up by adults are often boring. Although staff are paid to be bored in meetings and tend to get used to some occupational tedium, we do need to find the fun factor if young people are to stay on board.
3 *Young people need to get some personal benefit*: young people who have got involved in participatory activities frequently cite personal satisfaction as a key motivator. Satisfaction can come from knowing you are making a difference, having your voice heard, learning new skills, meeting new people and getting valuable experience that will help in future life and career choices. Adults can make a difference by considering what their young participants might want from the experience and taking steps to facilitate it.
4 *Incentives and rewards are important*: some participatory projects pay young people to be involved or provide other incentives such as tokens and cinema tickets. Payment can be important in helping to reach some young people and should always be considered when adults are being paid for similar services. However, payments are not the only incentive – a trip or a meal out for the group as a 'thank you' can be valued just as much.

---

5 *Young people need to feel valued and respected*: this is probably the most important motivating factor. Young people are very rapidly put off if they gain the impression that they are only there to make up the numbers or if their views are not really being listened to. This can frequently occur when adults, usually unintentionally, take over an event or meeting and the young people are gradually ignored. This often leads to young people withdrawing or becoming disruptive, but can usually be avoided if adults afford young people the same respect as they would other adults. Conversely, research has consistently shown how much young people appreciate genuine respect from adults.

6 *There needs to be results*: people of all ages want to see results for their efforts, but young people in particular can become demotivated if they do not see something changing as a consequence of their involvement. This presents a challenge to projects working towards longer-term outcomes, so it is important to build in some tangible results at the earlier stages.

7 *There needs to be feedback*: if short-term results aren't possible, young people still need to be given feedback about what will happen next and how their work will be used. This might mean being prepared to re-contact young people some time after their involvement to let them know what has happened.

CONCLUSIONS

In recent years, there has been a rapid growth in interest in how to involve children and young people in decision making and this has been reflected in the growing number of research reviews and practice accounts. These provide some important lessons for the development of young people's participation both individually and collectively. There are still some major gaps in the research (and in practice), including ways of involving younger children and socially excluded groups. Although we now know quite a lot about the processes of involvement, research into the outcomes of involvement is needed. Over the next few years, we need to consider whether the involvement of children and young people, in addition to being important in its own right, is actually having a beneficial impact on policy and practice development.

REFERENCES

Akpeki, T (2001) *Guide to Board Development: Involving Young People*. London: National Council for Voluntary Organizations.
Alderson, P. (1993) *Children's Consent to Surgery*. Buckingham: Open University Press.

Alderson, P. (1995) *Children, Ethics and Social Research*. Barkingside: Barnardo's.

Arnstein, S. (1969) Eight rungs on the ladder of citizen participation, *Journal of the American Institute of Planners*, 35(4): 216–24.

Boyden, J. and Ennew, J. (1997) *Children in Focus: A Manual for Participatory Research with Children*. Stockholm: Radda Barnen.

Boylan, J., Dalrymple, J. and Ing, P. (2000) Let's do it! Advocacy, young people and social work education, *Social Work Education*, 19(6): 553–63.

Brager, C. and Specht, H. (1973) *Community Organising*. New York: Columbia University Press.

Brannen, J. and O'Brien, M. (eds) (1996) *Children in Families*. London: Falmer Press.

Christensen, P. and James, A. (eds) (2000) *Research with Children: Perspectives and Practices*. London: Falmer Press.

Cohen, J. and Emanuel, J. (1998) *Positive Participation: Consulting and Involving Young People in Health-related Work – A Planning and Resource Guide*. London: Health Education Authority.

Connolly, M. and McKenzie, M. (1999) *Effective Participatory Practice: Family Group Conferencing in Child Protection*. New York: de Gruyter.

Cooper, P. (1993) Field relations and the problem of authenticity in researching participants' perceptions of teaching and learning in classrooms, *British Educational Research Journal*, 19: 323–38.

Davie, R. and Galloway, D. (1996) The voice of the child in education, in R. Davie and D. Galloway (eds) *Listening to Children in Education*. London: David Fulton.

Day Care Trust (1998) *Listening to Children: Young Children's Views on Child Care – A Guide for Parents*. London: Day Care Trust.

Fitzpatrick, S., Hastings, A. and Kintrea, K. (1998) *Including Young People in Urban Regeneration: A Lot to Learn?* York: Policy Press/Joseph Rowntree Foundation.

Gardner, R. (1987) *Who Says? Choice and Control in Care*. London: National Children's Bureau.

Gersch, I. (1996) Listening to children in educational contexts, in R. Davie, G. Upton and V. Varma (eds) *The Voice of the Child: A Handbook for Professionals*. London: Falmer Press.

Grimshaw, R. and Sinclair, R. (1997) *Planning to Care: Regulation, Procedure and Practice Under the Children Act 1989*. London: National Children's Bureau.

Hart, R. (1992) *Child's Participation: From Tokenism to Citizenship*. London: UNICEF International Child Development Centre.

Hart, R. (1997) *Children's Participation: The Theory and Practice of Involving Young Citizens in Community Development and Environmental Care*. London: UNICEF Earthscan Publications.

Hazlehurst, M. (2000) The involvement of young people in service development, *Representing Children*, 13(1): 15–23.

Hennessy, E. (1999) Children as service evaluators, *Child Psychology and Psychiatry Review*, 4(4): 153–61.

Hill, M. (1997) Participatory research with children, *Child and Family Social Work*, 2: 171–83.

Horgan, G. (1998) Involving children and young people in care planning, *Research Policy and Planning*, 16(3): 16–22.

Kirby, P. (1999) *Involving Young Researchers*. York: Joseph Rowntree Foundation.

Kitchin, H. (ed.) (2000) *Taking Part: Promoting Children and Young People's Participation for Safer Communities*. London: Local Government Information Unit.

Lansdown, G. (1995) *Taking Part: Children's Participation in Decision-making.* London: IPPR.

Lansdown, G. (1997) Children's civil rights in the family, *Child Care in Practice*, 4(2): 138–48.

Matthews, H., Limb, M., Harrison, L. and Taylor, M. (1998) Local places and the political engagement of young people: youth councils as participatory structures, *Youth and Policy*, 62: 16–29.

Mayall, B. (ed.) (1994) *Children's Childhoods Observed and Experienced.* London: Falmer Press.

McAuley, C. (1998) Child participatory research: ethical and methodological considerations, in D. Iwaniec and J. Pinkerton (eds) *Making Research Work: Promoting Child Care Policy and Practice.* Chichester: Wiley.

McGee, F. (2001) *Involving Young People in Community Safety.* London: London Borough of Camden Housing Department.

McNeish, D. (1999) *From Rhetoric to Reality: Participatory Approaches to Health Promotion with Young People.* London: Health Education Authority.

McNeish, D., Downie, A., Newman, T., Webster, A. and Brading, J. (2000) *The Participation of Children and Young People.* London: Lambeth, Southwark and Lewisham Health Action Zone.

Morgan, D. (1999) *Children and Young People's Rights and Participation: Implementing the UN Convention on the Rights of the Child in Milton Keynes.* Milton Keynes: Children's and Young People's Rights Service.

Morris, J. (1998) *Accessing Human Rights: Disabled Children and the Children Act.* Ilford: Barnardo's.

Morrow, V. (1998) *Understanding Families: Children's Perspectives.* London: National Children's Bureau/Joseph Rowntree Foundation.

Morrow, V. and Richards, M. (1996) The ethics of social research with children: an overview, *Children and Society*, 10: 90–105.

Neale, B. and Smart, C. (1998) *Agents or Dependants? Struggling to Listen to Children in Family Law and Family Research*, Working Paper No. 3. Leeds: Centre for Research on Family Kinship and Childhood, University of Leeds.

Newman, T. (1996) Rites, rights and responsibilities, in H. Roberts and D. Sachdev (eds) *Young People's Social Attitudes.* Barkingside: Barnardo's.

Pickford, J. (1996) *Youth Leisure Link Evalution Report.* Kirklees: Kirklees Metropolitan District Council/IYCE (Involving Young Citizens Equally).

Rhodes, J. (2000) *Friends: Supporting Young People*, progress report November/December 2000, Barnardo's Signpost Project, Wakefield: Ilford: Barnardo's.

Schofield, G. and Thoburn, J. (1996) *Child Protection: The Voice of the Child in Decision-making.* London: Institute of Public Policy Research.

Shier, H. (2000) Pathways to participation: openings, opportunities and obligations, *Children and Society*, 14: 111–17.

Sinclair, R. and Franklin, A. (2000) *Young People's Participation, Quality Protects Research Briefing.* London: Department of Health.

Speak, S. (2000) Children in urban regeneration: foundations for sustainable participation, *Community Development Journal*, 35(1): 31–40.

Thoburn, J., Lewis, A. and Shemmings, D. (1995) *Paternalism or Partnership? Family Involvement in the Child Protection Process.* London: HMSO.

Thomas, N. and O'Kane, C. (1998) *Children and Decision Making – A Summary Report.* Swansea: University of Wales Swansea.

Treseder, P. (1996) *Empowering Children and Young People.* London: Save the Children.

Wellard, S., Tearse, M. and West, A. (1997) *All Together Now: Community Participation for Children and Young People.* London: Save the Children.

Wheal, A. and Sinclair, R. (1995) *It's Your Meeting: A Guide to Help Young People Get the Most from Their Reviews.* London: National Children's Bureau.

Willow, C. (1996) *Children's Rights and Participation in Residential Care.* London: National Children's Bureau.

Willow, C. (1997) *Hear! Hear! Promoting Children and Young People's Democratic Participation in Local Government.* London: Local Government Information Unit.

PART 3

Promoting and protecting children's health

The World Health Organization has defined health as 'a complete state of physical, mental and social well-being'. This final section endorses an holistic understanding of health and addresses the well-being of children in three discrete but overlapping areas:

- the protection of children from abuse or neglect;
- the promotion of children's well-being through what can be broadly described as public health strategies; and
- the support that may be given to families by helping children overcome emotional and behavioural problems.

Our knowledge of what contributes to children's health and well-being has proved rather more extensive than our ability to bring it about. A speculator in the stock market of child welfare, who measured the return on their investment by gains in the physical, mental and social well-being of children, would have had mixed fortunes over the past half century. Shares in interventions that reduce mortality and physical morbidity would have performed strongly. Stock in the prevalence of child abuse can be best described as volatile. Most worryingly for our imaginary investor, children's emotional well-being has been something of a bear market, as the psychosocial health of children appears to have been in steady decline for several decades. This is particularly disappointing given that the political environment in which this degradation has taken place has been increasingly responsive to children's apparent needs. Children, by most objective measurements, have been placed more at the heart of the social agenda than at any other time in history. And yet up to a fifth of children may experience diagnosable emotional and behavioural disorders. This tide is unlikely to be reversed, as the contributors to this section would be the first to admit, purely by health and social welfare interventions, however well constructed and validated.

The range of interventions described in this section reflects this broad understanding of children's well-being. Reductions in child morbidity and mortality can only take place when the full range of factors that mediate childhood experiences are understood, the links between them are considered and the optimum balance between risk and opportunity is achieved.

10

GERALDINE MACDONALD

Child protection

KEY MESSAGES

- The development of effective child protection services requires clear evidence that beneficial outcomes for children and families arise from agency interventions.
- Randomized controlled trials are the most reliable source of evidence on the effectiveness of many social interventions.
- Robust and replicable research designs are necessary to enable us to make confident statements about cause and effect.
- Important questions about the protection of children cannot always be explored through randomized controlled trials. Quasi-experimental and single-case designs, surveys, cohort studies and client opinion studies are crucial sources of information, especially when they produce patterns of similar results.
- Current child welfare practice emphasizes values such as empowerment and client participation. The function of such values must be made explicit to clarify how exactly they contribute to positive outcomes for children.
- Experimental research on effective practice teaches us three important lessons:

  - that the *content* of practice – what practitioners do – strongly influences the outcomes for children;

> – that research findings on effective practice need to be
> disseminated to practitioners and accompanied by an
> implementation programme;
> – a failure to learn from robust findings on effective prac-
> tice is unethical and unprofessional.

INTRODUCTION

This chapter presents an overview of a range of interventions designed to help
protect children from abuse and neglect by adults and for which there is
evidence of their effectiveness. Child protection is a considerable challenge,
requiring effective legislation, procedures and organizational practices. Much
research has been undertaken regarding what constitutes effective organizational
and legal responses to child protection and about how best to manage risk,
and the trends identified here should be considered in this broader context.
Socio-economic factors make their presence felt in child maltreatment and
effective child protection undoubtedly requires macro-economic interventions,
such as those designed to abolish child poverty and to improve social housing.
The particular focus of this chapter, however, is on those interventions that
fall within the scope of individual practitioners and organizations with a remit
to intervene at an individual, group or community level. Although such interventions may not always directly address causal factors, they may nonetheless
be important strategies whereby families are enabled to cope in adverse circumstances and any damage to children's health, development and well-being is
minimized. Interventions aimed at helping children who have been abused or
neglected are not covered here (see Macdonald 2001).

In seeking to develop an evidence-based approach to practice, it is important to deal carefully with the findings of reviews about 'what works'. Even
systematic reviews only provide evidence of whether an intervention *can* result
in the kinds of changes that we might be seeking to bring about. When taking
the results and applying them to our own practice environments, we may find
that such interventions work less well, or perhaps even better, than expected.
This is because our clients may differ in key respects, we may have less expertise in the intervention we are seeking to deploy, or our team may be less well
resourced. We need, therefore, to monitor carefully what we do and how things
progress, making appropriate changes as the need arises. Most importantly,
we need to ensure that our choice of intervention is appropriate and that we
have the skills necessary to implement it effectively. The first requires that our
decisions are anchored in a sound assessment of the problems we are seeking to
ameliorate. Such an assessment entails a good, empirically based understanding
of the nature of the factors that interact to create abusive and/or neglectful
parenting, a detailed, empirically sound knowledge of child development, and

a sound approach to the assessment and monitoring of risk. The second may have implications for training and the organization of services. These topics are outside the scope of this chapter (see Macdonald 2001) but they are important. Attempts to deploy the interventions described here without due attention to these matters would probably result in premature and erroneous conclusions about the inapplicability of these interventions to practice and to the demoralization of both workers and service users alike.

INTERVENTIONS WORTH CONSIDERING

As well as being depressingly few in number, studies of interventions designed to address child abuse and neglect are fraught with a range of methodological problems (see Fink and McCloskey 1990; Oates and Bross 1995; Macdonald 2001). The inclusion criteria for interventions reviewed for this chapter were that they:

- made explicit their understanding of the issues with which they are concerned;
- provided information about the intervention (within the report or via reference elsewhere) that would permit replication;
- said clearly why and how the intervention is expected to impact upon the problem(s) of concern;
- provided a detailed account of the sampling procedures;
- made explicit the rationale for the choice of control group, where randomization was not used;
- demonstrated that the control group, if used, was matched on relevant variables;
- used measures of relevance;
- showed an appreciation of the limitations of the research design, including sample size, attrition, data analysis, and so on;
- were deemed to be of relevance to the UK (see below) and to the problems with which staff are concerned.

There are some areas of practice where no good evaluative research exists, but where the rationale of the project or intervention is explicit, enjoys an empirically based rationale and where early reports from staff and users suggest there is something worth developing and evaluating. In some instances, evaluations are in progress. There are many interventions in use for which there is no evidence base, so these are not included. They may, or may not, be effective. The challenge is whether, in the absence of good-quality evidence either way, we should continue with interventions about which we know so little. Most studies are American in origin and some may worry about their relevance and applicability to other policy contexts. The position adopted here is that if researchers were examining interventions that resembled those used in the UK, or which could be used, and were working with problems similar to those we routinely tackle, with clients who are similar, then these studies deserve careful consideration. Because we undertake so little rigorous evaluative research in the UK, we frankly do not have the luxury of choosing to ignore non-UK studies. To do so would, in any case, be foolish.

GROUPING STUDIES

KEY POINTS

- *Primary prevention*: interventions aimed at whole populations, irrespective of any known risk.
- *Secondary prevention*: interventions aimed at individuals who have been identified as being at high risk of abuse.
- *Tertiary prevention*: interventions that seek to ensure that abuse does not re-occur.

Societies seek to intervene to stop child maltreatment at several points and levels. A limited number of interventions are aimed at whole communities or populations irrespective of any known particular risk. These interventions are often referred to as concerned with the 'primary' prevention of child abuse and neglect. Others are aimed at individuals who are identified as being at high risk of abuse. These are usually referred to as interventions concerned with 'secondary' prevention; that is, they are designed to prevent the occurrence of abuse in circumstances where there is reason to think children are at increased risk, for example children of teenage mothers (rather confusingly, in some literature these are referred to as 'primary' prevention). 'Tertiary' prevention is the term used to refer to interventions aimed to ensure that abuse that has already occurred does not occur again. It includes the provision of help to children who have been abused and, for example, to parents whose children have been abused by others. The realities of research and practice mean that studies do not always fit neatly into these divisions, but it is difficult to imagine a tidier organizing principle.

WHAT WORKS IN PRIMARY PREVENTION?

KEY POINTS

- More resources should go into primary prevention. This would shift the emphasis of work towards children's overall well-being and encourage good parenting within supportive communities.

- Poverty is associated with child maltreatment. The prevention of child abuse and neglect requires economic and social reforms that target the root causes of poverty.
- Many effective social interventions aim to help families increase their incomes or limit the effects of poverty.
- Community-based projects may protect children by developing formal and informal support networks for parents and by helping professionals to work together.
- There is strong evidence that good-quality day care and pre-school education, with parental involvement, can protect children.
- Schools can play a key role in promoting attitudes that challenge violence and sexism and develop good interpersonal skills.
- Effective programmes to prevent the sexual abuse of children are characterized by length and intensity and include:

  - behavioural training in self-protection;
  - opportunities for repeated learning over time;
  - specific tailoring to their audience.

- Children from lower socio-economic groups seem to benefit most from preventive programmes.

In 1985, Gelles and Cornell identified several areas of activity as being particularly appropriate for the primary prevention of physical abuse. Their list included the reduction of socially determined, violence-provoking stress, such as poverty and inequality, the promotion of social organization and adequate networks of family support and educational programmes that reduce the likelihood of abuse and neglect. The latter includes tackling norms which legitimate and glorify violence and promote anti-sexist norms, values and expectations. We might add teaching alternative ways of solving problems without resorting to violence and increasing parental understanding of children's developmental needs. These areas of activity have formed the focus of many promising approaches, in terms of reported results. Although few primary prevention strategies have been rigorously evaluated, those that seek to intervene to limit the factors known to contribute to family violence and other forms of abuse need no justification in terms of their rationale. However, given their cost and the stakes involved, policy makers might be advised to take a more rigorous approach to evaluation than has hitherto been the case in the UK.

Economic and social interventions

Despite differing views about the magnitude of the impact of poverty and inequality on children's health and development, and the mechanisms whereby poverty has its effect, there is little disagreement that it is a key factor in bringing about poor outcomes in the health and development of children (see Davey-Smith and Egger 1986; Gelles 1992; Roberts 1997). It is not surprising, therefore, that a serious contender for primary prevention is a series of changes aimed at redressing inequality – or, minimally, improving the socio-economic contexts in which our poorer children are raised.

One hypothesis regarding the influence of poverty on child abuse is that its negative consequences are mediated by a range of factors. The first is the extent of community level social organization (Coulton *et al.* 1995) and the availability and quality of formal support services (see Bursik and Grasmick 1993; Pugh and McQuail 1995). It is this, some argue, rather than poverty *per se*, which distinguishes those neighbourhoods that are 'high risk' in terms of child abuse (Garbarino and Kostelno 1992a,b). The second, related factor, is the amount of social isolation among child-abusing families (Thompson 1994). Community-based interventions typically target both of these. There are many examples available in the literature of interventions designed to promote informal networks, to improve the availability and quality of formal support services and of interventions that seek to do both. Few, if any, have been rigorously evaluated.

In America, early findings from a group of 'comprehensive child development programmes' have been reported. These are community-based initiatives seeking to improve the lives of children and families in poverty by improving the range and coordination of health and welfare services. They are designed 'to address the pervasive needs of low-income children and families and to combat the fragmentation of existing programs that serve them' (Smith and Lopez 1994: 3). These programmes are legally required to provide, either directly or by contract, several core services for families:

1 Early childhood education and development services for all pre-school age children.
2 Early intervention for children with, or at risk for, developmental delays or disabilities.
3 Nutritional services for children and families.
4 Child care that meets state licensing standards.
5 Child health services (medical and dental).
6 Prenatal care for pregnant women.
7 Mental health services for children and adults.
8 Substance abuse education and treatment.
9 Parental education in child development, health, nutrition, and parenting.
10 Vocational training and other education related to obtaining employment or employment that pays more, has a benefit package, or both.
(Smith and Lopez 1994, cited in Striefal *et al.* 1998: 269)

Beyond this, projects develop in accordance with the needs of the local context and the wishes of participating families and community groups. This is more than *just* effective inter-agency working. The primary prevention focus means that a range of agencies are needed to plan and deliver a coordinated approach to the range of problems that can jeopardize children's optimum development. Evaluations of these programmes are not yet available, but are promising.

In the UK, such primary prevention strategies are generally the prerogative of the voluntary sector, where agencies endeavour to combine interventions relevant to the stress of poverty and social isolation with those that attempt to empower families to overcome some aspects of adversity. Broadly speaking, they aim to:

- alleviate social and economic pressure where possible;
- enhance informal and formal networks, thus reducing social isolation;
- offer help and opportunities for parents to improve particular, skills such as parenting, child management, social skills (so enhancing economic opportunities), literacy, and so on.

Such projects do not always explicitly identify the reduction of abuse and neglect among their aims, and the very limited number of evaluation studies makes it a particularly difficult area to summarize in terms of effectiveness. The rootedness of such programmes in local neighbourhoods emphasizes the importance of community development, an approach which has received renewed attention in recent years (see Cannan and Warren 1997). Judged by the value users place on them, community-based approaches merit development and further evaluation.

Day care and early education

There is now sufficient evidence of the effectiveness of good-quality day care and pre-school education in promoting a range of good outcomes for children, for it to be considered in terms of a major social intervention in the UK (see Sylva 1994; Zoritch and Roberts 1997). Evidence comes from a series of experimental evaluations of the impact of pre-school educational programmes on a range of outcomes for disadvantaged children in America. No such evaluations have occurred within the UK, but there is no reason to think that the benefits that have accrued to American children would not be repeated, given a faithful replication of the intervention.

The evidence suggests it is not simply that 'any educational experience' will produce good outcomes for disadvantaged children. Rather, it is the 'active-learning component' of particular pre-school programmes (e.g. plan/do/review) that appears to account for their effectiveness in providing children with long-lasting academic, cognitive and social gains. The following is Sylva's succinct description of the curriculum:

In the High/Scope curriculum children learn to be self-critical, without shame, to set high goals while seeking objective feedback. There is a deliberate encouragement to reflect on efforts and agency, encouragement to develop persistence in the face of failure and calm acceptance of errors.

(Sylva 1994: 142)

The positive experience of school which these programmes seem to engender appears to reduce the likelihood of early school failure and placement in special education, both key turning points in the lives of many children. This positive attitude to school has also been shown to be protective against later risk of maladjustment and delinquency.

Evidence for the effectiveness of these programmes and their potential impact on abuse and neglect is summarized in the following quote from two reviewers of early childhood programmes:

Parents made positive changes in their own educational and employment levels and showed reductions in child abuse and neglect. Early childhood programs clearly do help overcome the barriers imposed by impoverishment.

(Campbell and Taylor 1996: 78)

So, as a primary prevention strategy, early education may take a generation to make its mark on child protection, but it is not surprising that increasing a person's life changes appears to impact on their later ability to parent adequately. Parental involvement in early education appears to be an essential mediator of good outcomes for children from disadvantaged backgrounds, perhaps reflecting the kind of parental involvement that socially advantaged children take for granted. It emphasizes the importance of locating early education interventions in a broader framework of investment in family support.

Sexual abuse

KEY POINTS

- Sexually abused children may develop patterns of inappropriate sexual behaviour, be withdrawn and isolated, suicidal, self-harming or delinquent as adolescents.
- Evidence has been noted of a link between sexual abuse in childhood and greater likelihood of pregnancy in adolescence.
- Long-term health consequences include a higher incidence of physical complaints and psychiatric difficulties.

The task of identifying what works in relation to interventions aimed at the primary prevention of child sexual abuse is made easier by the existence of several carefully considered reviews (Carroll *et al.* 1992; Finkelhor and Strapko 1992; MacMillan *et al.* 1994b) and a recent meta-analysis (Rispens *et al.* 1997).

MacMillan and her colleagues (1994b) identified 19 controlled studies published in an English language journal between January 1979 and May 1993 inclusive. All were educational and included verbal instruction alone or with one or more of the following: behavioural training, film or video, play or skits. The effectiveness of the programmes was generally measured in relation to children's knowledge (via questionnaires) or skills thought to relate to prevention (assessed by verbal response to vignettes or to simulated conditions; e.g. stranger approach). Only two studies included data on child disclosure of sexual abuse. In their review, Rispens *et al.* (1997) arrived at similar conclusions, although somewhat different inclusion criteria were used. The overall conclusions are as follows:

- All studies yielded positive results at the end of the programme. Children of all ages benefit from these programmes in relation to improved knowledge and self-protection skills.
- At follow-up, these improvements are not maintained at their original, post-intervention level, but still represent significant changes.
- Programmes that include specific behavioural training in self-protection skills are more effective than those that do not.
- Longer and more intensive programmes achieve better results.
- Younger children generally demonstrate greater gains immediately following a programme, but these 'fade' at follow-up, adding weight to the argument that there should be more opportunity for repeated learning.
- Studies that provide data on socio-economic status (50 per cent) suggest that children from lower socio-economic groups benefit most from preventive programmes. However, there is also evidence of a 'fading' of effects over time. This suggests that, like age, low socio-economic status may be associated with poor retention of knowledge and skills.
- There is no evidence on the transferability of knowledge and 'proxy' skills to real-life situations in which children are at risk of sexual abuse.

The findings of one study suggest that behavioural skills training may be less confusing for pre-school children than 'feelings-based' programmes (Wurtele *et al.* 1989). More attention needs to be paid to developing programmes that are tailored to the developmental age of children, particularly their cognitive ability.

Such programmes have, with reason, been criticized for placing the responsibility of prevention on the shoulders of potential victims (see Cohn 1986; Melton 1992). There is some merit in these arguments, but there is also merit in equipping children in general self-protection skills, which will help them to cope in a social context that, *de facto*, contains threats of violence and intimidation (Asdigan and Finkelhor 1995).

WHAT WORKS IN SECONDARY PREVENTION?

KEY POINTS

- Effective secondary prevention depends on our ability to identify factors that place people at increased risk of abuse.
- Home visiting programmes are likely to be particularly effective when:
  - they use either professional visitors or well-trained lay people;
  - they are multi-dimensional, intensive and long term;
  - visiting starts before the child is born.
- Parenting programmes are most effective when:
  - they are group-based rather than individual-based;
  - they are behavioural in design rather than primarily based on relationship work;
  - they use modelling as a way of helping parents learn new skills.
- Parenting programmes do not work for everybody, particularly when the family is experiencing several problems.
- Anger-control training for parents offers a promising avenue for continued research.

At the level of secondary prevention, successful interventions are usually multi-faceted and are aimed at addressing a range of factors associated with enhanced risk, drawing on ecological models of child maltreatment (for an example, see Barth 1989). Programmes often comprise elements of education or parent-training, social and emotional support, and assistance to cope with the stresses of poverty or other social disadvantages. However, few interventions have been rigorously evaluated and, because they have been directed at factors *associated* with child abuse, they too have rarely collected data on abusive behaviour. Those that stand out are: home visiting, parent training and anger management.

Home visiting

Home visiting programmes vary enormously, but most focus on helping to shape parenting skills, to enhance the parent–child relationship and to improve relationships with informal and formal networks (for example, via social skills training). Visitors may be trained nurses, lay people or para-professionals. There have been several reviews of the effectiveness of these interventions (Olds and Kitzman 1993; MacMillan *et al.* 1994a; Clémant and Tourginy 1997). Methodologically, the most secure review remains that conducted by MacMillan and her colleagues. They focused on studies designed to prevent abuse and neglect, although of the 11 studies reviewed, only two reported outcomes directly relevant to child abuse and, of these, one was a primary prevention study as defined in this chapter (Hardy and Streett 1989). The other (Olds *et al.* 1994) was a fairly long-term programme of visiting by trained nurses, begun *during* pregnancy and designed to address several aspects of maternal and child functioning, including (Olds 1997: 133):

- outcomes of pregnancy for mother and child;
- the qualities of care-giving (including associated child health and developmental problems);
- maternal life-course development (helping mothers return to education or work and to plan future pregnancies);
- the prevention of child maltreatment.

The programme was grounded in an ecological framework, which conceptualized the adequacy of care provided by parents as a function of other relationships, and the wider social context. Home visitors, therefore, focused attention on the social and material environment of families. They sought to promote informal networks of friends and family members who could provide reliable sources of material and emotional support. In the course of its development, the programme has gradually paid more attention to theories of human attachment and to the perceived importance of self-efficacy theory – that is, that human behaviour is partly a function of how effective people perceive themselves to be. The latter resulted in an emphasis on behaviour rehearsal, reinforcement and problem solving, rather than a reliance on information. The former has had particular relevance to the process of helping, stressing the importance of:

- establishing an empathic relationship between mother and home visitor;
- reviewing with care-givers their own child-rearing histories;
- the development of an explicit focus on promoting a sensitive, responsive and engaged care giving in the early years of a child's life.

Mothers received an average of nine visits during their pregnancy and 23 visits from birth through the second year of the child's life. The results showed that, of those who received home visiting, only 4 per cent abused or neglected their children, compared with 19 per cent of those who did not receive this service. Between 24 and 48 months of age, children of home-visited women were 40 per cent less likely to visit a physician for an injury or ingestion (poisoning) than those in the comparison group. They lived in homes with fewer safety hazards and which were deemed more conducive to their intellectual and emotional needs (Olds *et al.* 1995). However, there were no differences noted in referrals for child maltreatment during this period. The authors pointed out that child maltreatment in the comparison group was likely to be under-detected, and that in the experimental group over-detected, because of the increased surveillance of child abuse and neglect afforded by the project, but that this 'washout' effect should not be minimized.

Further replications of the programme have had less striking results; the authors of these studies speculate that perhaps even longer periods of visiting are required to make a long-term impact on child abuse and neglect. Given (1) the changing demands that are placed on parents as their children develop, and the ongoing need to acquire new, age-appropriate knowledge and parenting skills, and (2) the long-standing nature of many of the problems faced by vulnerable families, it may well be that – as in many other areas of child protection work – longer-term interventions merit serious consideration.

The Child Development Programme is a UK-based programme (Barker 1988, 1994) that essentially makes available a source of social support for first-time mothers to help and encourage them in the task of parenting. This support was provided originally by specially trained health visitors, known as 'first parent visitors', but has subsequently been provided by experienced community mothers who receive support, some training and small financial recompense. The programme seeks to empower parents and to provide them with a sense of control over their lives and their children's upbringing. The visitors focus on all areas of a child's development, health and nutrition and use semi-structured methods to foster parents' development. Parents are encouraged to set themselves developmental, dietary, health or other tasks to carry out with their children in the coming month. As with the programme of Olds *et al.* (1994), there is an emphasis on the health and well-being of the mother, in her role as a woman with her own interests and future, and not merely the mother of her children. Some of the work is sometimes done in groups to promote social support and possibly to generate enhanced community involvement. Finally, enhancing the role of the father or partner is also taken seriously.

Two randomized controlled trials have been conducted of the effectiveness of this programme. The first focused on trained health visitors (Barker 1988); the second, more recent trial examined the effectiveness of the programme using specially trained community mothers (Johnson *et al.* 1993). Other evidence comes from analyses of longitudinal data gathered on the very large numbers of families served by the programme over several years. Results indicate improvement on a variety of home environment factors, including language and cognitive environments, the nutrition of intervention children and reductions in child abuse and neglect. Barker attributes the success of the project to the involvement of lay people – 'community mothers' – whom he believes are more acceptable to new parents and are more likely to be able to understand and assist them in relevant ways. This is a complex debate, with more opinions than data. There are pros and cons of using professionally trained staff or lay helpers and it is probably the case that the question should not be framed in terms of either/or, but that service providers should think carefully about what they are trying to do and who would therefore be most appropriate in terms of skills, efficiency and cost. For example, Olds and Kitzman (1993) also point out that it is those who are the most difficult to reach who require the most sensitive and persistent efforts to establish a relationship. Ironically, as is so often the case, they point out that most home visiting programmes have established policies that require the termination of efforts for those who are persistently 'not at home'.

Parenting programmes

Many things can make parenting exceptionally challenging, such as not having had a good experience of parenting oneself, thus being short of 'know-how', or having a child that is temperamentally difficult (Thomas *et al.* 1968) and/or behaviourally demanding. High negative emotion can distort a parent's judgements about their children's behaviour, increasing their negative expectations. Negative emotions, psychological or mental distress can also disrupt a parent's ability to monitor and attend to their children's behaviour, and disrupt their ability to problem-solve and think clearly about child-rearing conflicts (Patterson 1982; Dix 1991). Broadly speaking, parent training programmes endeavour to address these problem areas. Fundamentally, they aim to enhance parents' abilities to manage their children's behaviour, to reduce conflict and confrontation while increasing compliance, cooperation and pleasant interaction, and generally to alter the balance of reward and punishment in favour of the former. This may entail any combination of the following:

- providing information about child development, health, hygiene, safety, etc.;
- helping parents reconsider and reframe 'age-inappropriate' expectations and misattributions ('he's doing it to wind me up');
- enhancing the quality of child–parent relationships by, for example, teaching play skills and structuring the day so that they set aside some time for themselves and their children;
- developing parents' ability to monitor and track their children's behaviour and respond appropriately, including the management of challenging behaviour;
- increasing support networks.

However, there is great variation in the 'recipes' to be found in the literature (Polster *et al.* 1987; Smith 1996) and few programmes of any formula have been restricted to rigorous scrutiny (see Barlow 1997). Of these, only a handful involve work with parents deemed to be at 'high risk'.

In a systematic review, Barlow (1997) demonstrated the effectiveness of parent training programmes in improving behaviour problems in children aged 3–10 years. Overall, group-based programmes produced better results than individual programmes, and behavioural programmes produced better results than either Adlerian or parent effectiveness training programmes.

Cognitive-behavioural programmes enjoy considerable support in helping parents at risk of abusing or neglecting their children; the evidence for this is discussed in relation to tertiary prevention, as often studies combine parents known to have maltreated their children with those considered to be at risk of doing so. The results are, for the most part, encouraging. However, the evidence suggests that effective interventions for such families need a broader focus than purely child management and need to be provided on a longer-term basis (Patterson *et al.* 1982). What is also required is a more considered approach to the recruitment and retention of families who most need this kind of help and support. Evidence from studies conducted by Webster-Stratton and Herbert (1993, 1994) reinforce the importance of attending to the *process* of helping as well as to the content. Working collaboratively with parents and helping them to develop their self-esteem and self-efficacy are key components of success in these interventions. Before moving on to consider one particular cognitive-behavioural intervention – anger management – it is worth noting one further promising use of cognitive-behavioural approaches relevant to secondary prevention.

Applications for work with learning-disabled parents

Parents with learning disabilities face particular problems in parenting that are thought to contribute to neglect, developmental delay and behavioural problems in their children (Tymchuk and Feldman 1991; Feldman and Walton-Allen 1997). Learning-disabled parents are more likely to have their children removed from their care than other parents. This reflects prejudice and discrimination, but also indicates the parenting difficulties that may be encountered in the absence of appropriate support from informal and formal networks (Feldman 1998). Some studies have indicated that parents with learning disabilities experience high levels of stress and depression, which may contribute to their parenting difficulties (Feldman *et al.* 1997) and these may arise, in part, from the adverse social circumstances in which they often live. Children of learning-disabled parents are themselves at risk for developmental delay (Scally 1957; Reed and Reed 1965; Feldman and Walton-Allen 1997) and may need compensatory social and educational experiences, in addition to interventions aimed at improving their general level of care and stimulation.

Feldman describes a home-based parent training intervention designed to help parents with learning disabilities improve their parenting skills and reduce the risk of child neglect, developmental delay and behavioural problems. Trained parent education therapists visited participants' homes twice a week (more often if thought necessary and for newborns). In addition to parenting skills training, the staff provided ongoing counselling, stress management, community living and social skills training. The programme was sensitively and carefully structured and made use of direct observation, modelling, instruction and reinforcement. Training was pitched at the skills required for caring for a child at the age relevant to the family. Trainers saw their work as an essential component of a multi-agency approach.

The results of several evaluations testify to the promise of these programmes (see Feldman *et al.* 1989, 1992a,b, 1993). Feldman and his colleagues do not regard parent training as a panacea and are aware that other interventions, such as specialized pre-school programmes, may have more to offer some children. However, they rightly highlight the need for specialized and carefully tailored interventions. A problem with parent training as a 'one-off' is that the skills necessary to care for a 1-year-old baby will not suffice to meet the needs of a toddler or of an 8-year-old. Parents with learning disabilities may need long-term help and support that is shaped by the developmental needs of the child.

Anger management

Anger control training typically involves the following steps:

1 Teaching parents to identify cues that signal anger. These may be physiological – tension, shaking, 'going hot' – or situational – provocative situations such as the supermarket, where the parent feels particularly vulnerable. Some cues overlap both such as tiredness, pre-menstrual tension and financial worry.
2 Teaching parents how to relax when these cues are identified and to use various coping strategies. These include deep breathing, engaging in an alternative activity and changing the way he or she thinks about the situation, such as providing them with information about age-appropriate expectations of children.
3 Problem solving – teaching parents to generate alternative (non-aggressive) responses to circumstances in which their children provoke their ire and selecting the one that seems most suitable.

Whiteman *et al.* (1987) compared the relative effectiveness of three components of anger management both individually and in combination:

- *Cognitive restructuring*: aimed at rectifying misattributions of children's behaviour.
- *Problem-solving skills*: learning to think of alternative ways of resolving conflicts or dilemmas.
- *Relaxation*: staying calm so that the parent will be less likely to hit out.
- *A combination* of relaxation, cognitive restructuring and problem-solving skills.

The results of this small randomized controlled trial showed a reduction in anger measures for those in the experimental groups, with the composite group doing best. Unfortunately, this study relied rather heavily on self-report and role-play measures, rather than observed real-life situations.

Finally, a cautionary note. One of the dangers of résumés of effective strategies is that they tempt practitioners to adopt a 'tool-box' approach to intervention. If there is one thing that the better studies teach us is that careful assessment is imperative. Because the aim of anger management strategies is to help individuals identify the build-up of aggression from its earliest signs – when they are most likely to be able to intervene successfully – this approach is, by definition, contraindicated for those whose temper, coupled with physical violence, is 'instantaneous' and unpredictable.

WHAT WORKS IN TERTIARY PREVENTION?

KEY POINTS

- Cognitive-behavioural approaches are the most effective known interventions for preventing the recurrence of abuse and neglect.
- We can conclude from cognitive-behavioural studies that:
  - long-standing, complex problems may require longer-term programmes of support as well as intensive periods of task-centred activity;
  - the use of cognitive-behavioural approaches is best integrated within a broad-based and flexible approach.
- Parent training appears to be effective for parents with learning disabilities.
- Families in trouble are likely to need help with problems other than child management skills. Behavioural family therapy and eco-behavioural therapy are two effective broad-based approaches.
- The effectiveness of family therapy as an intervention in child protection is not yet clear but merits further investigation.
- The prevention of psychological maltreatment appears more effective when parents are involved in group work as well as individual parent training.
- In cases of serious maltreatment, programmes that combine family work and day care services show some promise.
- Direct work with children needs to focus specifically on the trauma of the abuse itself and the longer-term effects.
- There is some evidence that abuse-specific programmes that offer help to non-offending parents and to children at the same time are more helpful than those with either a focus on either parents or children alone.

There are scandalously few studies of the effectiveness of interventions in circumstances where physical abuse and neglect have already occurred. This, together with the accompanying methodological problems, means that it is difficult to conclude anything other than that the available evidence base underpinning what we shall term 'therapeutic' (as opposed to administrative or legal) interventions in child protection is wafer-thin. It is all the more serious, then, that what evidence *is* available is so rarely advocated, so rarely acted upon and so rarely taught.

One important emerging trend is that behavioural and cognitive-behavioural approaches have much to offer in dealing with the problems that need to be tackled if abuse and neglect are to be prevented from recurring (see Gough 1993; Wolfe and Wekerle 1993). These programmes typically combine parent training with self-management techniques (such as anger control) and problem solving and are increasingly delivered in contexts that also attend to the broader social context in which children and families live. Other sources of evidence of the effectiveness of such approaches include Wolfe and Sandler (1981), Wolfe *et al.* (1981, 1982), Egan (1983) and Crimmins *et al.* (1984).

Although there are more outcome studies of cognitive-behavioural approaches in tertiary prevention than there are studies of other approaches, controlled *group* studies are still relatively few in number and most have been conducted in the USA. One UK study that attempted a rigorous evaluation of the use of behavioural approaches in the tertiary prevention of abuse was that of Smith and Rachman (1984). They examined the 'value-added' of a behavioural approach to routine child protection services (i.e. monitoring, practical help and counselling). Over a 16 month period, all cases of child physical abuse were referred to the project, provided the families and social workers concerned were agreeable. The specific behavioural interventions varied according to the needs of the family, but included a variety of child management skills (such as the use of differential reinforcement, time out and token systems), relaxation training, assertion training, anger control, behavioural treatment of depression and structured approaches to problems involving social skills (e.g. job hunting, visiting dentists or family planning clinics). The results were not as encouraging as those conducted in the USA and a high attrition rate precluded a conclusive outcome.

A second UK-based study was conducted by Nicol *et al.* (1988), who undertook a randomized controlled trial examining the relative effectiveness of an intervention they termed 'brief focused casework' (and was essentially behavioural) and play therapy. Families were eligible to participate in the study if actual physical abuse had occurred, family life was marked by significant conflict and the family was typical of those worked with by child protection social workers. The study was a cooperative endeavour between a child psychiatry service and an NSPCC special unit. The authors believe it represented a move away from the 'long-term intensive support' traditionally provided by the latter agency. Again, attrition was high, with 45 per cent of families dropping out between assessment and follow-up. The results indicated that brief focused casework appeared to have improved rates of positive behaviour when family members are combined (rather than examined separately), but that this did not reach statistical significance. Brief focused casework also appeared to have reduced coercive behaviours. When family members were examined separately (that is, mothers, father and children), only one difference emerged, namely that after play therapy fathers evidenced *less* positive interaction with their children (perhaps they irritated them more by wanting to play). There were no significant differences in the final state of the problems.

These results are disappointing, but a common theme emerges from these and other studies. Many researchers (e.g. McAuley and McAuley 1977; Wolfe and Wekerle 1993) have suggested that long-standing, complex problems generally yield less positive outcomes and may well require long-term as well as intensive patterns of intervention. This is in contrast to the general trend in the psychotherapeutic literature, which suggests that if change is to occur, it usually does so within the first 12 weeks of an intervention; thereafter, the gains are marginal (see Rachman and Wilson 1980; Macdonald and Sheldon 1992). Task-centred approaches, while appropriate for many situations, may need to give way to longer-term, more broadly based programmes.

Broader-based cognitive-behavioural interventions

As well as encountering problems in child management, families in trouble are likely to need help with relationship problems, depression, low self-esteem, substance misuse and socio-economic troubles. An appreciation of the role played by these other factors in the aetiology and maintenance of family problems, including abuse, has influenced the development of two rather broad-based approaches to cognitive-behavioural assessment and intervention. The first is known as behavioural family therapy (see Griest and Wells 1983; Thyer 1989); the second is termed 'eco-behavioural'.

Behavioural family therapy is based on the premise that many factors conspire to produce abuse and neglect, that several of these factors are located within the family (or can be intervened with at the level of the family) and that cognitive-behavioural approaches are effective ways of intervening. The evaluation base of this approach, then, more often lies in reports of work directed at specific, relevant aspects of family functioning, from inter-parental conflict to alcohol misuse or depression. The evidence base of this approach is very broad, although we still lack sufficient studies that clearly explore the use of these techniques (and any other approach) with families in which abuse and/or neglect has occurred.

Family-based behavioural approaches have also been evaluated in the context of the broader, multi-systemic approach termed 'eco-behavioural'. These programmes target identified problems in a range of settings, including, but not restricted to, the family. Project 12-Ways is among the best known and best evaluated of these and derives its name from the 12 core services described in the original programme: parent–child training, stress reduction for parents, basic skill training for the children, money management training, social support, home safety training, multiple-setting behaviour management *in situ*, health and nutrition, problem solving, couples counselling, alcohol abuse referral and single mother services. Considerable importance was placed on *in-situ* assessment and delivery of services to maximize the generalization and maintenance of newly learned skills across behaviours, settings and time and to make it easier for families to participate.

The overall picture is that this is an effective intervention that reduces reports of abuse and neglect. A five year follow-up of more than 700 families, 352 of which had received services from Project 12-Ways, showed that project families had consistently lower rates of abuse across all years, except one – 1981 – when the rate was similar to that of the control group (see Lutzker and Rice 1987). In another study, Lutzker and Rice (1984) report that families who received services from Project 12-Ways were significantly less likely to be reported again for child abuse and neglect for up to four years; this was the case even though project families had more severe problems than their control counterparts. However, the authors note that, over time, the incidence of reported abuse increases for both groups, and the gap between them, while still statistically significant, looks clinically less impressive. In other words, there seems to be what they call a 'washout' effect over time. This may reflect the fact that some families either dropped out of the project or had not been successfully helped to resolve identified problems. Alternatively, it may point to a need for 'booster services' or additional support to these families to maintain the early differences between groups.

Family therapy

Judging by the popularity of training courses and the general literature, family therapy is a widely used intervention in secondary and tertiary prevention. However, it is rarely subjected to rigorous evaluation and, in relation to child abuse and neglect, there is only one study of acceptable methodological quality (Brunk et al. 1987), although even this study failed to include subsequent incidents of child abuse among its outcome indicators and had no follow-up.

Brunk and her colleagues compared the effectiveness of parent training and multi-systemic therapy – systemic family therapy that encompassed attention to the role of cognitive and extra-familial variables in maintaining problem behaviours, in this case child abuse and neglect. Eighteeen abusive and 15 neglectful families were randomly allocated to either parent training (run in groups) or multi-systemic family therapy (conducted in the home). Each programme operated for one-and-a-half hours a week for eight weeks. In brief, both interventions appeared to bring about statistically significant improvements in parental psychiatric symptomatology, overall stress and the severity of identified problems. Pre-versus post-test comparisons suggested that parent training was most effective in reducing identified social problems (perhaps because of the group format) and that multi-systemic family therapy had the edge on restructuring parent–child relationships; the latter also facilitated positive change in those behaviour problems that differentiate maltreating families from non-problem families (Crittenden 1981).

One limitation of this study is that Brunk and her colleagues should have compared 'parent training', a relatively simple intervention of proven effectiveness for child management, with multi-systemic family therapy, an intervention designed to address the multi-faceted nature of child abuse and neglect and which incorporates advice on child management. A more reasonable comparison might have been with a similarly broad-based intervention, behavioural family therapy or (because of its recognition that child abuse is located within a number of social systems) an eco-behavioural approach. Although these approaches currently enjoy limited support as effective strategies within tertiary prevention, this support is greater than that for systemic family therapy.

Social network interventions

Social network interventions are those that explicitly aim to address the problems of abuse and neglect by increasing the amount and quality of social support available to needy and socially isolated parents. Only one controlled study has been conducted to date, but it is methodologically quite secure and is one of the few studies that has targeted the needs of neglectful parents (Gaudin et al. 1990–91; Gaudin 1993). The intervention begins with a careful assessment of existing community formal support and an individual assessment of a family's informal support network, covering size, composition and supportiveness. This is followed by a psychosocial assessment aimed at identifying the range of problems facing a family, across a range of settings (school, home, housing, substance misuse, debt, etc.). Significant material and psychosocial barriers to the development of supportive networks are identified (e.g. lack of telephone, poor verbal and social skills, poor self-esteem or unresolved conflicts with family members of neighbours) and goals for intervention are agreed with the family. The intervention encompasses five discreet social network interventions, together with professional casework/case management activities that include extensive advocacy and brokering of formal services. The social network interventions include:

- *Personal networking*: direct interventions to promote family members' existing or potential relationships with family members, friends, neighbours or work associates.
- *Establishing mutual aid groups*: these focus on teaching parenting and more broadly based social skills to develop mutual problem sharing, problem solving and to enhance self-esteem.
- *Volunteer linking*: recruiting and training volunteers to do tasks akin to 'family aides' in the UK.
- *Recruiting neighbours as informal helpers*: these people are paid a small sum and receive support and weekly guidance from social workers.
- *Social skills training*.

Given the recognized difficulties in intervening effectively with neglectful families (Daro 1988), the results of this study are particularly encouraging.

Eighty per cent of those who received nine months of intervention or more improved their parenting from neglectful or severely neglectful to marginally adequate parenting (on the standardized parenting measures used in the study). Almost 60 per cent of cases were closed because of improved parenting. However, the authors point to a number of problems, partly with the study itself and partly in terms of implications for mainstream or routine practice.

First, in terms of the study, all the participants were volunteers, so it is doubtful whether the results would generalize to reluctant or resistant parents. Second, there was a high drop out rate due to the extreme mobility of the families involved. This is a characteristic of many neglectful families, but presents a particular challenge to this way of working. One of the major implications for mainstream practice within the UK is that this intervention requires frequent, consistent professional consultation for problem solving and support, and successful implementation depends on manageable caseloads of 20 or less and well-trained social workers with a combination of knowledge and skills that include case management, individual casework/counselling, group leadership, advocacy, mediation, supervision and consultation with volunteers, and community relations skills.

CONCLUSIONS

In the UK, considerable investment has been made in the legal and administrative infrastructures aimed at preventing child abuse and neglect. We now urgently need to focus our attention on the *content* of our services for such vulnerable children and their parents. The evidence base regarding 'what works' in helping parents to care more adequately for their children is not bewilderingly large or complex and has some clear messages. The evidence consistently points to a handful of approaches that merit consideration, but which are not routinely used in the UK. They are outlined above. There are many other interventions that enjoy no such evidence of effectiveness, but which are used. In working with vulnerable children and their parents, we owe a duty of care to deploy those interventions most likely to prove effective. To do so may not guarantee success; however, if success eludes us, then we have good reason to think we have done the best we can and seek other courses of action. Not to do so raises serious ethical questions.

REFERENCES

Asdigan, N.L. and Finkelhor, D. (1995) What works for children in resisting assaults?, *Journal of Interpersonal Violence*, 10(4): 402–18.

Barker, W. (1988) *The Child Development Programme: An Evaluation of Process and Outcomes*. Bristol: Early Childhood Development Centre.

Barker, W. (1994) *Child Protection: The Impact of the Child Development Programme*. Bristol: Early Childhood Development Unit.

Barlow, J. (1997) *Systematic Review of the Effectiveness of Parent-training Programmes in Improving Behaviour Problems in Children Aged 3–10 Years.* Oxford: Health Services Research Unit, University of Oxford.

Barth, R.P. (1989) Evaluation of a task-centered child abuse prevention program, *Children and Youth Services Review*, 11: 117–32.

Brunk, M., Henggeler, S.W. and Whelan, J.P. (1987) Comparison of multisystemic therapy and parent training in the brief treatment of child abuse and neglect, *Journal of Consulting and Clinical Psychology*, 55(2): 171–8.

Bursik, R.J. and Grasmick, H.G. (1993) *Neighbourhoods and Crime.* New York: Lexington.

Campbell, F.A. and Taylor, K. (1996) Early childhood programmes that work for children from economically disadvantaged families, *Young Children*, 51(4): 74–80.

Cannan, C. and Warren, C. (eds) (1997) *Social Action with Children and Families: A Community Development Approach to Child and Family Welfare.* London: Routledge.

Carroll, L.A., Miltenberger, R.G. and O'Neill, H.K. (1992) A review and critique of research evaluating child sexual abuse prevention programmes, *Education and Treatment of Children*, 15: 335–54.

Clémant, M.-E. and Tourginy, M. (1997) A review of the literature on the prevention of child abuse and neglect: characteristics and effectiveness of home visiting programs, *International Journal of Child and Family Welfare*, 1: 6–20.

Cohn, A.H. (1986) Preventing adults from becoming sexual molesters, *Child Abuse and Neglect*, 10: 559–62.

Coulton, C.J., Korbin, J.E., Su, M. and Chow, J. (1995) Community level factors and child maltreatment rates, *Child Development*, 66: 1262–76.

Crimmins, D.B., Bradlyn, A.S., St. Lawrence, J.S. and Kelly, J.A. (1984) In-clinic training to improve the parent–child interaction skills of a neglectful mother, *Child Abuse and Neglect*, 8: 533–9.

Crittenden, P. (1981) Abusing, neglecting, problematic and adequate dyads: differentiating by patterns of interaction, *Merrill-Palmer Quarterly*, 27: 201–8.

Daro, D. (1988) *Confronting Child Abuse.* New York: Free Press.

Davey-Smith, G. and Egger, M. (1986) Commentary: understanding it all – health meta-theories and morality trends, *British Medical Journal*, 313: 1584–5.

Dix, T. (1991) The affective organization of parenting: adaptive and maladaptive processes, *Psychological Bulletin*, 110(1): 3–25.

Egan, K. (1983) Stress management with abusive parents, *Journal of Clinical Child Psychology*, 12: 292–9.

Feldman, M.A. (1998) Parents with intellectual disabilities: implications and interventions, in J.R. Lutzker (ed.) *Handbook of Child Abuse: Research and Treatment.* New York: Plenum Press.

Feldman, M. and Walton-Allen, N. (1997) Effects of maternal mental retardation and poverty on intellectual, academic, and behavioral status of school-age children, *American Journal on Mental Retardation*, 101: 352–64.

Feldman, M.A., Case, L., Rincover, A., Towns, F. and Betel, J. (1989) Parent education project 111. Increasing affection and responsivity in developmentally handicapped mothers: component analysis, generalisation, and effects on child language, *Journal of Applied Behavior Analysis*, 22: 211–22.

Feldman, M.A., Case, L. and Sparks, B. (1992a) Effectiveness of a child-care training program for parents at-risk for child neglect, *Canadian Journal of Behavioral Science*, 24: 14–28.

Feldman, M.A., Case, L., Garrick, M. *et al.* (1992b) Teaching child care skills to parents with developmental disabilities, *Journal of Applied Behavior Analysis,* 25: 205–15.

Feldman, M.A., Sparks, B. and Case, L. (1993) Effectiveness of home-based early intervention on the language development of children of mothers with mental retardation, *Research in Developmental Disabilities,* 14: 387–408.

Feldman, M.A., Leger, M. and Walton-Allen, N. (1997) Stress in mothers with learning disabilities, *Journal of Child and Family Studies,* 6(4): 471–85.

Fink, A. and McCloskey, L. (1990) Moving child abuse and neglect prevention programs forward: improving program evaluations, *Child Abuse and Neglect,* 14: 187–206.

Finkelhor, D. and Strapko, N. (1992) Sexual abuse prevention education: a review of evaluation studies, in D.J. Willis, E.W. Holden and M. Rosenberg (eds) *Prevention of Child Maltreatment.* New York: Wiley.

Garbarino, J. and Kostelno, K. (1992a) Child maltreatment as a community problem, *International Journal of Child Abuse and Neglect,* 16(4): 455–64.

Garbarino, J. and Kostelno, K. (1992b) Neighbourhood and community influences on parenting, in T. Luster and L. Okagaki (eds) *Parenting: An Ecological Perspective.* Hillside, NJ: Lawrence Erlbaum Associates.

Gaudin, J. (1993) Effective interventions with neglectful families, *Criminal Justice and Behavior,* 20: 66–89.

Gaudin, J., Wodarski, J.S., Arkinson, M.K. and Avery, L.S. (1990–91) Remedying child neglect: effectiveness of social network interventions, *Journal of Applied Social Sciences,* 15: 97–123.

Gelles, R.J. (1992) Poverty and violence toward children, *American Behavioural Scientists,* 35: 258–64.

Gelles, R.J. and Cornell, C.P. (1985) *Intimate Violence in Families.* Newbury Park, CA: Sage.

Gough, R. (1993). *Child Abuse Interventions.* London: HMSO.

Griest, D.L. and Wells, K.C. (1983) Behavioral family therapy with conduct disorders in children, *Behavior Therapy,* 14: 38–43.

Hardy, J.B. and Streett, R. (1989) Family support and parenting education in the home: an effective extension of clinic-based preventive health care services for poor children, *Journal of Pediatrics,* 115: 927–31.

Johnson, Z., Howell, F. and Molloy, B. (1993) Community mothers' programme: randomized controlled trial of non-professional intervention in parenting, *British Medical Journal,* 306: 1449–52.

Lutzker, J.R. and Rice, J.M. (1984) Project 12-Ways: measuring outcome of a large-scale in-home service for the treatment and prevention of child abuse and neglect, *Child Abuse and Neglect,* 8: 519–24.

Lutzker, J.R. and Rice, J.M. (1987) Using recidivism data to evaluate Project 12-Ways: an ecobehavioral approach to the prevention and treatment of child abuse and neglect, *Journal of Family Violence,* 2: 283–90.

Macdonald, G. (2001) *Effective Interventions in Child Abuse and Neglect: An Evidence-based Approach to Planning and Evaluating Interventions.* Chichester: Wiley.

Macdonald, G. and Sheldon, B. with Gillespie, J. (1992) Contemporary studies of the effectiveness of social work, *British Journal of Social Work,* 22(6): 615–43.

MacMillan, H.L., MacMillan, J.H., Offord, D.R., Griffith, L. and MacMillan, A. (1994a) Primary prevention of child physical abuse and neglect: a critical review. Part 1, *Journal of Child Psychology and Psychiatry and Allied Professions,* 35(5): 835–56.

MacMillan, H.L., MacMillan, J.H., Offord, D.R., Griffith, L. and MacMillan, A. (1994b) Primary prevention of child sexual abuse: a critical review. Part 2, *Journal of Child Psychology and Psychiatry and Allied Professions*, 35(5): 857–76.

McAuley, R. and McAuley, P. (1977) *Child Behaviour Problems*. Basingstoke: Macmillan.

Melton, G.B. (1992) The improbability of prevention of sexual abuse, in D. Willis, E.W. Holden and M. Rosenberg (eds) *Prevention of Child Maltreatment: Developmental Perspectives*. New York: Wiley.

Nicol, A.R., Smith, J., Kay, B. *et al.* (1988) A focused casework approach to the treatment of child abuse: a controlled comparison, *Journal of Child Psychology and Psychiatry*, 29(5): 703–11.

Oates, R.K. and Bross, D.C. (1995) What have we learned from treating physical abuse?, *Child Abuse and Neglect*, 19(4): 463–73.

Olds, D. (1997) The Prenatal Early Infancy Project: preventing child abuse and neglect in the context of promoting child and maternal health, in D.A. Wolfe, R.J. McMahon and R. de V Peters (eds) *Child Abuse: New Directions in Prevention and Treatment Across the Lifespan*. Thousand Oaks, CA: Sage.

Olds, D.L. and Kitzman, H. (1993) Can home visiting improve the health of women and children at environmental risk?, *Pediatrics*, 86: 108–16.

Olds, D., Henderson, C.R. and Kitzman, H. (1994) Does prenatal and infancy nurse home visitation have enduring effects on qualities of parental caregiving and child health at 25–50 months of life?, *Pediatrics*, 93: 89–98.

Olds, D., Henderson, C.R., Kitzman, H. and Cole, R. (1995) Effects of prenatal and infancy nurse home visitation on surveillance of child maltreatment, *Pediatrics*, 95: 365–72.

Patterson, G.R. (1982) *A Social Learning Approach to Family Intervention: Coercive Family Process*. Eugene, OR: Castilia.

Patterson, G.R., Chamberlain, P. and Reid, J.B. (1982) A comparative evaluation of a parent training program, *Behavior Therapy*, 13: 638–50.

Polster, R.A., Dangel, R.F. and Rasp, R. (1987) Research in behavioral parent training in social work: a review, *Behavior Modification*, 1: 323–50.

Pugh, G. and McQuail, S. (1995) *Effective Organisation of Early Childhood Services*. London: National Children's Bureau.

Rachman, S.J. and Wilson, G.T. (1980) *The Effects of Psychological Therapy*. Oxford: Pergamon Press.

Reed, R. and Reed, S. (1965) *Mental Retardation: A Family Study*. New York: W.B. Saunders.

Rispens, J., Aleman, A. and Goudena, P.P. (1997) Prevention of child sexual abuse victimization: a meta-analysis of school programs, *Child Abuse and Neglect*, 21(10): 975–87.

Roberts, H. (1997) Children, inequalities and health, *British Medical Journal*, 314: 1122–5.

Scally, B.G. (1957) Marriage and mental handicap: some observations in Northern Ireland, in F.F. de la Cruz and G.D. La Veck (eds) *Human Sexuality and the Mentally Retarded*. New York: Brunner/Mazel.

Smith, A.N. and Lopez, M. (1994) *A Comprehensive Child Development Program: A National Family Support Program*, interim report to Congress. Washington, DC: US Department of Health and Human Services.

Smith, C. (1996) *Developing Parenting Programmes*. London: National Children's Bureau.

11

HELEN ROBERTS

Reducing inequalities in child health

KEY MESSAGES

- Compelling evidence links health and wealth.
- For us to make a difference to inequalities in health, we need to tackle not just health problems but the determinants of those problems.
- The health service on its own cannot tackle inequalities in child health.
- Some inequalities in child health appear to be widening.
- Some measures taken to improve health may widen inequalities.
- Although many interventions intended to improve matters for the poorest sections of the community are targeted, there is a strong public health argument for universal services. Most poor children do not live in poor communities.
- There is not an effective intervention for every problem. This makes it important to act on the basis of those interventions with good evidence of effectiveness and, where there is no good evidence, recognize that we are experimenting.
- Where we are experimenting, we need to evaluate well so that we can know whether we are doing good, doing harm or using resources that will leave matters much as they were.

Smith, J.E. and Rachman, S.J. (1984) Non-accidental injury to children – a controlled evaluation of a behavioural management programme, *Behaviour Research and Therapy*, 22(4): 349–66.

Striefal, S., Robinson, M.A. and Truhn, P. (1998) Dealing with child abuse and neglect within a comprehensive family-support program, in J.R. Lutzker (ed.) *Handbook of Child Abuse Research and Treatment*. New York: Plenum Press.

Sylva, K. (1994) School influences on children's development, *Journal of Child Psychology and Psychiatry and Allied Professions*, 35(1): 135–70.

Thomas, A., Chess, S. and Birch, H.G. (1968) *Temperament and Behaviour Disorder in Children*. New York: New York University Press.

Thompson, R.A. (1994) Social support and the prevention of child maltreatment, in G.B. Melton and F.D. Barry (eds) *Protecting Children from Abuse and Neglect*. New York: Guilford Press.

Thyer, B.A. (1989) *Behavioral Family Therapy*. Springfield, IL: Charles C. Thomas.

Tymchuk, A. and Feldman, M. (1991) Parents with mental retardation and their children: review of research relevant to professional practice, *Canadian Psychology*, 32: 486–96.

Webster-Stratton, C. and Herbert, M. (1993) What really happens in parent-training?, *Behavior Modification*, 17: 407–56.

Webster-Stratton, C. and Herbert, M. (1994) *Troubled Families–Problem Children. Working with Parents: A Collaborative Process*. Chichester: Wiley.

Whiteman, M., Fanshel, D. and Grundy, J.F. (1987) Cognitive-behavioral interventions aimed at anger of parents at risk of child abuse, *Social Work*, November/December: 469–74.

Wolfe, D.A. and Sandler, J. (1981) Training abusive parents in effective child management, *Behavior Modification*, 5: 320–35.

Wolfe, D.A. and Wekerle, C. (1993) Treatment strategies for child physical abuse and neglect: a critical progress report, *Clinical Psychology Review*, 13: 473–500.

Wolfe, D., Kaufman, K., Aragona, J. and Sandler, J. (1981) *The Child Management Program for Abusive Parents: Procedures for Developing a Child Abuse Intervention Program*. Winter Park, FL: Anna Publishing.

Wolfe, D.A., St. Lawrence, J.S., Graves, K. *et al.* (1982) Intensive behavioral parent training for a child abusive mother, *Behavior Therapy*, 13: 438–51.

Wurtele, S.K., Kast, L.C., Miller-Perin, C.L. and Kondrick, P.A. (1989) Comparison of programs for teaching personal safety to preschoolers, *Journal of Consulting and Clinical Psychology*, 57: 505–11.

Zoritch, B. and Roberts, I. (1997) The health and welfare effects of day care for preschool children: a systematic review of randomized controlled trials, *The Cochrane Library*, Issue 4. Oxford: Update Software.

- 'Strong' evaluation (rather than evaluation as justification) needs to be a routine part of ethical practice.
- In our search for ways of narrowing inequalities in child health, we can learn from children and young people, who have a unique perspective on what is it to be a child in an unequal society.

INTRODUCTION

Child, infant and maternal public health are potentially the most effective routes for tackling inequalities. The interventions likely to make the biggest difference lie in public policies, including fiscal policy, and there is some evidence in the UK of positive change in this direction. This chapter, however, is mainly concerned with *service* interventions, where those delivering education, housing and social welfare to families and children are in a key position to have an effect on reducing inequalities.

In common with other areas discussed in this book, we have evidence that some interventions are more effective than others. Our immediate needs are to create further evidence, disseminate that evidence and, most importantly, ensure implementation. To do this, those who use the services – children, parents and other carers – need to be closely involved not only in the final step (i.e. the delivery of services) but also in the earlier steps, including the generation of meaningful research questions.

This chapter describes some of the interventions in child health that appear to have good evidence of effectiveness, some recent policy and political initiatives that are likely to change the picture over the next few years, and some promising interventions that could be robustly evaluated to strengthen the evidence base.

Every child and every parent in the UK is familiar with the phrase 'It's not fair'. This theme was taken up at the end of February 2001 when the secretary of state for health told an audience at the Royal College of Physicians that:

> the biggest health improvement our country can make is to tackle ... unfairness ... Health at the beginning of life is the foundation for health throughout life. So our first health inequality target is: to reduce the health gap between children in different social classes.
>
> (Milburn 2001)

The sea change indicated by this approach to health issues in childhood cannot be underestimated. First, the minister's speech drew on sound evidence; second, inequalities in health were clearly recognized; and, third, the importance of abolishing child poverty was acknowledged.

WHAT ARE THE PROBLEMS?

Why is it that we expect interventions using grommets, transplant surgery and powerful drugs to be based on sound research evidence, but a hunch may be good enough before we introduce a social intervention? It can only be because there is a widespread and erroneous view that social interventions can do no harm.

Children born into poverty are more likely than their better off neighbours to die in the first year of life, be born small, be born early or both and be bottle fed. As they move through childhood, adolescence and adulthood, they are more likely to die from an accident in childhood, smoke and have a parent who smokes, have poor nutrition and die younger.

In the UK at the start of the twenty-first century, infectious diseases have all but disappeared as causes of death, although tuberculosis is making a comeback in some areas. It is now unusual for children to die from measles or pneumonia, although controversies over the measles, mumps and rubella (MMR) vaccine are likely to result in an upturn in measles deaths if immunization rates continue to fall. Deaths from accidental causes have become the greatest killer in childhood in the UK, with a very steep social class gradient illustrating that accidents do not happen by chance, but are a matter of who your parents are, how well off they are, whether you're a boy or a girl and where you are born. At a time of declining mortality among children, there remains an inequality gap that by some measures is increasing (Roberts and Power 1996).

WHAT CAN WE DO?

One of the first acts of the government which came to power in the UK in 1997 was to commission an independent inquiry into inequalities in health. The most important message to those of us working to reduce inequalities in childhood is that the areas identified for action are not 'medical' ones. Despite the fact that the inquiry was chaired by one of the country's most senior doctors, reporting to the secretary of state for health, most of what is covered by the recommendations is not a task for the National Health Service. There is no vaccine against poverty. Effective remedies involve tax and benefits, education, employment, housing, the environment, transport and pollution.

Of the recommendations in the report, ten are of particular relevance in reducing health inequalities for children and young people.

- Reductions in poverty in women of childbearing age, expectant mothers, young children and older people by increasing benefits in cash or kind.
- The development of high-quality pre-school education so that it meets, in particular, the needs of disadvantaged families.
- Measures to encourage walking and cycling and the separation of motor vehicles from pedestrians and cyclists.

- Policies that reduce poverty in families with children by promoting material support; removing barriers to work for parents who wish to combine work with parenting; and enabling those who want to be full-time parents to do so.
- An integrated policy for the provision of affordable, high-quality day care and pre-school education with extra resources for disadvantaged communities.
- Policies that improve the health and nutrition of women of childbearing age and their children, prioritizing the elimination of food poverty and the prevention and reduction of obesity.
- Policies that increase breastfeeding.
- Policies which promote social and emotional support for parents and children.
- Consideration of minority ethnic groups in needs assessment, resource allocation, health care planning and provision.
- Policies that reduce psychosocial ill health in young women in disadvantaged circumstances, particularly those caring for young children.

There is strong evidence that where practice is informed by robust evidence of effectiveness, and supported by a positive policy environment, child health inequalities can be substantially reduced (Roberts 2000). In what follows, some of this evidence is described.

EARLY LIFE

KEY POINTS

- At all ages in childhood, lower social class brings an increased risk of mortality.
- Babies born weighing under 2500 g in 1991 accounted for 59 per cent of neonatal deaths.
- In England and Wales, during 1989–91, the perinatal mortality rate for infants of mothers born in Pakistan was almost double the rate of infants born to UK-born mothers.
- Despite efforts to encourage breastfeeding, the level in the UK has remained static for the last 20 years, with strong social class differences.

Inequalities in health start early, at or before birth. Poor parents are at greater risk of a stillborn baby, and babies born to poor parents are more likely to die in the first week of life (neonatal deaths) and the first year of life (infant deaths). They are more likely to be born early and at a low birthweight. Despite improved obstetric and neonatal care, babies born early and babies born small are at risk of a range of poor outcomes both immediately and in later life. Having a premature or very small baby also means an anxious start to parenthood.

Social support in pregnancy

A study by Oakley *et al.* (1990) demonstrated the effectiveness, appropriateness and safety of social support provided by midwives to women with a high-risk pregnancy. In this study, women with a history of low birthweight were randomly assigned to receive either a social support intervention in pregnancy in addition to standard antenatal care or standard antenatal care only. Social support was given by four research midwives through 24 hour contact telephone numbers and a programme of home visits. During these visits, the midwives provided a listening service for the women to discuss any topic of concern to them, gave practical information and advice *when asked*, carried out referrals to other health professionals and welfare agencies as appropriate, and collected social and medical information.

Babies of the intervention group mothers had a mean birthweight slightly higher than that of control group babies and there were fewer very low birthweight babies in the intervention group. Interestingly, as follow-up has continued, differences between the intervention and control groups have been maintained, with more positive results in the intervention group. At 7 years, there were fewer behaviour problems among the children and less anxiety among the mothers in the intervention group (Oakley *et al.* 1996).

Some babies are at increased risk of poor outcomes. Mothers and babies from minority ethnic groups, including travellers, refugees and asylum seekers, frequently have particular risks at and around the time of birth. In the 1980s, the Department of Health and Save the Children engaged in the Asian Mother and Baby Campaign (AMBC), a joint initiative to improve the health of mothers and babies. This included a programme of publicity and health promotion and the provision of link workers. An evaluation of the campaign found that publicity had limited success in making Asian women aware of the scheme (Rocheron and Dickenson 1990). The link worker scheme was associated with several improvements to quality and continuity of care, although it was less successful in terms of imparting health education knowledge (Mason 1990). The evaluation suggested that the campaign was weakened by a lack of specific objectives, which initially allowed structural racism to be ignored. Protests by the community and growing evidence of racism led the campaign to place greater emphasis on these problems (Garcia *et al.* 1994).

Reducing postnatal depression

Depression in the first few weeks and months of motherhood is painful for the mother and her family and is associated with a range of unwanted outcomes for children. At least one mother in ten experiences a period of medically diagnosable depression in the early months following birth (Cooper *et al.* 1991). Treatment programmes have been developed and evaluated in Edinburgh, Staffordshire, Lewisham and Cambridge (Cox *et al.* 1987; Holden *et al.* 1989; Gerrard *et al.* 1993; Cooper and Murray 1997). These programmes use a simple screening questionnaire (The Edinburgh Postnatal Depression Scale) to detect depression during home or clinic visits. Mothers found to be at risk are offered counselling. Health visitors in the Cambridge study were also trained to offer help in using problem-solving skills to overcome depressive thoughts and to deal with difficulties in responding to their babies' needs. The programmes are delivered in the home.

The Cambridge study compared mothers who were diagnosed as depressed and were supported by specially trained health visitors with a control group of mothers who were diagnosed as depressed in the months just before the health visitors were trained and who received conventional care. The rate of difficulties with the mother–baby relationship halved for the treatment group of mothers, but remained the same for the control group. A second study of depressed mothers who received similar treatment found mothers reporting significantly fewer behaviour problems with their children by the time they were aged 18 months, compared with mothers who had routine care (Seeley *et al.* 1996; Cooper and Murray 1997; Utting 1999).

MIDDLE CHILDHOOD

Child injury

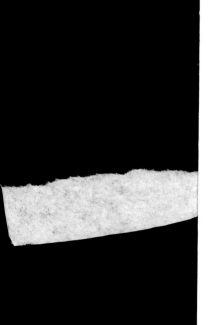

KEY POINTS

- Child accidents are the main cause of death in childhood after the age of 12 months in the UK.
- Child accidents are a cause of considerable morbidity in children and anxiety in adults.
- There is a steeper social class gradient for child accidents than for any other cause of death.
- A child from the lowest social class is 16 times more likely to die in a house fire than a child from a well-off home.
- The gap between the least and the most well-off in this area is growing.

Unintentional injury is the most important cause of child death in the UK and has a steeper social class gradient than any other cause of death. Although there is a considerable industry addressing child protection in the sense of child abuse, it is far less common for authorities to systematically address the dangers to children in the wider domain, through accidental injury (McNeish and Roberts 1995). There is a need to develop children's service plans which aim to reduce accidental injury to children, as well as abuse, particularly as the latter probably presents rather less scope for effective detection, prevention and treatment.

The steep social gradient in child accidents was highlighted 20 years ago by those preparing the Black Report, and the inequalities they signalled were targeted as important issues for action and investigation (Working Group on Inequalities in Health 1980). Accidents have traditionally had a relatively low profile and a low priority as a threat to children's well-being, although the introduction of a national accident reduction target in 1999 as one of four key public health targets (Department of Health 1999) is helping to focus attention on child accidents.

There are effective ways to keep children safe and the evidence base for interventions in this area is improving.

Preventing household fires

In terms of the difference between the best off and worst off children, house fires are a major contributor to life and death inequalities. Among children aged 0–14 years in England and Wales, house fires are a leading cause of death, with a very steep social class gradient. It has been suggested that smoke alarm ownership is associated with a reduced risk of fire injury or death. A systematic review by DiGuiseppi and Higgins (2000) summarized well-designed interventions in this area in a way that serves to illustrate the danger of simply deciding 'smoke alarms are good, let's have some'. If money is to be spent effectively, we need to know which smoke alarms will work for whom, and whether at the end of the day they have the expected effect on reductions of injuries and deaths from smoke inhalation or burns.

Many smoke alarms delivered to households do not get fitted; many of those that do are disabled because of nuisance alarms or other calls on the battery. How do we make sure they are installed properly and how do we make sure they are not disabled for causing a nuisance every time the toast is burned? Are some kinds of smoke alarm more likely to be functioning after the passage of time than others? Does it make a difference if the battery has a long life? As part of a Health Action Zone in Camden and Islington, a Single Regeneration Bid in West Euston and a trial funded by the Medical Research Council (MRC), an exploration of the effectiveness of different kinds of smoke alarm is being tested. This involves a randomized controlled trial with a qualitative element exploring what the users, installers, recruiters and children of the households in the study area say about their experiences of different kinds of alarm.

Robust statistical methods have been used to determine which alarms are working best at the end of the trial, while the qualitative work enables us to understand more about why some people won't accept them at all, why alarms get disabled and what persuades people to replace batteries. Interviews and focus groups were held with the people recruiting to the trial, the people installing alarms, people receiving alarms and children in the neighbourhood.

Drawing on children's and parents' safe-keeping strategies – or what are people doing right?

We have relatively limited data on how parents manage to keep their children safe most of the time and why these strategies sometimes fail. Even in a high-risk area, safety is a dominant social value and good practice will draw on this. Towner *et al.* (1993) reviewed health promotion approaches to child accidents. Important data on keeping children safe in very localized environments and strategies for improving the safety of an area form part of a largely untapped reservoir of knowledge held by ordinary parents and children.

Drawing on evidence from the Nordic countries, where the incidence of child injuries is much lower than in the UK, the most promising approaches appear to be those based on the separation of children from traffic. Also important are 'passive' measures, such as thermostats on water systems preventing scalding.

Three observations (Roberts *et al.* 1995) underlie the effective reduction of accidents to children in the context of the family and the community.

1 *Most accidents occur in hazardous environments.* Spatial and socio-economic disparities in accident rates are a reflection of differences in the incidence of risky environments. Effective accident prevention is concerned as much with environmental change as with behaviour modification. Road traffic accidents can be 'planned out' of particular urban areas through the use of road layout, chicanes and off-street parking. Other accidents can be reduced by attention to housing design and the provision of safe places for children to play. In practice, between a third and a half of all accidents may be preventable through specific engineering, environmental or legislative measures (Stone 1993).

2 *Parents and children living in particular environments are experts in identifying local risks.* At present, much of the information used by those trying to prevent child accidents is insufficiently localized. Moreover, there are no records of child accidents, only of child injuries. These data tend to describe the consequences of an accident rather than the accident itself and its antecedents. Although people living with local risks may become used to them, and even find ways of avoiding them most of the time, on the whole they know what these risks are – the broken fence beside the railway line or the cars that don't stop at the lights even when the green man is showing. Children as young as 7 years who took part in a Safe School project (CAPT and Roberts 1993) were able to identify risks and dangers and suggest practical measures to alleviate them. Effective accident prevention draws on the specialist local knowledge of children and parents.

3 *Strategies among parents for keeping their children safe are more apparent than irresponsible risk-taking.* Just as local people are well-placed to recognize local risks, they are also likely to have strategies for avoiding these, most of which will work most of the time. Prevention policies need to explore the ways in which safety behaviours are integrated into everyday life and played off against other household routines ('Do I leave my children alone while I go down two floors to hang out my washing, or take them with me down the stone steps?'). Effective prevention policies recognize that people living in risky communities are knowledgeable, imaginative and cost-conscious and use this expertise.

Children as experts

In carrying out research into child accidents in Rochdale, children were involved in their role as experts as well as research respondents. In addition to being consulted by means of group discussion in school, during Child Safety Week a group of school children conducted their own traffic survey on the main road near the school. They monitored the traffic lights at the school crossing for an hour and found that 31 drivers went through when the lights were red, 73 at amber. The school crossing attendant confirmed: 'This isn't unusual. I regularly nearly get run over'. One child described an experience that others confirmed: 'The green man was on and a car just came zooming past and I stopped, and after the car went past, I crossed the road'. In the light of this, their suggestions for improvement were directed towards engineers and drivers, rather than their own behaviour:

Drivers in Wardleworth have to make their cars slower . . .

It would be safer for children by keeping traffic low and policemen and ladies walking around . . .

You can make a bridge going over the road . . . (McNeish *et al.* 1995: 29)

LATER CHILDHOOD AND YOUNG ADULTHOOD

KEY POINTS

- Although it is never too early to make a difference to the lives of young people, and early life is the best time to intervene effectively, it is never too late.
- The desire to 'do something' can mean that interventions with vulnerable groups are not properly thought out and may be ineffective or worse.

Education

- The best remedy for a disadvantaged start is a good education.

Unwanted teenage pregnancy

- A good general education is strongly associated with low rates of teenage pregnancy. A range of life choices may make early pregnancy in less than ideal circumstances, less attractive.

Looked after children and young people

- Looked after children and young people get a particularly poor deal.
- The Quality Protects initiatives offer a way to start to monitor and improve the looked after experience for children.

Education

Data from the National Survey of Health and Development, one of the UK cohort studies, indicate that the most important protective factors for children from poor socio-economic circumstances are:

- Parental interest in, and enthusiasm for, their education. Children fortunate enough to have this help display a strong tendency to do better in cognitive tests and in educational attainment (Douglas 1986). In due course, such children, as adults, were more likely than others to be enthusiastic about their own children's education (Wadsworth 1986, 1991).
- Parental enthusiasm also helps to fend off the risk to educational attainment presented by parental divorce and separation (Wadsworth and Maclean 1986).
- The importance of educational attainment is seen in all aspects of the findings on adult life. Those who gained qualifications at 'A' level (or training equivalents) or above had much better chances in health (Braddon *et al.* 1988; Kuh and Cooper 1992; Mann *et al.* 1992; Kuh and Wadsworth 1993) as well as in occupation and income (Kuh and Wadsworth 1991; Wadsworth 1991).

For people reading this book, the ability to read and write has been empowering. It has helped us explore other worlds, find employment and enjoy leisure. The ability to read is a liberating experience for children. Supporting parents who have had a poor educational experience themselves to enter their child's school without feeling intimidated and to be in a position to give their child a hand with school work, appears to be beneficial to children's well-being and have positive long-term outcomes (Wadsworth and Maclean 1986).

PRACTICE EXAMPLE

'Boox* on the Move'
Castle Project, Leeds

This partnership between Barnardo's, a local health authority and a library service aims to develop basic, life-long learning, communication and information technology skills. The service uses a bus as an alternative to the care setting. As well as providing a range of activities that promote the value of reading, the initiative also creates opportunities for health promotion.

* The title was derived from a national project and was also the choice of the young people involved.

Contact: The Castle Project: 0113-2583300

Pregnancy prevention

The most important data available on the effectiveness of interventions designed to reduce unintended teenage pregnancies are contained in the review produced by the NHS Centre for Reviews and Dissemination (1997) at the University of York and the review from the Social Science Research Unit, University of London Institute of Education (Peersman *et al.* 1999a,b). In their overview of effectiveness, the Health Education Authority (HEA, now the Health Development Agency) suggests that tightly focused local interventions targeting vulnerable groups are likely to be more effective (Meyrick and Swann 1998). The groups they identified are:

- young people living in deprived areas;
- young people who do not attend school;
- young people who are looked after by, or leaving, local authority care services;
- young people who are homeless; and
- young people who are the children of teenage parents.

While 'health education' or 'sex education' is sometimes seen to be the key, there is stronger evidence that the best protection is a good basic education, providing as it does a route into different life choices for young women (Centre for Reviews and Dissemination 1997).

The UK has the highest rate of teenage pregnancy in western Europe, although it has been relatively stable for some decades. What has changed has been the numbers of young women giving birth to children outside marriage. Among the reasons (Kubba and Carr 1999: 88) are:

- low expectations (no reason not to become pregnant) – in the UK, only 75 per cent of 15- to 19-year-olds are in education or training; and
- mixed messages (it sometimes seems that sex is compulsory but contraception is illegal).

A report from the Social Exclusion Unit on teenage pregnancy (SEU 1999; www.cabinet-office.gov.uk/seu/1999/Teenpar/index.htm) and a recent empirical study (Churchill *et al.* 2000) indicate that teenage pregnancy is not just about a lack of sex education. Some young people may see no reason *not* to get pregnant and have low expectations.

Given that by no means all teenage pregnancies are unintended, unwanted or unplanned, supporting teenage mothers and their children is as important as preventing unwanted pregnancies. Many young mothers do well (Phoenix 1990), including some young mothers leaving care. The results of a small-scale qualitative study of young people leaving care in Wales (Hutson 1997) suggest favourable outcomes in terms of stability and maturity for those who were early mothers. Although it is difficult to draw conclusions from small numbers, the young mothers appeared less poor and, in some ways, less isolated than the young people newly moved into single person's schemes. Despite the enormous challenge of having and looking after a baby, these young women seemed more closely drawn into mainstream life.

One young mother in Hutson's (1997) research gets up at 6 am every day. She gets herself and her 2-year-old daughter ready and catches the bus at 8 am to a college ten miles away. While her daughter is in the crèche, she studies. She wrote in a feedback letter: 'The government copy America in all their ideas, so why don't they copy them and provide schools/crèches with free colleges like America?'

Given what we know about the effectiveness of early education, good support to young parents and their children in the early years for those who do become parents, and for their children, is likely to be effort well invested.

In the light of the above, it is likely that the following would be positive moves:

- Treating young mothers as people who have made a positive choice, albeit from a limited range of choices, and focus on using their experience to learn how best to provide support, not as a dreadful warning to others of the folly of premature maternity.
- Recognizing that male partners may have a greater role than is apparent and may have financial disincentives to being more involved in the lives of their children.
- Working with colleges on the logistical arrangements and support that is necessary to enable young parents to remain in education.

A recent European review (Mielck *et al.* 2001) looked at a whole range of issues across Europe on reducing inequalities in health; Table 11.1, adapted from their work, summarizes some of these.

PRACTICE EXAMPLE

Sally Jenkins at the Barnardo's Marlborough Road Project in Cardiff manages a cluster of supported accommodation and one of the housing units is for young parents. These young people are unlikely to have any family support and often have a history of abuse. The focus of her work is on supporting young parents, not pregnancy prevention as such, although encouraging lifestyles that make a second early pregnancy less likely is part of her work. She points out that:

- The young people she works with are not, overall, in need of sex education – their pregnancies were not due to ignorance or unavailability of contraception. In many cases, it was a matter of positive choice or a normative act given their backgrounds.
- Young women who avoid second pregnancies are the ones who succeed in education. Where routes into education are made easier for young mothers by providing crèches, transport to college and support that extends over several years, this will be a more probable route. Crèches that finish too early or poor transport to colleges in the suburbs can be major obstacles to young people.
- Fathers are more involved than often reported but can be rendered 'invisible' by benefit traps that penalize couples for openly co-habiting.

CAUTIONARY TALES...

Fluoridation

In using evidence, we need to be aware of context and changes in the evidence base over time. In a previous review of strategies that can reduce child health inequalities (Roberts 2000), my view was that fluoridation of water was a strong contender for inclusion. However, in October 2000, the Centre for Reviews and Dissemination at the University of York published a review of the literature on fluoridation. This high-quality review concluded:

> Given the level of interest surrounding the issue of public water fluoridation, it is surprising to find that little high quality research has been undertaken. As such, this review should provide both researchers and commissioners of research with an overview of the methodological limitations of previous research conducted in this area.
> (Centre for Reviews and Dissemination 2000: 4)

The evidence of a benefit of a reduction in caries should be considered together with the increased prevalence of dental fluorosis. The research evidence

Table 11.1 Interventions primarily aimed at children and adolescents (adapted from Mielck et al. 2001)

Health problem	Target population	Intervention	Effect of the intervention	Evidence	Reference
Malnutrition	Deprived 7- and 8-year-olds	Provision of free school milk	Height gain: 2.9 mm higher in experimental group	RCT	Baker et al. 1980
Mental health problems		Training in active problem solving	Increased self-initiated health enhancing activities, best effect in low SES children	Controlled experiment	Arborelius/ Bremberg 1988/1992
Accidental injuries	Deprived areas, general population	Community interventions; feedback of local data to authorities in charge of local environmental injury risks	Reduction of accidental injuries	Qualitative work and controlled experiments	Roberts et al. 1993 Svanström et al. 1995
Road traffic accidents (pedestrian and cyclist)	Children	Introduction of 20 mph zones in residential areas	Pedestrian and cyclist accidents fell by 70% and 48% respectively (67% overall: no 'accident migration' to other areas)	Controlled before/after study	Webster/ Mackie 1996
Mental health problems	Low SES families, general population	Child-centred quality day care	Reduction of behavioural and social problems, effect size increases by age of child	Observation studies	Andersson 1992 Broberg et al. 1997 Zoritch et al. 2000

Table 11.1 *(Cont'd)*

Health problem	Target population	Intervention	Effect of the intervention	Evidence	Reference
Mental health problems	Low SES district	Structured schooling; clear and realistic targets for the students, feedback from teachers to students, headteacher leadership, etc.	Fewer behavioural problems, improved social adjustment	Observation study	Rutter et al. 1979
Mental health problems	General population	Schools with fewer than 500 students	Fewer behavioural problems, improved social competence	Observation study	Rutter 1983
Accidental injuries	General population	Building of separate bicycle lanes	20% reduction of accidental injuries	Observation study	Sabey 1995
Accidental injuries	Families in deprived areas	Separation of residential areas from motor traffic	Reduction of fatal injuries	Observation study	Sharples et al. 1990
Accidental injuries	General population	Child-resistant containers for drugs	Reduction of accidental injuries	Time series	Lawson et al. 1983
Tobacco smoking	General population	Increased tobacco tax	Reduced smoking in low income group	Time series	Pekurinen 1989

is of insufficient quality to allow confident statements about other potential harms or whether there is an impact on social inequalities. This evidence on benefits and harms needs to be considered along with the ethical, environmental, ecological, costs and legal issues that surround any decisions about water fluoridation. All of these issues fell outside the scope of this review, which concluded 'any future research into the safety and efficacy of water fluoridation should be carried out with appropriate methodology to improve the quality of the existing evidence base' (NHS Centre for Reviews and Dissemination 2000: 4).

Clearly, if interventions are to be imposed on whole populations, without the requirement for consent, the evidence needs to be particularly strong.

Educating people out of danger

We also need to be aware that some interventions that appear benign may have no effect, or even have an adverse effect, and that self-evidently effective interventions may be unpopular. A common intervention in child accident prevention has been the use of leaflets, pamphlets and health education. Surprisingly, there is little evidence to support the use of educational materials and some to suggest that it may be hazardous, increasing anxiety among mothers without reducing risks to children (Roberts *et al.* 1993). A good deal of evaluation in the child safety area has looked at whether or not the message has been received and remembered rather than whether behaviour has changed (let alone whether the child accident rate is affected). The emphasis of road safety work, moreover, has traditionally focused on the child's behaviour rather than the behaviour of motorists. Seventy per cent of car drivers exceed the 30 mph limit in built-up areas. For a child pedestrian, chances of survival are 5 per cent if struck at 40 mph, 45 per cent at 30 mph but 95 per cent at 20 mph. Even so, proposals to reduce speed in built-up areas, or enforce current limits more effectively, do not meet universal approval.

Transferability

Finally, initiatives which may work well in one context may not transfer easily. Home visiting schemes, well-designed and well-delivered, appear very promising as an intervention. However, a recent paper from a group which has worked very extensively on the effectiveness of this intervention (Eckenrode *et al.* 2000) cautions against its use in circumstances of severe domestic violence. On the basis of a 15 year follow-up of a randomized controlled trial of home visitation to reduce child maltreatment, the authors found that in families with high levels of domestic violence, the intervention did not significantly reduce child maltreatment. They concluded that the presence of domestic violence may limit the effectiveness of interventions to reduce the incidence of child abuse and neglect. Another commentator (Graham Vimpani, personal communication, September 2000) suggests that we also need to know more about its effectiveness in relation to learning-disabled parents, substance-misusing parents and in the presence of parental mental illness.

This serves to emphasize the need, even in interventions where the evidence of effectiveness is good, to look at contextual factors and explore the effectiveness of apparently effective interventions in different situations.

AND FINALLY . . .

We should not become so focused on children's futures that we forget that what is happening to children in the here and now is important also.

> Health is not bought with a chemist's pill
> Nor saved with a surgeon's knife
> Health is not only the absence of ills
> But the fight for the fullness of life
> (Piet Hein)

ACKNOWLEDGEMENTS

I am grateful to several colleagues who helped me think about this chapter, in particular Tony Newman, who offered critical comment, ideas and support throughout. David Utting allowed me to use his work on the evidence that can be used by trailblazers in Sure Start; Andreas Mielck, Sven Bremberg and Hilary Graham and their editors allowed me to adapt their work for Table 11.1.

REFERENCES

Andersson, B.E. (1992) Effects of day-care on cognitive and socio-emotional competence of thirteen-year-old Swedish schoolchildren, *Child Development*, 63(1): 20–36.

Arborelius, E. and Bremberg, S. (1988) It is your decision – behavioural effects of a student centred school health education model for adolescents, *Journal of Adolescence*, 11: 287–97.

Arborelius, E. and Bremberg, S. (1992) How do teenagers respond to a consistently student-centred programme of school health education at school? *Health Promotion in Action*, ESSOP Congress. Valencia, Spain, 1992: 69.

Baker, I.A., Elwood, P.C., Hughes, J. *et al.* (1980) A randomised controlled trial of the effect of the provision of free school milk on the growth of children, *Journal of Epidemiology and Community Health*, 34(1): 31–4.

Braddon, F.E.M., Wadsworth, M.E.J., Davies, J.M.C. and Cripps, H.A. (1988) Social and regional differences in food and alcohol consumption and their measurement in a national birth cohort, *Journal of Epidemiology and Community Health*, 42: 341–9.

Broberg, A., Wesselt, H., Lamb, M. and Hwang, C. (1997) Effects of care on the development of cognitive abilities in 8-year-olds: a longitudinal study, *Developmental Psychology*, 33: 62–9.

CAPT and Roberts, H. (1993) *A Safe School is No Accident*. London: Child Accident Prevention Trust.

Centre for Reviews and Dissemination (1997) *Preventing and Reducing the Adverse Effects of Unintended Teenage Pregnancies*, 3(1). York: University of York.

Centre for Reviews and Dissemination (2000) *Systematic Review of the Safety of Public Water Fluoridation*. York: University of York.

Churchill, D., Allen, J., Pringle, M. *et al.* (2000) Consultation patterns and provision of contraception in general practice before teenage pregnancy: case-control study, *British Medical Journal*, 321: 486–9.

Cooper, P.J. and Murray, L. (1997) The impact of psychological treatments of post-partum depression on maternal mood and infant development, in L. Murray and P.J. Cooper (eds) *Postpartum Depression and Child Development*. New York: Guilford Press.

Cooper, P.J., Stein, A. and Murray, L. (1991) Postnatal depression, in J. Seva (ed.) *The European Handbook of Psychiatry and Mental Health*. Zaragos: Anthropos.

Cox, J.L., Holden, J.M. and Sagovsky, R. (1987) Detection of postnatal depression: development of the 10-item Edinburgh postnatal depression scale, *British Journal of Psychiatry*, 150: 782–6.

Department of Health (1999) *Getting Family Support Right: Inspection of the Delivery of Family Support Services*. London: Department of Health.

DiGuiseppi, C. and Higgins, J.P.T. (2000) Interventions to promote smoke alarm use: systematic review of controlled trials, *Archives of Disease in Childhood*, 82: 341–8.

Douglas, J.W.B. (1986) *The Home and the School*. London: MacGibbon and Kee.

Eckenrode, J., Ganzel, B., Henderson, C.R. *et al.* (2000) Preventing child abuse and neglect with a program of nurse home visitation: the limiting effects of domestic violence, *Journal of the American Medical Association*, 284: 1385–91.

Garcia, J., France-Dawson, M.F. and Macfarlane, A. (1994) *Improving Infant Health*. London: Health Education Authority.

Gerrard, J., Holden, J.M., Elliott, S.A. *et al.* (1993) A trainer's perspective of an innovative programme teaching health visitors about the detection, treatment and prevention of postnatal depression, *Journal of Advanced Nursing*, 18: 1825–32.

Holden, J.M., Sagovsky, R. and Cox, J.L. (1989) Counselling in a general practice setting: a controlled study of health visitor intervention in the treatment of postnatal depression, *British Medical Journal*, 298: 223–6.

Hutson, S. (1997) *Supported Housing: The Experience of Young Care Leavers*. Barkingside: Barnardo's.

Kubba, A. and Carr, S. (1999) Teenage pregnancy or sex by any other name?, *Public Health Medicine*, 1(3): 88–9.

Kuh, D.J.L. and Cooper, C. (1992) Physical activity at 36 years: patterns and childhood predictors in a longitudinal study, *Journal of Epidemiology and Community Health*, 46: 114–19.

Kuh, D.J.L. and Wadsworth, M.E.J. (1991) Childhood influences on adult male earnings in a longitudinal study, *British Journal of Sociology*, 42: 535–55.

Kuh, D.J.L. and Wadsworth, M.E.J. (1993) Physical health status at 36 years in a British national birth cohort, *Social Science and Medicine*, 37: 905–16.

Lawson, G.R., Craft, A.W. and Jackson, R.H. (1983) Changing pattern of poisoning in children in Newcastle, 1974–81, *British Medical Journal*, 287(6384): 15–17.

Mann, S.L., Wadsworth, M.E.J. and Colley, J.R.T. (1992) Accumulation of factors influencing respiratory illness in members of a national birth cohort and their offspring, *Journal of Epidemiology and Community Health*, 46: 286–92.

Mason, E.S. (1990) The Asian Mother and Baby Campaign: the Leicestershire experience, *Journal of the Royal Society of Health*, 110: 1–9.

McNeish, D. and Roberts, H. (1995) *Playing it Safe*. Ilford: Barnardo's.

Meltzer, H. (1994) *Day Care Services for Children*. London: HMSO.

Meyrick, J. and Swann, C. (1998) *Reducing the Rate of Teenage Conceptions: An Overview of the Effectiveness of Interventions*. London: Health Education Authority.

Mielck, A., Graham, H. and Bremberg, S. (2001) Children, an important target group for the reduction of socioeconomic inequalities in health, in J. Mackenbach and M. Bakker (eds) *Reducing Inequalities in Health: A European Perspective*. London: Routledge.

Millburn, A. (2001) Speech by Rt. Hon. Alan Milburn MP to Long Time Medical Conditions Alliance Conference, Royal College of Physicians. Reported in press notice, 'Health Secretary announces new plans to improve health in poorest areas', 28 February. London: Department of Health.

Oakley, A., Hickey, O. and Rajan, L. (1996) Social support in pregnancy: does it have long term effects?, *Journal of Reproductive Infant Psychology*, 14: 7–22.

Oakley, A., Rajan, L. and Grant, A. (1990) Social support and pregnancy outcome, *British Journal of Obstetrics and Gynaecology*, 97: 155–62.

Peersman, F., Oakley, A. and Oliver, S. (1999a) Evidence based health promotion: some methodological challenges, *International Journal of Health Promotion and Education*, 37(2): 59–64.

Peersman, G., Sogolow, E., Harden, A. and Mauthner, M. (1999b) *The Role of Theories of Behaviour Change in the Development of Effective Interventions for the Prevention of HIV Infection*, The Cochrane Collaboration, Issue 1. Oxford: Update Software.

Pekurinen, M. (1989) The demand for tobacco products in Finland, *British Journal of Addiction*, 84(10): 1183–92.

Phoenix, A. (1990) *Young Mothers*. Cambridge: Polity Press.

Roberts, H. (2000) *What Works in Reducing Inequalities in Child Health?* Ilford: Barnardo's.

Roberts, H., Smith, S.J. and Bryce, C. (1993) Prevention is better . . . , *Sociology of Health and Illness*, 15(4): 447–63.

Roberts, H., Smith, S. and Bryce, C. (1995) *Children At Risk? Safety as a Social Value*. Buckingham: Open University Press.

Roberts, I. and Power, C. (1996) Does the decline in child injury mortality vary by social class? A comparison of class specific mortality in 1981 and 1991, *British Medical Journal*, 313: 784–6.

Rocheron, Y. and Dickenson, R. (1990) The Asian Mother and Baby Campaign: a way forward in health promotion for Asian women?, *Health Education Journal*, 49(3): 128–33.

Rutter, M. (1983) School effects on pupil progress: research findings and policy implications, *Child Development*, 54: 1–54.

Rutter, M., Maughan, B., Mortimore, P. and Ouston, J. (1979) *Fifteen Thousand Hours*. London: Open Books.

Sabey, B. (1995) Engineering safety on the road, *Injury Prevention*, 1(3): 182–6.

Seeley, S., Murray, L. and Cooper, P.J. (1996) The outcome for mothers and babies of health visitor intervention, *Health Visitor*, 69(4): 135–8.

Sharples, P.M., Storey, A., Aynsley-Green, A. and Eyre, J.A. (1990) Causes of fatal childhood accidents involving head injury in northern region, 1979–86. *British Medical Journal*, 301(6762): 1193–7.

Social Exclusion Unit (1999) *Teenage Pregnancy*. London: The Stationery Office.

Stone, D. (1993) *Costs and Benefits of Accident Prevention: A Selective Review of the Literature*. Glasgow: Public Health Research Unit, University of Glasgow.

Svanström, L., Ekman, R., Schelp, L. and Lindström, Å. (1995) The Lidköping accident prevention programme – a community approach to injury to preventing childhood injuries in Sweden, *Injury Prevention*, 1(3): 169–72.

Towner, E., Dowswell, T. and Jarvis, S. (1993) *The Effectiveness of Health Promotion Interventions in the Prevention of Unintentional Childhood Injury: A Review of the Literature*. London: Health Education Authority.

Utting, D. (1999) *Sure Start: A Guide to Evidence-based Services, 'Trailblazer' edition*. London: Sure Start Unit.

Wadsworth, M.E.J. (1986) Effects of parenting style and preschool experience on children's verbal attainment: a British longitudinal study, *Early Childhood Research Quarterly*, 1: 237–48.

Wadsworth, M.E.J. (1991) *The Imprint of Time: Childhood, History and Adult Life*. Oxford: Oxford University Press.

Wadsworth, M.E.J. and Maclean, M. (1986) Parents' divorce and children's life chances, *Children and Youth Services Review*, 8: 145–59.

Webster, D. and Mackie, A. (1996) *A Review of Traffic Calming Schemes in 20 mph Zones*, TRRL report 215. Crowthorne: Transport and Road Research Laboratory.

Working Group on Inequalities in Health (1980) *The Black Report*. London: Department of Health and Social Security.

Zoritch, B., Oakley, A. and Roberts, I. (1998) The health and welfare effects of day care: a systematic review of randomized controlled trials, *Social Science and Medicine*, 47(3): 317–27.

Zoritch, B., Roberts, I. and Oakley, A. (2000) *Day Care for Pre-School Children. The Cochrane Library 2002, Issue 1*. Oxford: Update Software.

ANN BUCHANAN

12

Family support

KEY MESSAGES

- Strategies and programmes work best when the community, child and family want to be involved and want the intervention to work. Motivating the family and child may be as important as the intervention itself.
- Interventions may be at the community level or at the level of the individual.
- Most strategies and programmes will only work in a percentage of cases.
- Some programmes cross the Atlantic, but we need to be careful that they are culturally appropriate in the UK.
- At different times in the life cycle, families and children are more open to change, for example around the birth of a child or early in adolescence. These are the best times for prevention projects.
- Generally, difficult children are trying to communicate their distress; to solve a problem rather than be one.
- The 'avalanche' factor is important – a little change can set off big changes. An intervention does not need to 'cure all'.
- Parents and children need skills and strategies.

INTRODUCTION

> Parenting is probably the hardest job an adult will undertake, but also the one for which the least amount of training and preparation is provided. By learning the most effective approaches, parents can reduce behaviour problems before they get out of control.
>
> (Webster-Stratton 1992: 3)

Here I argue that a central focus in supporting families is helping 'troubled' children become less 'troubled'. First, I provide a brief outline of the causes of, and consequences for, children's emotional and behavioural problems. Next, I summarize ideas for prevention projects with proven efficacy and, finally, provide an overview of interventions for children and young people with particular difficulties. Although such interventions cannot be assured 'to work' in every case, there is research evidence to suggest that they have 'the best chance' of helping families cope with a troubled child or young person.

SUPPORTING FAMILIES

Supporting families is about the 101 things that can be done by friends, neighbours and social care professionals to help families manage the essential task of bringing up children. Such are the stresses of family life; most of us at some time need a little help. Parenting is a challenging task. Some children appear to cope with major adversities without crisis; other children by their very nature are likely to have more problems.

Children are at their most troubled or troublesome when they are in distress. Children's psychological well-being is like a barometer of how a family is coping. Directly or indirectly, troubled children are at the centre of the more serious problems in family life. Whatever difficulties a family may be experiencing, these are multiplied many times over once children become distressed. It is therefore not surprising that such families constitute the vast majority of referrals to family support services. It is also not surprising that a main focus in supporting families is helping children become less troubled.

In England and Wales, local authorities, under the Children Act 1989, have legal responsibilities both to assess the number of children who may be 'in need' in their area, as well as to provide services for individual children in need. If a child is designated as 'in need', both the child and their family are entitled to services. A child is in need if:

(a) He is unlikely to achieve or maintain, or to have the opportunity of achieving or maintaining, a reasonable standard of health or development without the provision for him of services by a local authority under this Part;

> **Case vignettes presented by senior social workers in one local authority of families 'in need'**
>
> Following domestic violence, a mother and her three young children lived in a refuge. Mother and children severely traumatized by experiences.
>
> A lone mother is at the end of her tether and feels she could harm the children. She cannot get children aged 6 and 7 to bed at nights.
>
> Oldest boy over-chastized. Now copying behaviour of father on younger brothers and sisters.
>
> A 15-year-old girl is becoming out of control at home. She is verbally and physically assaulting her mother.

(b) his health or development is likely to be significantly impaired, or further impaired, without the provision for him of such services; or
(c) he is disabled. (Children Act 1989: Section 17)

Section 17(11): 'development' means physical, intellectual, emotional, social or behavioural development and 'health' means physical or mental health.

The definition is very broad and inevitably different local authorities have prioritized different categories of children and families who may be 'in need'. The deliberate aim of the legislation, however, is to direct services towards supporting families before children suffer 'significant harm'. The summary of over 20 research studies brought together in the Department of Health (1995) publication *Child Protection – Messages from Research* found that most children who enter the child protection process exit after the early stages of the investigation and receive no subsequent support or service. The report concluded that social service departments needed to change their thresholds and re-focus more services to support children and families in need.

The Children Act Report (Department of Health 2001) estimates that, at any one time, 3 per cent of the 11 million children in England and Wales are 'children in need'. The 'Framework for the Assessment of Children in Need' (Department of Health 2000) separates 'vulnerable children' – children who may be at risk because of difficult family situations – from 'children in need' – children with recognizable health, educational or behavioural needs. Even so, the 3 per cent 'in need' are likely to be just the tip of the iceberg. In some inner-city areas, for example, up to a quarter of children may have significant emotional and behavioural difficulties (see Buchanan and Hudson 2000).

Difficult behaviour at home

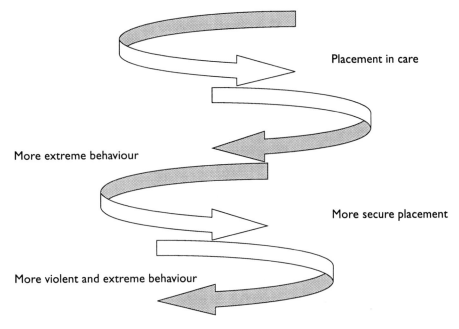

Placement in care

More extreme behaviour

More secure placement

More violent and extreme behaviour

Figure 12.1 The 'spiral' effect.

THE SPIRAL EFFECT

The anxiety about children with emotional and behavioural problems is that whatever may have been the cause of a child's initial difficulties, once serious difficulties present, and in particular once a child becomes separated from their family, emotional and behavioural difficulties can escalate. Apart from the tragedy for the child, the cost as more and more care is required can also escalate out of control (Figure 12.1).

THE INCREASING NUMBER OF CHILDREN WITH EMOTIONAL AND BEHAVIOURAL PROBLEMS

There is considerable evidence that the number of children with 'troubled behaviour' is rising (Rutter and Smith 1995), particularly in inner-urban areas where services are already stretched. Although more psychiatric and psychological services are required, a report from the Maudsley Hospital (Goodman 1997a) suggests that most children with 'troubled behaviour' need social and educational solutions rather than health interventions. Indeed, the report goes

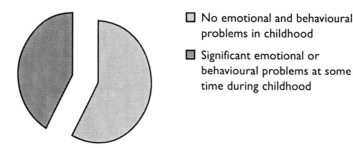

No emotional and behavioural problems in childhood

Significant emotional or behavioural problems at some time during childhood

Figure 12.2 Children with significant emotional and behavioural problems some time in their childhood (from Buchanan *et al.* 2000a).

so far as to say that, in some cases, psychiatric intervention may be counter-productive. Labelling a child a 'psychiatric case' can be more damaging than the disorder itself. The best people to help a 'troubled' child may be those who know the child best.

MANY CHILDREN HAVE EMOTIONAL OR BEHAVIOURAL PROBLEMS AT SOME STAGE. MOST CHILDREN 'RECOVER' – BUT THEY MAY NEED A LITTLE HELP

Recent research (Buchanan and Hudson 2000) using data from the National Child Development Study (NCDS) has shown that nearly 50 per cent of all children have 'difficult' behaviour at some stage (see Figure 12.2). About half of the children who had difficult behaviour at the age of 7 had grown out of it by 11; similarly, half of those who had problems at 11 had recovered by age 16. Very few of these children had formal treatment. It is likely that the natural process of development is responsible for many of these changes, but other children are helped to modify their behaviour by the actions of parents, teachers and friends.

This picture will be familiar to many parents who use a range of strategies to support their children through a 'difficult patch'. The problem is that the parents with the most difficult children may not have the necessary skills, or may be so weighed down by their own problems that they do not have the strength to cope. These families will need a little extra expertise.

WHAT ARE THE CONSEQUENCES OF EMOTIONAL AND BEHAVIOURAL DIFFICULTIES?

In the last 50 years, our understanding of both the causes and consequences of emotional and behavioural difficulties in children has developed considerably.

Table 12.1 Some possible consequences of emotional and behavioural problems

In childhood
- Poorer family relationships
- Lower school achievement
- Greater risk of school suspension/expulsion
- Links with offending behaviour
- Fewer qualifications
- Poorer employment prospects
- Social exclusion

In adult life
- Poorer relationships with partners and own children
- Links with mental health problems in adult life
- Possible links with a range of serious physical illnesses

When it comes to the consequences of emotional and behavioural difficulties, there is now good evidence, especially from longitudinal studies, that such problems can significantly affect a child's life course (Table 12.1). What appears to happen is that there is a chain effect. Emotional and behavioural difficulties in the pre-school period become associated with poorer school progress, fewer educational qualifications, poorer job opportunities – perhaps leading to adult depression – and another whole cycle of sub-optimum parenting in the next generation (for a full review, see Buchanan and Hudson 2000).

WHAT CAUSES EMOTIONAL AND BEHAVIOURAL PROBLEMS?

In the past, different theorists held very differing views about the causes of emotional and behavioural problems in children. More recently, the 'ecological' model has brought together some of the earlier theories (Figure 12.3). Life-history research and findings from longitudinal studies in the UK and elsewhere give support to the model (Bronfenbrenner 1979). Broadly speaking, a developing child, whatever their genetic inheritance, interacts with the different systems with which they come into contact – the child both influences these systems and is influenced by them. Life-history research has shown us that, in each domain, there is a range of risk factors for emotional and behavioural problems and a range of protective factors – that is, factors that may protect a child from maladjustment.

RISK AND PROTECTIVE FACTORS FOR EMOTIONAL AND BEHAVIOURAL PROBLEMS

The following summary (Table 12.2) comes from an extensive review of the literature undertaken by Buchanan and Hudson (2000). Some things cannot

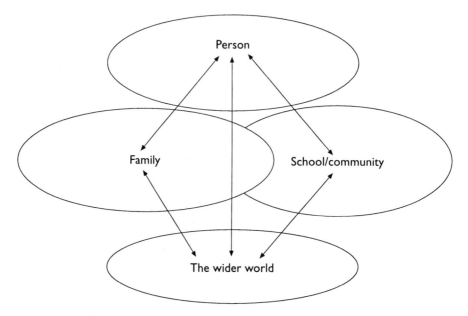

Figure 12.3 The ecological framework.

be changed, but there is evidence (Buchanan and Hudson 2000) that children's emotional well-being can be improved if you *reduce* the number of risk factors, particularly family adversities and *increase* the number of protective factors. In effect, if you manipulate the environment, or set up a compensatory programme, the child may overcome their emotional or behavioural problems. In effect, this is what much of family support as practised in social care agencies is about.

Family adversities, particularly family tensions, have a strong association with both emotional and behavioural difficulties. On the other hand, where families are involved with their children, do things together and are interested in their education, children are protected against psychological difficulties. This has practical implications. Although some children may be vulnerable because of personal characteristics, they are less likely to have behavioural problems if their parents take an interest in their education. 'Involved' fathers or father figures can also be very helpful.

Personal and family characteristics also interact with risk and protective factors in the child's school. For children with difficult home lives, schools and education are the great escape route. If a child reads well, this opens many educational doors. Those who 'look after' children in the state system know that young people need to attend school to benefit from education, but frontline workers may be less aware that frequent changes in schools can be just as destructive as not attending. Bullying is another serious problem in schools, which can devastate a child's emotional health and life chances (Katz *et al.* 2000).

Table 12.2 Risk and protective factors

Factors in the person	Factors in the family	Factors in the school/community	Wider world
Risk	*Risk*	*Risk*	*Risk*
• Biological factors making the child more vulnerable to emotional and behavioural problems, e.g. inherited mental illness • Temperament • Impulsiveness • Physical illness or disability • Mental disabilities	• Family adversities • Poverty • Mental illness in parents • Alcoholism, criminality • Conflict with and between parents • Lax inconsistent discipline • Punitive, authoritarian/ inflexible parenting	• Poor reading/low school attainment • Poor rates of achievement in schools • Bullying in schools • Disadvantaged community/ neighbourhood crime • Racial tension/ harassment • An experience of public 'care'	• Economic recession • Unemployment • Housing shortage • Family change: increasing family breakdown • Long working hours/job insecurity
Protective	*Protective*	*Protective*	*Protective*
• Biological resilience • Good health and development • Good problem-solving skills/high IQ	• Good relationships with parents • Supportive grandparents • Lack of domestic tensions • Family involvement in activities • Being brought up in a birth family	• Supportive community • Schools with good rates of achievement, good 'ethos', lack of bullying • Opportunities for involvement and achievement	• 'Inclusive' policies

Source: Buchanan and Ten Brinke (1998)

Cultural, social and economic changes are responsible for some of the increase in numbers of emotionally disturbed children. The latest figures show that 4.5 million children in the UK were living in poverty (Child Poverty Action Group 2001) and racism is still a serious cause of concern in many areas. Any child who has been looked after by the state carries a significant risk of maladjustment; to a lesser extent, this also applies to children brought up in poverty (Buchanan *et al.* 2000b). Figure 12.4 compares emotional and behavioural outcomes for children brought up in different circumstances.

For example, children who have had some experience of being looked after (care) as well as being brought up by a step-family carry the greatest risk of emotional and behavioural problems; at the other end of the spectrum, boys and girls brought up by birth parents carry the lowest risk. It may, of course, be that the behaviour of some 'looked after' children was extremely troubled before entering care, but there is growing evidence (Buchanan 1995) that the

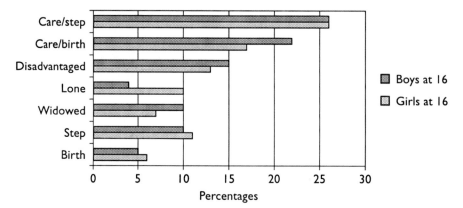

Figure 12.4 Percentages of boys and girls with maladjustment by family background (*Source*: National Child Development Study).

experience of public care may in itself do something to children's self-esteem and identity that magnify their difficulties. If this is true, supporting troubled children in their own homes wherever possible is a better option.

RESILIENCE – THE X FACTOR?

A central finding in the literature on psychosocial adversities is that some children, despite prolonged and severely negative experiences, survive intact. What is this 'X' factor? What can be done to promote resilience? Recent research has taken some of the mystery out of resilience. Certainly, personal attributes play a part ('the born survivor'), but there is also much that can be done to *promote* resilience.

The Christchurch longitudinal study compared two groups who scored highly on a family adversity index. Assessed at age 15–16 years, the resilient group had low ratings on self-reported offending, police contact, conduct problems, alcohol abuse and school drop-out, whereas the non-resilient group had higher ratings on each of these factors. In this high-risk group, the resilient young people had significantly lower adversity scores. Those with multiple problems usually had the highest scores. Resilient young people tended to have higher IQs at 8 years, had lower rates of novelty seeking at age 16 and were less likely to belong to delinquent peer groups. Girls were no more resilient than boys. There was little difference between the two groups on parental attachment; other individual features were not linked to the variations in resilience (Fergusson and Lynskey 1996).

What are the implications of this study? First, even with children who experience multiple adversities, lightening the load may free up energy that can be used productively. Second, in adolescence, the key influence is not so much the family but the peer group. Common-sense strategies to divert young people away from delinquent peer groups seem to be supported by research.

Rutter *et al.* (1998), in a review of research, hypothesized that resilience in young people may be promoted in several ways:

KEY POINTS

- *Reducing sensitivity to risk*: giving young people opportunities to succeed in challenging *activities*.
- *Reducing the impact of the risk*: parental supervision, positive peer group experience, avoidance of being drawn into parental conflict and opportunities to distance oneself from the deviant parent.
- *Reducing negative chain effects*: resulting, for example, from suspension from school, truancy, drug and alcohol abuse.
- *Increasing positive chain effects*: eliciting supportive responses from other people; for example, linking a young person with someone who may help in getting them a job.
- *Promoting self-esteem and self-efficacy*: giving young people opportunities to succeed in tasks and success in coping with manageable stresses.
- *Compensatory experiences* that directly counter the risk effects; for example, where a child has witnessed domestic violence, positive models of non-violent men.
- *Opening up of positive opportunities*: for example, through education and career opportunities.
- *Positive cognitive processing of negative experiences*: for example, not feeling sorry for yourself or letting other people feel sorry for you, viewing negative experiences positively, being constructive.

WHAT HELPS? THE VIEWS OF YOUNG PEOPLE

The exciting new research on resilience suggests that we need to get into young people's heads, or to perceive the world as they see it if we want to help them. The following are comments from two national studies that elicited the views of over 4000 young people aged 13–19 years throughout the UK. These views are their *perceptions*; we do not know to what extent they relate to what we may call their reality. The girls' study took place in 1996, that of the boys in 1998 (Katz *et al.* 1997, 1999).

If you want to help me, you need to see the world as I see it.

Many of us worry about family relationships, fear parents breaking up and are stressed by family conflict. These family difficulties affect how we feel about ourselves and lower our self-esteem. These are everyday stresses for us.

Those of us who need it most may have less emotional support from parents.

We feel good about ourselves when parents [these may be step-parents or foster carers] listen, talk about things that concern us and give us guidance. We also feel good about ourselves when we do things together with the family and when fathers or father figures take an interest in us. But as we get older, we need to learn how to make decisions. This may involve letting us make mistakes.

We worry about the effects of drugs on others and on ourselves. For some, this is an important source or stress.

Good experiences in school make all the difference to our self-esteem. We need teachers who know us as people, courses that are delivered well, teachers who don't make us feel stupid if we don't understand something and good career advice.

More important, we need schools where we are not bullied, that have anti-bullying policies that work and where we are not threatened with violence.

PRINCIPLES INVOLVED IN SUPPORTING FAMILIES AND INTERVENING IN CHILDREN'S AND YOUNG PEOPLE'S LIVES

Every intervention can make things better, make no difference or do harm. 'Do no further harm' is perhaps the first principle that should govern all interventions. How does one ensure that? We can, of course, never be certain, but the following principles should ensure better practice.

KEY POINTS

- Every social care professional involved in supporting families and intervening in children's and young people's lives needs to be mindful of the rights and needs of young people; as far as possible, this means working in partnership and being open about the likely consequences of any intervention.
- To be aware of the legal obligations, such as consent to treatment.
- To be sensitive to ethics and values.
- To be aware of their own competence and lack of competence. Social care professionals should be aware of what type of interventions they are *competent* to undertake and which cases they should refer on. In this chapter, suggested interventions are at Tier One and Tier Two

(Health Advisory Service 1995) – that is, within the competence of a trained social worker.

- As far as possible, only to use evidence-based interventions.
- To take a 'benchmark' at the beginning of an intervention and then compare the progress made against this benchmark.

ASSESSMENT

Assessment can be at many levels. Central to an assessment is obtaining a benchmark. At a primary prevention level, there may be an assessment of the risk and resources present in the community. For example, in setting up the Sure Start initiative, each community involved was required to undertake an assessment of the needs of parents and young children under 4 years in their areas, so that interventions could be put in place at community level to meet these needs. Later progress can be monitored against the original benchmarks.

At an individual level, it is also essential to undertake an assessment to establish benchmarks, so that progress can be measured. Identifying risk and protective factors in the four systems of the person, family, community school and wider world can help plan a 'compensatory programme' (Bronfenbrenner 1979). From this, an individual audit of the strengths and needs of children and their families can be established (Buchanan 1996). The Department of Health (2000) guidance, *A Framework for Assessment of Children in Need*, should also be followed.

A very useful measure is the Goodman Strengths/Difficulties Questionnaire (Goodman 1997b), which can be downloaded free from the internet (www.sdqinfo.co.uk). This questionnaire provides a useful baseline on a child's emotional and behavioural well-being, against which progress in individual cases can be measured.

Ecograms can be used to assess the importance of 'significant others'. For behavioural programmes, an ABC assessment of precipitating factors, and the consequences of both negative and positive behaviours, can be useful. This means:

A   the factors that cause anxiety
B   the child's response
C   the consequences

Finding out what the child is doing when they are *not* having a temper tantrum can often be more revealing than monitoring what is happening when they are. Another useful tool, often used in the probation service in cases involving alcohol or drug abuse, is 'motivational interviewing' (Prochasta and Di Clementi 1982; Buchanan 1999). This tool can be used to help parents and children decide where they are in the cycle of change. Do they want to change their behaviour? What are the benefits or losses of changing behaviour? This step may be needed before starting any formal intervention.

EVIDENCE-BASED INTERVENTIONS

Table 12.3 summarizes a range of interventions that have been evaluated and which, to varying extents, show evidence of effectiveness. Most of these ideas are at the primary level of intervention – that is, they are available to all families or to groups of families and children who may have a particular need.

Projects for vulnerable children

Some children are at more risk because of the circumstances in which they live or because of their current experiences. These children broadly fall into the Department of Health classification of 'vulnerable children'. Table 12.4 lists projects that could be directed to this group of children and young people.

Individual interventions: children aged 3–10

Problem behaviour among young children in its many forms adds stress to an already fraught family situation (Table 12.5). Some problems, such as soiling and bedwetting, may place children at serious risk of abuse.

Table 12.3 Prevention projects

Type of intervention	What it does	Further information
Peri-natal home visiting	Home visit by nurses and health visitors before and around the birth and up to 5 years	***Olds et al. (1997); currently being researched in the UK
Working with fathers	A range of projects being developed all over the UK. Based on growing evidence of the beneficial effects on children of father involvement	**Richardson (1998); ***Flouri and Buchanan (2001)
Targeted pre-school programmes	US models: Headstart and Perry Pre-school programme. Now replicated in some Sure Start projects	***Schweinhart and Weikart (1993)

Table 12.3   *(Cont'd)*

Type of intervention	What it does	Further information
Pre-school home visits with an educational focus	Home visits by a parent–educator. Education focus sometimes more acceptable to parents	***Classic study of Pfannensteil and Seltzer (1985); similar interventions developing in UK
Parent training programmes	Behavioural orientated most successful, but parents need to be carefully recruited or drop-out can be a problem	***Classic programmes by Webster-Stratton (1998); now being used all over the UK
Home visiting by volunteers	Trained volunteers are attached to a family and provide practical support	**Home-Start
Problem solving in pre-school and primary years	Teachers are trained to give the curriculum to the whole class. The goal is to teach children to problem solve and cope with frustration	***US study of Spivack et al. (1976); models developing in the UK
Social awareness and problem solving in primary schools	Curriculum includes teaching children self-control, turn taking, regulation of emotions and improved communication, and problem solving. There are also programmes for parents to help children's learning to be reinforced at home	***US study of Elias and Clabby (1989); Family Links programme in Oxford replicates some of the ideas and is currently being evaluated
Anti-bullying strategies in schools	Children and young people are often the subject of severe bullying (Katz et al. 2000). Whole-school anti-bullying policies can help, but they need to be monitored to ensure that they work	***Olweus (1993)
Teaching life skills to adolescents	Local staff train college students who coordinate programmes and recruit high school student-leaders to lead a GOAL programme	***Danish et al. (1992); programmes led by trained volunteer young people are developing in this country

*There is substantive practitioner case study support for the intervention.
**The research evidence consists of descriptive studies.
***There is research evidence involving a comparative or control group to support the findings.

Table 12.4 Interventions for vulnerable children

Vulnerable group	Type of intervention	Further information
Children whose parents are separating	Programmes geared to different ages given by teachers to whole school classes. The aim is to foster coping and resilience should parents separate	***US study of Pedro-Caroll and Cowen (1985); recent research (Buchanan et al., 2001) shows that children need more information and help when parents are separating
Living with domestic violence	Studies have shown that professionals can help by being alert to women's experience of violence from their partners. Children are damaged not only by being involved in violence, but also by observing violence	**Hester et al. (1996), Hester and Radford (1996), Buchanan et al. (2001).
Young carers	Growing research evidence that young carers need support. Several useful examples of Young Carers projects in the UK	**Frank (1995)
Children living with parental mental Illness	*Crossing Bridges* is a useful UK pack that explores assessment and intervention in this difficult area	**Falkov (1998)
Work with runaways	Around 43,000 young people ran away in England and Scotland in 1990. Most were aged 14–17 years, but 7 per cent were under 11	**Abrahams and Mungall (1992) provide some ideas of possible strategies to help these young people
Children at risk of exclusion	Several projects now in the UK to try and keep children in school	For example, Barnardo's LeCropt Project (Hamill and Hewitt 1993)

*There is substantive practitioner case study support for the intervention.
**The research evidence consists of descriptive studies.
***There is research evidence involving a comparative or control group to support the findings.

Table 12.5 Effective individual interventions for children aged 3–10 years

Type of programme	How it works	Further information
Bedtime programmes*	A bedtime chart is set up (with young children using drawings) outlining the bedtime routine. The child receives stickers for each successful bedtime or part of a sticker for a partially successful bedtime. Parent is given a routine to adopt when the child gets out of bed	***Webster-Stratton (1992), *Buchanan (1999)
Focused morning activity	Getting children to school often leads to rows and arguments. Similar to the bedtime contract, a programme is set up with the child and parent outlining what has to happen each morning with the child having clear duties: get up; clean teeth; find school bag; eat breakfast, and so on. Again, there is a reward at the end	*Buchanan (1999)
Modifying aggressive behaviour	This programme uses cognitive-behavioural principles. That is, the child is helped to become aware of their own anger and is given a strategy, such as a traffic light (red for anger, orange for cooling down, green for go) to remind them to stay calm. Some children can use this to take themselves off to cool down	*Buchanan (1999)
Stopping stealing	Stealing among young children is very common. The card with the happy face in the window and the sad face behind bars, which the child is encouraged to carry in their pocket, is a cognitive-behavioural strategy to remind the child of the consequences of taking things	**Buchanan (1999)
School phobia	Some school phobics have an equally phobic parent. After careful assessment of the child's situation and fears, parents may need help in planning to be strong; that is, choosing a day when they have all the necessary support to ensure that the child goes to school	*Buchanan (1999)

Table 12.5   (*Cont'd*)

Type of programme	How it works	Further information
Eating problems	The basic strategy, unless there are major medical concerns – in which case the child should be under a doctor – is to avoid getting into a dispute about food and simply allow the child to eat what they like until they are eating properly	***Iwaniec (1995), *Buchanan (1999)
Wetting and soiling	Wetting and soiling may have a medical basis and this needs to be checked out. Wetting can now be treated effectively by behavioural principles using the bed pad and buzzer. School nurses often have a supply of these. Soiling is more complicated. Very often this is associated with constipation and this needs to be treated. Soiling can also be helped by a behavioural programme focused on successful defecation. It must not focus on being clean, as this can increase the problem as the child retains and becomes more constipated	***Buchanan (1993)

*There is substantive practitioner case study support for the intervention.
**The research evidence consists of descriptive studies.
***There is research evidence involving a comparative or control group to support the findings.

Slight modifications in a child's behaviour may keep a difficult family situation together while a more complex package of support is put in place. In other cases, a slight modification in a child's behaviour can set off a surprising avalanche of change: the children get to bed at night, parents feel better as they get more sleep, family arguments decrease, a child's behaviour improves at school.

When putting a behavioural programme in place, it is important to understand the basic principles. First, no programme will work unless both the child and the parent are involved. Second, you need to find out how often the behaviour occurs, when and where it occurs, and what reinforces it. After this, you need to establish the desired outcomes, such as getting to bed on time or avoiding tantrums. The next step is to find out what the child likes to do and what they are good at. This may be used to motivate him or her. Finally, you need clearly to specify the behaviour that is the target for change. Several good books are available outlining in simple steps the basic principles. Webster-Stratton's (1992) *The Incredible Years* is fun to read and can be shared with parents.

Common adolescent emotional and behavioural problems

The key difference between children under the age of 10 and those entering adolescence is that the primary influence in their life is less the parent and more the peer group. One of the simplest interventions when a young person is developing emotional and behavioural problems is to adjust the peer influences. In cases of severe bullying, this may mean changing schools; in cases of antisocial activities, it may be a question of filling the time with an equally attractive but socially preferable activity (Table 12.6).

Some young people may still have specific problems for which they need help. Essentially, these are about teaching the young person coping strategies rather than involving them in formal therapy. Harm reduction is often the key objective. Substance abuse and offending behaviour are not discussed in this chapter; however, the possibility of substance misuse being part of the problem should be considered.

Table 12.6 Effective individual interventions for adolescents

Type of problem	Possible intervention	Further reading
Feeling down and depressed	Mood swings are common in young people. When sleeping, eating and a normal way of life are threatened, they may need specialist help for depression. Less severe negative styles of thinking can be helped by cognitive-behavioural techniques. Young people are taught to identify and monitor their emotions, self-reinforce or reward themselves by pleasurable activities when targets (e.g. exam revision) have been reached. Difficulties with social relationships can also be responsive to cognitive-behavioural principles	***Wood et al. (1996)
Recognizing suicidal behaviour	The volatility of young people's emotions can be very frightening. Suicide is a risk in cases of depression, unusual social stresses, alcohol and substance abuse, custody, bullying, isolation, physical and sexual abuse, previous deliberate self-harm, family problems and conflicts. Once a young person has undertaken an act of deliberate self-harm, they should be assessed by their local child psychiatric service	Kingsbury (1994), Royal College of Psychiatrists (1982)

Table 12.6 *(Cont'd)*

Type of problem	Possible intervention	Further reading
Managing fears and anxieties	Cognitive-behavioural techniques also work well in helping young people manage more severe anxieties. Here it is useful to assess the young person by using an ABC framework. The young person is then helped to develop a strategy to manage the anxiety	Ronan and Deane (1998)
Managing anger	Similarly, cognitive-behavioural therapy is useful in anger management programmes. The technique is to help the young person recognize that they may be getting out of control and then suggest strategies to divert or manage the anger better	***Novaco (1975)
Loss and bereavement	Kane has shown that, at different ages, children respond differently to loss and bereavement. Recent research has shown that different people also respond differently to loss and bereavement. Some may feel better able to cope by not talking about it or only talking about it when they choose. Listening, being available, giving permission for the child to talk or not talk about their sadness and the person they have lost appear to be the best strategies	Kane (1979), Buchanan (1999)
Post-traumatic stress disorder	Following major emotional upheavals (including sexual abuse), a high proportion of children experience several distressing reactions, including flash backs, fear and depression (Herbert 1996). Where a child experiences more than two of the following symptoms, they may need medical help: exaggerated startle response/ hyper-alertness, sleep disturbance, guilt feelings about survival, memory/ concentration problems, avoidance of activities that remind them of the trauma, intensification of symptoms when reminded of the trauma	Yule *et al.* (1990)

*There is substantive practitioner case study support for the intervention.
**The research evidence consists of descriptive studies.
***There is research evidence involving a comparative or control group to support the findings.

CONCLUSION

There is now a growing body of information on interventions and strategies that have been shown to help troubled children and thus support families. To date, many of the more reliable studies have been undertaken in the USA and there is a concern to what extent such projects and strategies cross the maritime and cultural divide.

In the UK, the reluctance to assess 'what works' is being overcome. More evaluations are becoming available, but very few of these are full randomized controlled trials. To date, most evaluations remain descriptive, with no comparison groups. When applied to children's programmes, one cannot tell from these studies whether, with the normal process of growing up, children have simply grown out of their problems or whether, as hoped, the interventions have made some difference. Given the expense involved in many projects and the focus on best value, this is a curious economy. Much will be learnt from the new longitudinal studies if and when follow-up sweeps are undertaken.

Political expediencies dictate and elected governments inevitably look for short-term solutions. The worry is that, without adequate controlled trials, we will not be sufficiently confident as to whether an intervention makes a difference, no difference or actually does harm. Ethically, this is rather uncomfortable. On the positive side, however, there is still much we can build on. In helping troubled children become less troubled, we will be also be supporting their families.

REFERENCES

Abrahams, C. and Mungall, R. (1992) *Runaways: Exploding the Myths. An Evaluative Report*. London: NCH/Police Federation.

Bronfenbrenner, U. (1979) *The Ecology of Human Development: Experiments in Nature and Design*. Cambridge, MA: Harvard University Press.

Buchanan, A. (1993) *Children Who Soil: Assessment and Management*. Chichester: Wiley.

Buchanan, A. (1995) Young people's views on being looked after in out-of-home care under the Children Act 1989, *Children and Youth Services Review*, 17(5/6): 681–91.

Buchanan, A. (1996) *Cycles of Child Maltreatment*. Chichester: Wiley.

Buchanan, A. (1999) *What Works for Troubled Children?* Ilford: Barnardo's.

Buchanan, A. and Hudson, B. (eds) (2000) *Promoting Children's Emotional Well-being*. Oxford: Oxford University Press.

Buchanan, A. and Ten Brinke, J.-A. (1998) *'Recovery' From Emotional and Behavioural Problems. Report to NHS Executive Anglia and Oxford*. Oxford: Department of Applied Social Studies and Research, University of Oxford.

Buchanan, A., Flouri, A. and Bream, V. (2000a) In and out of behavioural problems, in A. Buchanan and B. Hudson (eds) *Promoting Children's Emotional Well-being*. Oxford: Oxford University Press.

Buchanan, A., Flouri, A. and Ten Brinke, J.-A. (2000b) Parental background, social disadvantage, public 'care' and psychological problems in adolescence and adulthood,

Journal of the American Academy of Child and Adolescent Psychiatry, 39(11): 1415–23.

Buchanan, A., Hunt, J., Bretherton, H. and Bream V. (2001) *Families in Conflict: Parents' and Children's Perspectives of Welfare Reporting*. Bristol: Policy Press.

Child Poverty Action Group (2001) *An End in Sight: Tackling Child Poverty in the UK*. London: CPAG.

Danish, S., Mash, J., Howard, C. *et al.* (1992) *Going for Goal: Leader Manual and Student Manual*. Richmond, VA: Department of Psychology, Virginia Commonwealth University.

Department of Health (1995) *Child Protection – Messages from Research*. London: HMSO.

Department of Health (2000) *The Framework for the Assessment of Children in Need*. London: The Stationery Office.

Department of Health (2001) *Children Act Report, 1995–2000*. London: The Stationery Office.

Elias, M.L. and Clabby, J.F. (1989) *Social Decision-Making Skills: A Curriculum Guide for the Elementary Grade*. Rockville, MD: Aspen.

Falkov, A. (1998) *Crossing Bridges*. Brighton: Pavilion Press.

Fergusson, D.M. and Lynskey, M.T. (1996) Adolescent resilience to family adversity, *Journal of Child Psychology and Psychiatry*, 9(4): 483–94.

Flouri, E. and Buchanan, A. (2001) Fathertime, *Community Care*, 42: 4–10 October.

Frank, J. (1995) *Couldn't Care More: A Study of Young Carers and Their Needs*. London: Children's Society.

Goodman, R. (1997a) *Child and Adolescent Mental Health Services: Reasoned Advice to Commissioners and Providers*, Maudsley Discussion Paper No. 4. London: Institute of Psychiatry.

Goodman, R. (1997b) The Strengths/Difficulties questionnaire, *Journal of Child Psychology and Psychiatry*, 38(5): 581–6.

Hamill, P. and Hewitt, C. (1993) *Barnardo's LeCropt Project: Evaluative Study*. Strathclyde: University of Strathclyde.

Health Advisory Service (1995) *Child and Adolescent Mental Health Services: Together We Stand*. London: HMSO.

Herbert, M. (1996) *Post-Traumatic Stress Disorder in Children*. Leicester: The British Psychological Society.

Hester, M. and Radford, L. (1996) *Domestic Violence and Child Contact Arrangements in England and Denmark*. Bristol: Policy Press.

Hester, M., Kelly, L. and Radford, J. (1996) *Women, Violence and Male Power*. Buckingham: Open University Press.

Iwaniec, D. (1995) *The Emotionally Abused and Neglected Child: Identification, Assessment and Interventions*. Chichester: Wiley.

Kane, B. (1979) Children's concepts of death, *Journal of Genetic Psychology*, 134: 141–5.

Katz, A., Buchanan, A. and Ten Brinke, J.-A. (1997) *Can-Do Girls*. London: Young Voice.

Katz, A., Buchanan, A. and McCoy, A. (1999) *Leading Lads*. London: Young Voice.

Katz, A., Buchanan, A. and Bream, V. (2000) *Bullying in Britain*. London: Young Voice.

Kingsbury, S. (1994) *Suicide Prevention – The Challenge Confronted*. London: HMSO.

Novaco, R.W. (1975) *Anger Control: The Development and Evaluation of an Experimental Treatment*. Lexington, MA: D.C. Heath.

Olds, D.L., Eckenrode, J., Henderson, C.R. *et al.* (1997) Long term effects of home visitation on maternal life course and child abuse and neglect: fifteen-year follow-up of a randomized trial, *Journal of the American Medical Association*, 278: 637–43.

Olweus, D. (1993) *Bullying in School: What We Know and What We Can Do*. Oxford: Blackwell.

Pedro-Caroll, J.L. and Cowen, E.L. (1985) The children of a divorce intervention program: an investigation of the efficacy of a school-based prevention programme, *Journal of Consulting and Clinical Psychology*, 14: 277–90.

Pfannensteil, J. and Seltzer, S. (1985) *New Parents as Teachers Project: Evaluation Report*. Overland Park, KS: Research and Training Associates.

Prochasta, J.O. and Di Clementi, C.C. (1982) Trans-theoretical therapy: toward a more integrated model of change, *Psychotherapy: Theory, Research and Practice*, 19: 276–88.

Richardson, A.J. (1998) *Father's Plus: An Audit of Work with Fathers Throughout the North East of England*. Newcastle-upon-Tyne: Children North-East.

Ronan, K.R. and Deane, F.P. (1998) Cognitive behavioural interventions with children, in P. Graham (ed.) *Cognitive-Behaviour Therapy for Children and Families*. Cambridge: Cambridge University Press.

Royal College of Psychiatrists (1982) The management of parasuicide in young people under 16, *Bulletin of the Royal College of Psychiatrists*, October, pp. 182–5.

Rutter, M., Giller, H. and Hagell, A. (1998) *Antisocial Behaviour by Young People*. Cambridge: Cambridge University Press.

Rutter, M. and Smith, D. (1995) *Psychosocial Disorders in Young People*. Chichester: Wiley.

Schweinhart, I. and Weikart, D. (1993) *A Summary of Significant Benefits: The High/Scope Perry Pre-School Study Through to 27*. Ypsilanti, MI: High/Scope Press.

Spivack, G., Platt, J.A. and Shure, M. (1976) *The Problem-Solving Approach to Adjustment*. San Francisco, CA: Jossey-Bass.

Webster-Stratton, C. (1992) *The Incredible Years – A Trouble Shooting Guide for Parents of Children Age 3–8*. Toronto: Umbrella Press.

Webster-Stratton, C. (1998) Adopting and implementing empirically supported interventions, in A. Buchanan and B.L. Hudson (eds) *Parenting, Schooling and Children's Behaviour*. Aldershot: Ashgate.

Wood, A.J., Harrington, R.C. and Moore, A. (1996) Controlled trial of a brief cognitive-behavioural intervention in adolescent patients with depressive disorders, *Journal of Child Psychology and Psychiatry*, 37: 737–46.

Yule, W., Udwin, O. and Murdoch, K. (1990) The 'Jupiter' sinking: effects on children's fears, depression and anxiety, *Journal of Child Psychology and Psychiatry*, 31: 1051–61.

DIANA McNEISH
TONY NEWMAN

Last words: the views of young people

The contributors to this book are all experts in their field and have applied their knowledge of relevant research to describe the elements of effective practice in welfare services for children and young people. Using research to highlight 'what works' is fraught with difficulties: all of the chapters contain some uncertainty and ambiguity and, while in some areas of practice we can assert with confidence that some things work better than others, in others the evidence is incomplete and uncertain. Nevertheless, the contributors to this book have highlighted several key messages for the practitioner, manager or policy maker to take into account and these messages constitute a fair summary of the best available research to date.

So what do young people themselves make of these messages? This final chapter gives young people the last word. It is based on interviews with about a hundred young people aged 12–18 years during the spring and summer of 2001, the aim of which was to highlight the policy and practice priorities of young people themselves (Barnardo's 2001). All the young people were service users of Barnardo's at the time of interview, involved with projects providing support to care leavers, young parents, young carers and young disabled people. As such, they can all lay claim to the description 'socially excluded' and have insider's knowledge of what that means in terms of lived experience.

YOUNG PEOPLE'S VIEWS ON THE LOOKED AFTER SYSTEM

Experiences of life in care and leaving care have an enormous impact and many young people expressed very strong views about what does and does not 'work' in the looked after system. Drawing on the issues raised by young people during the interviews, we have highlighted the factors that seem to make the difference between a negative care experience and a more positive one. So, if you are an adult involved in supporting young people through the care system, here are some of the things you could be doing to make a difference:

Be reliable and trustworthy

Young people's experiences of social workers, foster carers, residential staff and teachers appear to be highly variable. Social workers, in particular, are frequently criticized for being unreliable:

> When I was 14–15 my social worker was like, 'I'll see you next week'. He rang up 3 months later . . . fair enough you may have more people to see, but you may depend on them doing something.

> They make an appointment to see you and then they phone up to cancel and I think everyone builds up their hopes of seeing their social worker . . . and they were always phoning up and cancelling.

> There's two things about social workers: they're either an hour late, or an hour goes by and they ring you up and say they're not coming, or all day you're waiting and they don't turn up and then you get a phone call the next day saying 'I couldn't come'.

> On the rare occasion I have bumped into some really nice social workers. But the other 99.9% of the social workers are ignorant or complete xxxxxers.

Many young people have positive and enduring relationships with their foster carers. However, some young people have less positive experiences. Two themes emerge in particular. First, that young people feel that some foster carers' prime motivation is money. Second, that they feel unfairly treated in comparison with foster carers' own children:

> Their house was spectacular, but it was from the money they were getting from social services. It should have been our money. We couldn't have what we wanted but they could have whatever they wanted.

> What annoys me is when you go to review meetings your foster parents are all lovey dovey to you and you go home and they grill you.

Teachers also come in for some criticism, particularly for a lack of sensitivity and negative attitudes towards young people in care:

> They [teachers] automatically say 'oh you're in a children's home that's why you do that'.

> Schools think because you're in children's homes you're a problem tag not because of your proper family background.

However, despite these criticisms, some young people had very positive experiences of adults. Several attributes were repeatedly mentioned, including the ability of a worker to have a laugh, to communicate informally and to demonstrate commitment to the young person. An essential ingredient, however, was the young person feeling as if the adult genuinely cared – that they were there for them and not just doing their job:

> I found my key worker, he helped me a lot, we were really compatible, so if I was having any problems he'd help me, say with homework, and if I passed a test he'd get cake or something, that's how he'd celebrate it.

> I mean I was really lucky and the staff that I had there, and I didn't want to leave, I mean I still keep in touch now, I phone them as often as I can. He was really, really funny, he cared ... Most of the other staff were pretty much like him as well, but I don't know, there was just something about him because he was really like a father to me. I mean after I moved out he used to come down on the weekends, pick me up, take me out for a drink and I used to stay at his house with him and his wife and all that.

> When I left care, then I had [name of key worker] and he was good because when he was young he was in care, and he's been in the same position as I have, and he's turned out to be a carer or whatever.

> I just want to give credit as well to the residential workers because I do think that they do try, I know that, they usually say that if the child's not helping themselves then you can't help them, but even though they do say that they do still try, so I just want people to know that they do try their best.

> Aye, every social worker I've had has been brilliant like ... I love all my social workers ... They've just treated me, like an individual, they don't treat me as if I'm someone in care and someone, that's, you know.

Provide young people with information

Young people described having little or no information about their entitlements and services available to them. Some also described being given little explanation for the decisions made about their lives:

> 'Cos, I won't tell you all my details, but I was taken away from my father and nothing was explained to me. I know I was 11 years old, but there are certain ways you can explain stuff to a child.

> All that I was told was there was an after-care team, but that was it. I wasn't told where it was, nothing like that.

> [Things should be] explained to you ... what they can do for you and what you're entitled to.

I think that foster children should know what they're entitled to while they're in care as well as when they've left . . . Because we were never told.

Really listen to young people and be prepared to act on what you hear

Young people often described feeling as if their views did not count. Although there are processes for listening to young people in reviews and so forth, some young people found these tokenistic rather than genuine:

The care system, they should listen to the young people more, what they're saying to them. If they're unhappy in a home or something, they should move them.

Social workers choose not to hear you.

They try to make your decisions for you.

They might say 'well let's hear what the young person says' you know, 'let's hear what they want'. But at the end of the day they just don't, they put what they want to say, and they just go ahead with what they want and what they think's right.

[in the LAC review forms]. It always says in your form 'who do you think should be at your review?' and 'who don't you'. But see, if you say who you don't want to be there, they won't listen to it.

They sit and say 'Oh, I think you should do this' and 'I think you should do that'. I'd rather just get on with it. I'm 18, I'm an adult and I'll do whatever I want to do at the end of the day. Actually, they've made some very wrong decisions for me, the worse decisions. I'm not going to go into . . . well, I hate them, and they know I hate them and that's why, because they made decisions for me that weren't right.

I think they do listen to you, but they don't do anything about it . . . It's just a waste of their time and ours. If they want our points of view, they should listen, take it in, take it back and do something about it, not just listen to us, pretending they're doing something.

Don't rush young people into leaving care before they are ready

Many young people interviewed had left care at 16 and felt unprepared:

I think I needed more support from them when I actually left care than when I was in care . . . it was a bit rushed [leaving care]. I was asked, well obviously I mean because they have things for where you're supposed to live next and I had an interview at the time they said well we'll put you down our list and I said 'well I'm not really ready to leave care for the moment and I was enjoying it there as well', but they said it's alright because it'll probably take about a year before we find you something anyway. So I said 'well, alright then' and like we found a place about four or five months later and then . . . I didn't have much time for preparation to move out and before I knew where I was, I was living on my own and I wasn't ready for it.

Once they're 16 they're expected to live on their own even though you're not classed as an adult until you're 18. Once they're 16 they're expected to be able to live on their own, get a job, pay a mortgage.

I think you should stay at a placement until you're ready to move out, because they will . . . you should be able to like come up and say like, I'm ready to move out and not when you're 16. When I was 16, I wasn't ready for the move.

I always said that, well if I was living at home I wouldn't be chucked out, but that is the rule, I don't know why but that is the rule that you go out when you're 18 unless, I think there's disability or they think you need to stay on, and then there's still an age on that and that's 21 . . .

Don't abandon young people once they've left care

Having left care, the support experienced by young people was variable and often grossly inadequate:

When I left care, they forgot about me, like.

We don't get any training schemes, like, we don't get to hear about it because we haven't got, you know, parents . . . If it wasn't for here [Barnardo's project] we wouldn't have a clue . . . we wouldn't know where to get all our grants from, we wouldn't know nothing.

You're just a little project and once it's done with that's it.

I've been told when I was in the children's home . . . it cost £60,000 for one child for a year . . . When you're in a children's home compared to like what we are, we're in now, it's like royalty really . . . But things all change when you hit the age of 17, 18.

So I mean I was 16 and I wasn't ready at all. I think it's worked out for the worse because I've been homeless. Because I moved out earlier my social worker wasn't keeping in contact I mean, luckily we've had [name of project worker] and he's really good and he's helped me get myself back together. But there wasn't the after-support. They [the local authority] sort of make all these promises but they never do it.

YOUNG PEOPLE'S VIEWS ON SOCIAL EXCLUSION

The term 'socially excluded' has become a commonly used, some might say over-used, phrase in recent years. It has turned into modern short-hand for an amalgam of more old-fashioned terms such as 'poor', 'disadvantaged', 'discriminated against'. The problem with such handy phrases is that they tend to depersonalize what for many people is a deeply personal experience. All the young people interviewed have experience of social exclusion affecting them personally in their daily lives and we have highlighted the following factors as being important to them.

The experience of stigma

Many young people described scenarios in which their sense of exclusion was further heightened by the insensitive behaviour of adults. Young people in care, for example, were acutely aware of being 'different' and of being subject to negative stereotyping:

> They make you feel very different. You know, these people here have got real mummies and daddies, even if they're probably divorced or something, they've still got their mummy and daddy. And we've got taken away from our mums and dads and are living with total strangers. And people in school didn't actually understand that. Umm, they did ask an awful lot of questions why, and you felt that you had to tell them why. So, just by even asking and putting you on the spot, it just wasn't nice at all.

> In care, you get labelled differently: They're walking past [the project] looking in as if we were pieces of shit on the floor . . . That's their problem, obviously, but it's not nice to be done.

> Yeah definitely, as I say they found out it was a children's home and it's more or less it's a young offenders or a detention centre . . . They think you've done something really bad to go in there and there are people just trying to find out details about you or what these children in residential homes are actually about because there's a stigma.

> I think, I don't know how you deal with that, it's . . . Living in care it's a very difficult thing. You shouldn't be treated too differently. We shouldn't be treated with any more or less respect. But the problem is that not enough schools understand, just because we live in care doesn't mean we're hooligans. Doesn't mean we're off the wall.

> Your record, from care. People know where you've been and who you're with. Once they've looked at the record, they totally look at you differently from a normal person. See how I have to use normal person, you

know what I mean. That's why I have to use the normal word, because they look at us as if we are not normal.

Young parents described similar experiences:

Everyone mocks young mothers . . . [People judge you] . . . just because you're a young mum. It's not fair, they think that all you does is sit on your backside, like there is some young mums that do want to do things with their life. And that's what people need to realize . . . they think we only get pregnant to get a house.

Disabled young people also experienced stigma:

They pick on people with disabilities, I always find.

And then people stare if people are in a wheelchair or something they stare.

You find people who do stick up for you. But you get other people saying 'you should be dead'.

You've gotta feel sorry for these people 'cause they're just uneducated and they just got the way they've been brought up. They must have been just taught like that.

It's grown-ups, you find it's grown-ups more than what it is like people our age.

Some described experiencing similar stigma by having a parent or sibling who is disabled or has a mental health problem:

You've got all these nosy neighbours sitting around the wall watching while the police had to take my mum away 'cause she was really bad then, depressed and all that . . . the neighbours were talking and I'm melting with shame. People would deliberately stand nearby watching while she was [taken away], shouting you're mum's a psycho and all that.

Me parents carry the cane and my dad's got a hearing aid to show he's deaf and you know you get people walking past saying 'oh, disgusting' . . . really slagging them off and that. I look after my nan who's got emphysema and she can't walk, she's in a wheelchair, so if you go out with the wheelchair you're getting more abuse thrown back in your face.

The importance of education

Many of the young people interviewed had experienced serious disruption to their education. Some had experienced both mainstream and specialist provision but what mattered to them was not so much where they were educated, but the quality of education they received and attention to their individual needs:

At mainstream I found it quite difficult because I had the situation at home and that, I was having problems at home. I had behavioural difficulties at school because of the issues at home. And I found that they could only take so much in mainstream, so the school excluded me, which I agreed with anyhow because it was probably the best thing that could be done at that time. And then I went to a residential school and I was deprived of the grades that I could have got . . . And that was because of the residential school teachers. They weren't pushing you like they do in mainstream. Like, they didn't give you homework unless you asked for it, they weren't pushing you to do as well as you could do. And even though I was having a difficult time of it, if I'd had my school work to concentrate on, then it might have been a bit better for me, you know, to cope with everything else. They just didn't push me to do anything.

At the end of the school you should go back and then teachers can help you with your own way . . . just help you through it until you get used to doing whatever they're doing.

The young people's general experience of school was that:

Teachers do not have time to devote attention to individual pupils.

You know if you ask a teacher to help they think you're being sarcastic, they think you're just being idle because you asked them a question. Our mate asked questions and the teacher goes 'I've explained already', but she needed a bit more help and they just don't give it to her.

I think there should be more teachers in the room. One teach one group and one teach another group and explain it to two groups instead of one teacher going around the classroom.

You get 30–40 in a class and not everyone is being seen to.

I left school last year. First year you say 'look, I don't like this, I don't like that, I want something done about it'. Second year, nothing's done about it, third year, fourth year and I'm leaving school by fifth year and they've done nothing and they wonder why we don't like school?

Some teachers don't understand if you've had a really bad day and they start shouting over the little . . . I remember I got kicked out by my mum and I just wasn't in the mood for a teacher and all of a sudden it was like 'you've got lip-gloss on'. And I was like – I'd been through the worst time and all he could pick on was me lip-gloss.

See what annoys me is if kids who aren't even that bad get kicked out of school. What are they gonna do?

For some young people, bullying in school is a particularly important issue:

Bullying should . . . have like support ways if you go through bullying or anything like that . . . you should have cameras to see what's going on . . . on the playgrounds so you can see bullying when that happens.

With bullies, they'll expel them from the school for being bullies, but they should look and see why they're bullying. There's gonna be a reason for why they're being bullies themselves. I think they just don't understand. They should be sat down and talked to.

Try and get someone [who has been bullied themselves] . . . if they haven't been bullied they don't know how you feel, they can just turn round and say 'yeah I've been through it'. You know that they've actually felt the way you're feeling, which is better.

The importance of social spaces and activities

Many young people describe feeling excluded from social activities and a common plea is for more places for young people to go where they can have fun but also feel safe:

It's nowhere for kids to go, so they go in gangs on the streets and that.

I think we need more community services for young people.

It should be on a Friday or a Saturday because everyone is on the street corners getting bullied and there's nowhere to go.

Something concrete like building, like some sort of sport centre where it was cheaper to get in or you know. Send them out ice skating, something for young people to do without standing on street corners and getting drunk.

What about a gym? I would enjoy going to a gym.

I work for a youth club . . . and at first you've got people going in there enjoying themselves, getting away from the problems, they can be themselves. And then you get other people coming in saying 'look I'm older than you' and then saying this and saying that and you just say 'I'm not coming back here' and then you go off.

When I used to go to youth clubs I used to get bullied, but I went to one and I didn't make any friends, so I didn't bother going after that.

For disabled young people, the issue of accessible social activities is particularly important:

It's about the physical environment, communication, the resources and the attitudes whether you're in McDonald's or a youth club or a college, every organization needs to have those kind of strategies.

At xx sports centre you have to get changed in like a stock cupboard because a wheelchair can't get through the door. They're just starting a new one which is separate.

America's got it right. Nearly all their shops are wheelchair accessible and people more ready to help. We need to start thinking about it over here, especially international companies with plenty of money should get their finger out.

How can anyone in a wheelchair get through a revolving door!

And it's not just about people who are in wheelchairs, it's about people with visual impairment, people with hearing difficulties or learning disabilities. Those barriers are really about communication.

The importance of accessible and informal services

Many young people felt that it is difficult to find out about support that is available. In addition, they pointed out that most support is currently crisis-based. The young people were also aware of the inequity in support currently available. For example, homeless care leavers may have more readily accessible support than other homeless young people. They wanted to see more information being made available that was not full of jargon, but written in a format accessible to all. They also felt that services should be more inviting, taking an informal approach.

Drop-in service with young people, sort of, running it. Say like, you've got a problem and you want to speak to someone, it's not always easy to speak to adults, is it? You'd rather speak to someone your own age who's in the same position as you, so I reckon there should be more drop-ins, easier access . . . Because it all seems to be formal, the way you've got to do it like. I think it should be more informal.

He's never been in care but half the support he's tried to get, he's never been able to get it and he really does need it. Just as much as we do.

I think they should just listen to what you have to say and like find out what you need and then they should just help you, innit? Because if they don't . . . I don't know . . . they just treat you like you're the same as everyone else. If someone's got your problem they automatically assume that you need the same thing as them. Everyone's different, they've all got their own needs, like.

YOUNG PEOPLE'S VIEWS ON HEALTH AND SAFETY

Many of the young people interviewed had experienced threats to their health or personal safety at some point in their lives. Some young people made reference to experiences of abuse, many others talked about bullying or feeling unsafe in their environment, or the importance of health education for themselves and for others.

Many of the older teenagers interviewed felt that things were getting worse, that younger people were more likely to be involved in drugs or alcohol misuse than even a few years previously.

> If you go up the road, you'll see 10- and 11-year-olds smoking spliffs and all that and it ain't funny.

> I looks at them as if to say, and I was born and brought up down here, and you didn't see none of that. And I moved away, and if you walk down there and there's heroin, people looking for crack, and they're asking 13-, 14-year-olds for it. And it ain't funny, I just say to myself, 'I've got to get out of here'.

Keeping safe in a dangerous environment

The young people interviewed currently had few places to go other than the streets. They spoke about how they cope in a rough environment. Their experience shows:

> . . . the intimidation of gangs on streets . . .

> You've got gangs on the street corners drinking and everything – if you walk past as innocent as anything, they just jump on you thinking that you're an easy target.

> And you can't even go to the pictures or walk about an area or even to McDonald's or something without getting the crowd on the corner, you know, giving you snotty looks and the rest of it.

> . . . their dealings with the police . . .

> You've got to go out in a big gang yourself, but then if you go out in a big gang you're gonna be stopped, you know what I mean? But you can only do it 'cause if you're in a big gang, they won't pick on you, you know what I mean?

> The police came and took pictures of myself and we were just walking down the road, we weren't doing anything. And then the gangs on the corners they were too scared to go over to the gangs.

Every person under 18 has got a title and their title is 'trouble'. And it's not right at all.

>...the effects of peer pressure...

People do say that 'just say no and walk away and it's easy and all that', but then when you're with your mates ... it's not as much the peer pressure it's just to do it. Do you know what I mean? Just to be.

I think mainly as a teenager it's getting accepted and stuff. There's groups of people and boys and you know what I mean. Trying to find yourself.

When I used to go out with my mates, they'd say 'come out' and then there'd be a big gang of us and then we'd start shouting at someone in the street and that. I'd be like – I wouldn't know what to do but I still liked the people, do you know what I mean?

Got kicked out of school for smoking and I know it was wrong, but you're hardly gonna stay out of smoking when everybody else was doing it.

I can't wait to be an adult 'cause you're getting rid of that pressure then.

Health education

Many young people felt they had insufficient health education or that the adults responsible for their care were inadequately informed about health issues:

I think there should be more crime prevention things in schools and maybe foster carers to be taught, like parents, sex education, easier access ... to family planning, drug and alcohol misuse, you know.

It shouldn't be vulgar, it should be more like the information side.

It should be easier to discuss it as well.

We should be taught more about health and that, we don't get taught nothing about health in school and why you shouldn't go on a diet our age. We get told we're too young to diet because that can do something to your body but we don't know why.

[Need] more awareness of [mental health] and that it's not something to be ashamed of.

It's harder to be healthy when you have little money

Some young people who are struggling to live independently on a low income or who are young parents illustrated how difficult it is to maintain a healthy lifestyle with little money without making many personal sacrifices:

> I used to buy loads of healthy food and all, but since the baby . . . it's just I've got no time to cook with the baby, she's always just there, there, everywhere.

> I was selfish before the baby and I said to [boyfriend] 'I'm too selfish to have a baby', but I couldn't get rid of it because I don't believe in it. And then I had it and I just adapted to spending money on her, it's hard not to buy stuff for yourself. I just wanted to go out and buy new clothes, but I can't, you just got to think of her [child] first. I manage alright though . . . I think I does quite well myself, considering I'm alone. For a single mother on welfare I does quite well, don't I? She's [child] got everything.

CONCLUSIONS

A clear theme emerging from these interviews with young people is the importance of the relationship between a young person and the adults who are providing support and care. Unfortunately, research cannot provide us with the precise ingredients of the ideal social worker, teacher, foster carer or residential worker. And although research evidence can help us weigh up the pros and cons of different approaches to service provision, it can never give the definitive answer to what might be best for young Wayne in his particular circumstances. The evidence-based practitioner needs to apply the knowledge derived from research in conjunction with their knowledge of the individual young person, their knowledge of the current context and their assessment of the future. And all this needs to be combined with commitment, care and compassion.

Although young people do not use the language of 'effectiveness' or 'evidence-based practice', some of their messages have a lot in common with those outlined by the contributors to this book. Many young people who have experience of the care system, for example, concur with the messages in Part 1 of this book about the importance of listening to young people and providing support during and after care. These young people and others can also speak eloquently about the experiences of social exclusion highlighted in Part 2 and many of the issues concerning health and safety in Part 3 are also echoed by young people. Of course, the views of young people, however carefully collected, are themselves only one source of evidence. To pretend that young people have all the answers would be both foolish and patronizing. But they provide a source of knowledge that has frequently been overlooked and, combined with other sources, they offer an essential addition to the evidence base for practice.

ACKNOWLEDGEMENTS

The authors would like to thank the young people who provided the information for this chapter. We also thank the Barnardo's projects and staff who facilitated access to young people, carried out interviews and collated information, especially Sarah Blackburn, Atalanta Christopher, Pam Hibbert, Kristin Liabo, Simone Sadiq, Jo Stephens, Patricia Thompson and Claire Turner.

REFERENCE

Barnardo's (2001) *Whose Government is it, Anyway?* Ilford: Barnardo's.

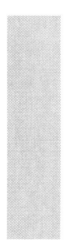

Name index

Ainscow, M., 131–2

Barker, W., 218
Barn, R., 93
Beresford, B., 154
Berridge, D., 89–90
Biehal, N., 63, 65, 66, 70, 71–2, 74–5, 96
Boykin, A.W., 134–5
Brunk, M., 225–6
Buchanan, A., 256, 257–8, 259
Bullock, R., 87–8

Carr, S., 242–3
Cheung, Y., 64, 65
Cleaver, H., 43
Colton, M., 88–9
Connors, C., 149–50
Cook, R., 65

Devine, C., 51, 52
DiGuiseppi, C., 238

Farmer, E., 95–6
Feldman, M.A., 220
Festinger, T., 62
Finch, N., 153
Fisher, T., 22
Fitzpatrick, S., 197

Gartner, A., 131
Gaudin, J., 226
Gibbs, I., 96–7

Hart, R., 190
Heath, A., 64, 65
Henderson, P., 112
Higgins, J.P.T., 238
Hudson, B., 256, 257–8
Hutson, C., 243

Jackson, S., 50

Katz, A., 261–2
Kubla, A., 242–3

Lipsey, M., 168
Lipsky, D.K., 131
Little, M., 90–1
Lopez, M., 212
Lutzker, J.R., 225

McGuire, J., 168–9
MacMillan, H.L., 215
Meyrick, J., 242
Mielck, A., 245–6
Miers, D., 177
Minnis, H., 51, 52
Mitchell, W., 151
Morris, J., 158–9, 160

Newman, T., 84
Nicol, A.R., 223–4

Oakley, A., 236
O'Donnell, C.R., 174

O'Kane, C., 194
Oldman, C., 154
Olds, D., 217

Parker, R., 87
Perry, F., 157–8
Pithouse, A., 52
Pollock, S., 95–6
Priestley, M., 149–50

Rachman, S.J., 223
Rice, J.M., 225
Rispens, J., 215
Roberts, H., 84, 239–40
Rowe, J., 89
Russell, J., 88
Rutter, M., 260

Sellick, C., 19–20
Sinclair, I., 19, 96–7

Sinclair, R., 85
Slavin, R., 132
Sloper, P., 151
Smith, A.N., 212
Smith, D., 85
Smith, J.E., 223
Stalker, K., 149–50
Stein, M., 69–70, 74–5
Stone, J., 16–17
Swann, C., 242
Sylva, K., 214–15

Thoburn, J., 19–20
Thomas, N., 50, 194
Triseliotis, J., 20, 23–4, 88, 91–2

Wade, J., 70, 74–5, 96
Wadsworth, M.E.J., 241
Wang, M.C., 134
Watson, N., 149–50
Whiteman, M., 221

Subject index

abusive behaviour, 95–6
accidents, 237–8
    prevention, 238–40, 245, 246, 247
    see also road accidents, prevention
accommodation, for care leavers, 77–8
Action Plan Orders, 176–7
adolescents, *see* young people
adopters, assessment, 30
adoption
    and age, 32, 45
    outcomes, 28, 88
    and placement stability, 44–5
    and service provision, 30
    see also permanent family placement;
        placement breakdown
age
    and adoption, 32, 45
    and placement breakdown, 25, 28
aggression, interventions for, 267
anger management
    for child protection, 221–2
    for emotional and behavioural
        difficulties, 270
Anti-Poverty Strategy, Barnardo's, 112
anxiety
    interventions for, 270
    see also school phobia, interventions
        for
area regeneration, *see* regeneration
Asian Mother and Baby Campaign,
    236

assessment
    of adopters, 30
    of care leavers' needs, 74–6
    of disabled children, 154–5, 160
    for family support, 263–4
    of foster carers, 20–1
    of young offenders, 168, 169–70,
        180–1
attachment patterns, in looked after
    children, 47

banking model, of education, 135
Barnardo's
    Anti-Poverty Strategy, 112
    'Boox on the Move' project, 242
bedtime problems, 267
bedwetting, interventions for, 268
behavioural difficulties, *see* emotional
    and behavioural difficulties
behavioural family therapy, 224
behavioural interventions, *see* cognitive-
    behavioural interventions
bereavement, support in, 270
birth families
    contact with
        by care leavers, 77
        and placement breakdown, 29, 32
        and placement stability, 43
    placement with, and placement
        stability, 43–4, 49
black care leavers, problems, 61, 66–7

black foster carers, 18
'Boox on the Move' project, 242
brief focused casework, in tertiary
    prevention, 223–4
Brownlow Community Trust, 112
bullying, 91, 150, 258, 265, 282

care leavers, 59–60
    accommodation for, 77–8
    assessment of needs, 74–6
    consultation with, 74–5
    contact with birth families, 77
    contingency plans for, 78
    disabled, 67–8, 75–6
    early parenthood, 65–6, 243
    education and training, 76
    educational attainment, 63–4, 93–4
    emotional and behavioural difficulties,
        67, 68
    employment, 65, 76
    financial support, 76
    health, 68, 75–6
    homelessness, 63, 67
    information for, 276–7
    mental health problems, 67, 68
    outcomes, 60–8
    personal advisers for, 74
    poverty levels, 65
    young people's experiences, 277–8
    see also leaving care services
care system
    and outcomes for care leavers, 61
    and placement turnover, 41
    see also foster care
carers
    ideal characteristics, 91–2, 100, 275–6
    see also foster carers; social workers
Child Development Programme, 218–19
child protection, 207–8
    and children's homes, 95
    parenting programmes for, 219–21,
        225
    and participation, 197–8
    see also primary prevention; secondary
        prevention; tertiary prevention
childhood
    definition, 109
    see also early years, health inequalities
        in; middle childhood, health
        inequalities in; young people

children, participation, see consultation;
    participation
Children Act (1989), 73, 158–9, 188,
    253–4
children in care, see looked after
    children
Children (Leaving Care) Act (2000),
    73–4, 76
children in need, 253–4
Children in Need Programme (Children's
    Society), 157–8
Children's Hearing System, Scotland,
    167
children's homes
    and child protection, 95
    compared with adoptive homes, 88
    compared with foster care, 88–90
    and education, 87, 89, 91, 93–4, 275,
        281
    and minority ethnic groups, 92–3
    outcomes, 62, 87–8, 89, 92, 97
    population, 86, 87
    quality factors, 97, 99–100
    research reviews, 86–8
    and runaways, 96
    and specialist services, 100
    staff, ideal characteristics, 91–2, 100,
        275–6
    state of research, 97–9
    stigma of, 86
    young people's views, 90–2, 96–7,
        279
Children's Society, Children in Need
    Programme, 157–8
cognitive-behavioural interventions
    for emotional and behavioural
        difficulties, 267, 268, 269, 270
    in secondary prevention, 219–20, 221
    in tertiary prevention, 223–5
    for young offenders, 172–3, 175
communities
    children's participation in, 196–7
    and emotional and behavioural
        difficulties, 258
    engagement with schools, 139–40
    see also social exclusion
Communities that Care, 181–2
community development, 107
    benefits for children, 111–12
    with children, 113–17

evaluation, 118–21
research needs, 117–18, 121–2
definitions, 108, 109–11
and diversity, 109–10
international perspectives, 112–13,
114–16
and social research, 113
see also regeneration
'community mothers', and home visiting,
218
community safety, children's
involvement in, 115–16, 240
community-based interventions
for child protection, 212–13
for young offenders, *see* young
offender programmes
concurrent placement, 32
consultation
and accident prevention, 239, 240
with care leavers, 74–5
with children, on placement
breakdown, 41
and participation, 191
see also participation
contingency plans, for care leavers, 78
continuity, *see* stability
court proceedings, and placement
turnover, 42, 49
Crime and Disorder Act (1998), 167,
176–8
curriculum development, and inclusive
education, 137

day care, and child protection, 213–14
decision making, *see* individual decision
making, children's participation in;
participation
depression, 236–7, 269
disability, medical model, 158
disabled care leavers, 67–8, 75–6
disabled children
access to information, 154–5
access to leisure activities, 150–1, 153,
156–8, 283
access to transport, 152–3
assessment, 154–5, 160
housing for, 153–4
inclusive education, 129, 133
participation, 116, 154–5, 157
play, 151, 154, 156–7

rights, 159
sense of stigma, 280
short-term care, 149, 161–2
and social exclusion, 147–50
and the Children Act (1989), 158–9
effects, 151–5
policy development, 158–60
practice implications, 160–2
prevention, 156–62
research needs, 155, 158
discretionary leaving care services, 73,
76
diversity, and community development,
109–10
divorce, *see* family breakdown, support
in
domestic violence
and emotional and behavioural
support, 266
home visiting in, 247
drug misuse, young people's views, 284

early education
and child protection, 213–14
and emotional and behavioural
support, 264, 265
early years, health inequalities in, 235–7
eating problems, 268
eco-behavioural therapy, 224–5
ecological framework, for emotional and
behavioural difficulties, 257–60
education
banking model, 135
for care leavers, 76
in child safety, effectiveness, 247
and children's homes, 87, 89, 91,
93–4, 275, 281
and emotional and behavioural
difficulties, 258–9, 264, 265, 266
and health inequalities, 241–2, 244
of young offenders, 173
young people's views, 280–2
see also early education; health
education; inclusive education;
pedagogy; schools
education system, and inclusion,
136–40, 141–2
educational attainment
of care leavers, 63–4, 93–4
and placement turnover, 40, 46–7

educational continuity, for looked after
    children, 46–7
emotional and behavioural difficulties
    of care leavers, 67, 68
    and education, 258–9, 264, 265, 266
    effects, 256–7
    interventions, 264–70
    of looked after children, 19, 48, 95–6,
        259–60
    protective factors, 257–62
    risk factors, 257–60
    spiral effect, 255
    statistics, 255–6
    training for foster carers, 21, 52
    young people's views, 261–2
    see also abusive behaviour;
        attachment; mental health
employment, of care leavers, 65, 76
empowerment
    definition, 111
    see also consultation; participation
encopresis, see soiling, interventions for
England, National Curriculum, 137
enuresis, see bedwetting, interventions
    for
environmental change, and accident
    reduction, 239
environmental issues, work with
    children, 115
ethnicity, see minority ethnic groups;
    race relations, involvement of
    children; racism, in children's
    homes
evidence-based practice
    critique, 2–5, 84
    see also research methodologies
exclusion, see school exclusion; social
    exclusion

Fairbridge, 175
families
    children's participation in decision
        making, 193–5
    engagement with schools, 139–40
family breakdown, support in, 266
family characteristics, and emotional and
    behavioural difficulties, 258, 259,
    260
family contact, see birth families, contact
    with

family group conferences, for young
    offenders, 176
family placement, 13–15
    see also adoption; foster care;
        placement
family support, 252–5, 262–3
    and assessment, 263–4
    see also emotional and behavioural
        difficulties
family therapy, 171, 224–6
fathers, work with, 264
fear, see anxiety; school phobia
fees, for foster carers, 21, 23, 49–50,
    275
financial support
    for care leavers, 76
    see also funding
fire prevention, 238–9
fluoridation, research into, 244, 247
foster care
    compared with children's homes,
        88–90
    kinship, 17–18, 26, 45
    outcomes, 62, 65, 89
    and placement stability, 45, 50–2
    and Quality Protects, 15
    temporary, 15–19, 23–4, 26–7, 33
    for young offenders, 171–2
    see also permanent family placement;
        placement; specialist foster care
foster carers
    assessment, 20–1
    characteristics, 17–18
    fees for, 21, 23, 49–50, 275
    ideal characteristics, 275–6
    and placement stability, 51–2
    recruitment, 19–20, 24
    retention, 20, 22, 23
    support for, 17, 21–3, 24
    training, 21, 51–2
fostering agencies, independent,
    17
friends, see relationship continuity
functional family therapy, for youth
    crime prevention, 171
funding
    and inclusive education, 137–8
    see also financial support

gangs, young people's views, 284–5

health
    of care leavers, 68, 75–6
    definitions, 205
    and poverty, 286
    see also drug misuse; mental health;
        smoking
health care continuity, for looked after
    children, 47
health education, 242, 244, 285–6
health inequalities, 232–3
    in early life, 235–7
    and education, 241–2, 244
    independent inquiry, 234–5
    interventions, 244–8
    in middle childhood, 237–40
    and teenage pregnancy, 242–4
    in young people, 240–4
health visitors, and home visiting,
    218
home visiting, 216–19, 247, 264, 265
homelessness, of care leavers, 63, 67
household fires, *see* fire prevention
housing
    for care leavers, 77–8
    for disabled children, 153–4
human rights, 159, 188

identity problems, of looked after
    children, 61, 66–7
incentives, for participation, 200–1
inclusion, *see* inclusive education;
        inclusive schools; social exclusion
inclusive education, 127–8
    and curriculum development, 137
    definition, 130
    of disabled children, 129, 133
    and the education system, 136–40,
        141–2
    pedagogy of, 133, 134–6
    research needs, 141
    and social inclusion, 129, 133, 140–1
    and social policies, 139, 140–1
inclusive participation, 199–200
inclusive schools, 130–4, 138–40
independent fostering agencies, 17
Independent Inquiry into Inequalities in
    Health, 234–5
individual decision making, children's
    participation in, 154–5, 192, 193–5,
    277

inequality, *see* health inequalities; social
        exclusion
information
    for disabled children, 154–5
    for looked after children, 276–7
    and participation, 191
injuries, *see* accidents
instability in care, *see* placement
        breakdown; placement turnover
integrated provision, *see* 'joined-up'
        services

'joined-up' services
    in community-based interventions,
        212–13
    for disabled children, 161
    and inclusive education, 139

kinship care, 17–18, 26, 45

ladder of participation, 119
learning disabled parents, parenting
        programmes for, 220–1
leaving care services, 69–70
    best practice, 73–8
    discretionary, 73, 76
    outcomes, 71–2
leisure activities
    access of disabled children, 150–1,
        153, 156–8, 283
    young people's views, 282–3
    see also physical activities; play
life skills training, 69–70, 75, 265
lifting and handling, and provision for
        disabled children, 161–2
local authorities, and inclusive
        education, 138–9
long-term care, *see* permanent family
        placement
looked after children
    attachment patterns, 47
    continuity for, *see* placement
        breakdown; placement turnover;
        stability
    educational performance, 63–4, 93–4
    emotional and behavioural difficulties,
        19, 48, 95–6, 259–60
    experience of stigma, 279–80
    identity problems, 61, 66–7
    information for, 276–7

participation in decision making, 194, 277
statistics, 11
views on looked after system, 274–8
see also adoption; care leavers; children's homes; foster care
Looking after Children materials, 53–4
loss, support in, 270

male foster carers, 18
malnutrition, interventions for, 245
manual handling, see lifting and handling, and provision for disabled children
medical model of disability, 158
mental health problems
in care leavers, 67, 68
interventions for, 245–6
of looked after children, 48
in parents, 266, 280
see also depression; post-traumatic stress disorder; suicidal behaviour
mentoring, of young offenders, 173–4, 179
middle childhood, health inequalities in, 237–40
minority ethnic groups
in children's homes, 92–3
perinatal risks, 236
and placement breakdown, 29
see also Asian Mother and Baby Campaign; black care leavers; black foster carers; race relations; racism
mixed race care leavers, 61, 67
morning activities, support for, 267
motivation, see incentives, for participation
motor projects, for young offenders, 175–6
multi-agency working, see 'joined-up' services
multi-systemic therapy
for tertiary prevention, 224–6
for youth crime prevention, 171

National Curriculum (England), 137
networks, see social network interventions, for tertiary prevention

offending, see young offenders, assessment of; youth crime

'Open File on Inclusive Education' (UNESCO), 136–7

parenting programmes
for child protection, 219–21, 225
and emotional and behavioural support, 265
for youth crime prevention, 170–1
see also home visiting
parents
mental health problems, 266, 280
see also fathers, work with
participation, 186–7
attitudinal factors, 197–8
benefits, 188–9
characteristics, 189–92
and child protection, 197–8
in communities, 196–7
in community safety, 115–16, 240
development of, 188–9
of disabled children, 116, 154–5, 157
drawbacks, 189
inclusive, 199–200
in individual decision making, 154–5, 192, 193–5, 277
ladder of participation, 119
levels of, 190–2
of looked after children, 194, 277
motivation for, 200–1
in policy development, 193
processes for, 198–9
in race relations, 116
in regeneration, 114–15
in research, 192
in service development, 192, 195–6
see also community development, with children; consultation
partnership, and participation, 191
pathway planning, for care leavers, 74–5
payments, see fees, for foster carers
pedagogy, of inclusive education, 133, 134–6
peer groups, and emotional and behavioural difficulties, 260, 269
peer pressure, young people's views, 285
peer support, for foster carers, 22–3
permanent family placement, 24–6, 31–2
outcomes, 26–9
and placement delays, 31

and service provision, 30
see also adoption
personal advisers, for care leavers, 74
physical activities, for young offenders,
174–5
placement breakdown
and age, 25, 28
and birth family contact, 29, 32
and consultation with children, 41
and educational continuity, 46
and ethnicity, 29
and experienced foster carers, 51
rates, 27
risk of, 18–19, 22, 28–9, 40
and school exclusion, 46
see also placement stability; placement
turnover
placement choice, 17–18, 31–2
outcomes, 26–9
and stability, 44–5
placement stability, 43–5, 48–52
see also placement breakdown
placement turnover
causes, 41–2, 43, 49
costs, 48
and educational achievement, 40,
46–7
and mental health problems, 48
rates, 39–41
placements
and characteristics of the child, 25
concurrent, 32
delays in, 31
length, 19
of siblings, 29
unplanned, 18–19
see also adoption; children's homes;
foster care; permanent family
placement
play
for disabled children, 151, 154,
156–7
see also leisure activities
police, young people's views, 284–5
post-traumatic stress disorder, 270
postnatal depression, 236–7
poverty
anti-poverty strategies, 112
in care leavers, 65
and child protection, 211–13

and emotional and behavioural
difficulties, 259
and health, 286
see also health inequalities; social
exclusion
pre-school education, *see* early education
pregnancy
social support during, 236
teenage, 243–5
see also teenage parents
prevention
of accidents, 238–40, 245, 246, 247
of child abuse, *see* child protection;
primary prevention; secondary
prevention; tertiary prevention
of social exclusion for disabled
children, 156–62
of youth crime, *see* young offender
programmes; youth crime,
prevention
primary prevention, 210–15
problem solving, for emotional and
behavioural support, 265
Project 12-Ways, 224–5
PTSD, 270

Quality Protects, and foster care, 15

race relations, involvement of children,
116
racism, in children's homes, 93
randomized controlled trials, 84
recruitment, of foster carers, 19–20,
24
regeneration
role of schools, 140–1
work with children, 114–15
relationship continuity
for disabled children, 151
for looked after children, 47–8, 77
relatives, *see* birth families; kinship care
reparation orders, 176–7
representation, and participation, 191
research
children's participation in, 192
and community development, 113
implementation of results, 208–9
research methodologies, 84–5, 98–9,
118–19, 209–10
see also evidence-based practice

residential care, 83
  and placement stability, 45
  see also children's homes
residential schools, young people's
    experiences, 281
resilience, promotion of, 260–2
respite care, *see* short-term care
restorative justice, 176–7
retention, of foster carers, 20, 22, 23
rewards, *see* incentives, for participation
rights, *see* human rights
risk assessment, of young offenders, 168,
    169–70, 180–1
risk factors
  for emotional and behavioural
    difficulties, 257–60
  for offending, 169–70, 181
road accidents, prevention, 239, 240,
    245, 246
runaways, 96, 266

safety
  young people's views, 284–5
  see also accidents; child protection;
    community safety, children's
    involvement in
school exclusion, 46, 266, 281–2
school phobia, interventions for, 267
school-age parents, *see* teenage parents
schools
  and area regeneration, 140–1
  engagement with families, 139–40
  see also bullying; education; inclusive
    schools
Scotland, Children's Hearing System,
    167
secondary prevention, 216
  and anger management, 221–2
  definition, 210
  and home visiting, 216–19
  and parenting programmes,
    219–21
self-efficacy, and child protection,
    217
self-help groups, for foster carers,
    22–3
self-identity, *see* identity problems, of
    looked after children
self-management (by children), and
    participation, 191–2

separation, *see* family breakdown
    support in
service provision
  for children in residential care, 100
  children's participation in, 192,
    195–6
  for disabled children, 160–1
  and permanent family placement,
    29–30
  young people's views, 283
  see also 'joined-up' services; leaving
    care services
sexual abuse, prevention, 214–15
short-term care, for disabled children,
    149, 161–2
siblings, placement, 29
single foster carers, 18
smoke alarms, research into, 238–9
smoking, prevention, 246
social activities, *see* leisure activities
social class
  and health inequalities, 234
  and injury rates, 237–8
social exclusion
  and child protection, 211–13
  and inclusive education, 129, 133,
    140–1
  young people's views, 279–83
  see also disabled children, and
    social exclusion; poverty; school
    exclusion
social network interventions, for tertiary
    prevention, 226–7
social research, *see* research
social workers
  and adoption support, 30
  and foster carer support, 22–3
  ideal characteristics, 275–6
soiling, interventions for, 268
SPACE, 157
specialist foster care, 45, 88–9
Spice Group: PACT Yorkshire, 157
sport, *see* leisure activities; physical
    activities
stability
  for looked after children, 37–9, 42–3,
    45–8
  see also placement breakdown;
    placement stability; placement
    turnover

staff
  training, for inclusion of disabled
    children, 156
  see also carers; children's homes, staff,
    ideal characteristics; social workers
stealing, interventions for, 267
stigma, young people's experiences, 86,
  279–80
street children, work with, 116
Student Scheme: PACT Yorkshire, 157
Suffolk Partnership Achieving Choice
  and Experience, 157
suicidal behaviour, interventions for,
  269
supplementary foster care, *see* temporary
  foster care
support
  for adoptive families, 30
  in bereavement, 269
  for care leavers, 74–8, 277–8
    see also leaving care services
  for children with mentally ill parents,
    266
  during family breakdown, 266
  during pregnancy, 236
  for foster carers, 17, 21–3, 24
  for inclusive schools, 138–40
  for participation, 197, 199
  for teenage parents, 66, 243–4
  for young carers, 266
  see also family support; social
    network interventions, for tertiary
    prevention

Take 10: PACT Yorkshire, 157
talent development model, of pedagogy,
  134–5
teenage parents, 65–6, 243–4, 280, 286
teenage pregnancy, prevention, 242–4
teenagers, *see* young people
temporary foster care, 15–19, 23–4,
  26–7, 33
  see also foster carers; placement
    stability
tertiary prevention, 222–3
  cognitive-behavioural approaches,
    223–5
  definition, 210
  family therapy, 224–6
  social network interventions, 226–7

theft, *see* stealing, interventions for
tokenism, in participation, 190
training
  of foster carers, 21, 51–2
  for participation, 196
  see also education; life skills training;
    staff, training, for inclusion of
    disabled children
transferability, of health interventions,
  247–8
transport, for disabled children,
  152–3
transracial placements, outcomes, 29
troubled behaviour, *see* emotional and
  behavioural difficulties

UNESCO, 'Open File on Inclusive
  Education', 136–7
United States, Communities that Care,
  181–2
unplanned placements, 18–19

wetting, *see* bedwetting, interventions
  for
'wilderness' programmes, for young
  offenders, 174–5

young carers, 266, 280
young offender programmes, 165–6
  cognitive-behavioural interventions,
    172–3, 175
  education, 173
  foster care, 171–2
  mentoring, 173–4, 179
  motor projects, 175–6
  parenting programmes, 170–1
  physical activities, 174–5
  principles for effectiveness, 168–70,
    179
  research needs, 178–81
  restorative justice, 176–7
young offenders, assessment of, 168,
  169–70, 180–1
young people
  emotional and behavioural support,
    269–70
  experience of stigma, 86, 279–80
  health inequalities in, 240–4
  views of children's homes, 90–2,
    96–7, 279

views on emotional and behavioural
  support, 261–2
views on health, 285–6
views on looked after system,
  274–8
views on safety, 284–5
views on social exclusion, 279–83
see also runaways; street children,
  work with; teenage parents
'Youth at Risk' programme, 173–4
youth clubs, *see* leisure activities

youth crime
  government policies, 167, 180
  prevention, 177–8
  protective factors, 170
  risk factors, 169–70, 181
  statistics, 166–7
  see also young offender programmes
Youth Justice and Criminal Evidence Act
  (1999), 167, 177
Youth Offending Panels, 167, 177
youth offending teams, 180